SOTHIS PRESS

Sothis Press aims to completely reimagine the public domain book with an emphasis on universal access to captivatingly designed print editions. We believe that technology will enable every single book ever published to be perpetually accessible in beautiful print form. Sothis is beauty in ubiquity.

www.sothis.press
1 Waterhouse Square, London, ECIN 2ST

The Flora Homoeopathica

Or Illustrations and Descriptions of the Medicinal Plants Used as Homoeopathic Remedies

Edward Hamilton

SOTHIS PRESS

ISBN 978-1-0365-1006-0

The Flora Homoeopathica
is in the public domain.

THE FLORA HOMŒOPATHICA.

THE

FLORA HOMŒOPATHICA;

OR,

Illustrations and Descriptions

OF THE

MEDICINAL PLANTS USED AS HOMŒOPATHIC REMEDIES.

BY

EDWARD HAMILTON, M.D., F.L.S.,

MEMBER OF THE BRITISH HOMŒOPATHIC SOCIETY; PHYSICIAN TO THE LONDON HOMŒOPATHIC HOSPITAL, ETC. ETC.

IN TWO VOLUMES.

VOL. I.

LONDON:
H. BAILLIERE, 219, REGENT STREET; AND
290, BROADWAY, NEW YORK, (U. S.)
WM. HEADLAND, 15, PRINCES STREET, HANOVER SQUARE.
EDINBURGH: GEORGE ALLSHORN. MANCHESTER: H. TURNER.
LIVERPOOL: THOMPSON & Co.

1852.

K

"With wise intent
The hand of Nature on peculiar minds
Imprints a different bias.
* * * * * *
To some she taught the fabric of the spheres,
* * * others by the hand
She led o'er vales and mountains, to explore
What healing virtue swells the tender veins
Of herbs and flowers; or what the beams of morn
Draw forth, distilling from the clifted rind
In balmy tears."

AKENSIDE.

LONDON:
THOMAS HARRILD, PRINTER, SILVER STREET,
FALCON SQUARE.

TO

FREDERICK FOSTER QUIN, ESQ., M.D.,

President of the British Homœopathic Society,

ETC. ETC. ETC.

THIS WORK IS DEDICATED,

WITH FEELINGS OF ESTEEM AND REGARD,

BOTH FOR HIS WORTH AS A FRIEND, AND FOR HIS VALUABLE LABOURS

IN PROMULGATING

THE DOCTRINES OF HAHNEMANN

IN THIS COUNTRY.

PREFACE.

In undertaking the publication of the present work, the Author is actuated by a double motive. In the first place, he considers that the actual position of the cause he advocates renders it most desirable that those interested in homœopathy should be in possession of some regular account or history of the medicines employed; and, in the second place, because a great number of persons entertain a mistaken notion that homœopathic medicines vary from those used in the allopathic school, both as being different in kind, of a highly poisonous nature, and therefore most deleterious to the human frame.

This unfounded prejudice, the Author regrets to find, is frequently promulgated and held *in terrorem* over timid persons by many medical opponents, who thus endeavour to discourage and suppress a system of practice contrary to their own opinions, by intimidation rather than by argument. It is hoped that the error of these conclusions will be made apparent, and that it will be proved that the medicines are precisely the same as those adopted by the opponents of homœopathy, and gathered either from the surface of the earth, or extracted from its interior recesses; but with this great difference, that in homœopathy they are so prepared, that no mistake can render them dangerous in their action, when, through want of coincidence with the disease, they fail to produce benefit; while, in the practice of allopathy, the carelessness of a chemical preparation, the ignorance or thoughtlessness of an assistant, may produce consequences the most lamentable and dangerous. And let it be remembered, that *all* medicines, in large doses, act poisonously upon the human system, modified by idiosyncrasy and other causes, from common irritation of the membranes, to ulceration, paralysis, and death.

In arranging the notices of each plant under different heads, the Author has given: 1st, its botanical characteristics. 2nd, its history, as well as the uses of the plant in allopathic practice, for the purpose of comparison. 3rd, a botanical and general description to identify the species. 4th, the geographical distribution and localities, as far as they are known, according to the latest authors. 5th, the physiological effects on man and animals; a most important study in connection with our investigation of the pathogenetic effects of medicine on the human organism. 6th, the parts of the plant used, and the mode of preparation. 7th, the general uses of the plant, homœopathically considered; and from Hahnemann's useful and instructive remarks much valuable knowledge may be gained. Noack and Trinks's clinical observations will be found interesting, in comparing the various diseases for which each drug has been given under the different systems of medicine.

The Author gladly seizes this occasion to offer his cordial thanks to those kind friends who have assisted him in the illustrations of his work, both as regards the original drawings and the lithographic execution. To Mr.

Kippist, the librarian of the Linnean Society, his thanks are especially due, for the kind and efficient aid he has given towards the necessary investigations.

In committing his work to the press, the Author is sensible that he has to ask indulgence for frequent errors and omissions, arising from the many interruptions and conflicting interests of an arduous profession, and which he hopes will be admitted in his excuse. He has aimed, with what degree of success others can best determine, to introduce to the public, and especially the professional mind, his views on this most interesting and instructive subject, in connection with the study of homœopathy; while he is very diffident as to his capabilities of doing justice to the theme.

The Author is anxious to attract the attention of every philosophical inquirer after Science and Truth, who will discover in the pursuit of this branch of study unbounded suggestiveness, and ever-expanding views of Creative Wisdom, which has thus concealed in the unassuming and often unattractive forms of the plants beneath our feet, many of its divinest secrets. These can be developed only by patient and laborious research. Let us then continue, with unabated ardour, to penetrate more and more deeply into the beneficent arcana of Nature. The reward is certain; for what consciousness can be so gratifying as that of success, in adding to our treasury new means of encountering the Demon of Disease, and bringing back the Angel of Health?

LONDON, *May*, 1852.

INTRODUCTION.

Botany, and more particularly Medical Botany, is of very ancient origin; the first idea of applying plants for medicinal purposes having, it is said, originated with the Chaldeans (the priests or learned men of Babylonia), who from their earliest youth devoted themselves to the examination of the laws of Nature, and who made the study of the properties of plants available for relieving the diseases of mankind. This knowledge was transmitted by them to the Egyptians, from whom it descended to the Greeks, and for a long time remained in the hands of the priests of the mythological god of medecine, Æsculapius; to them we must ascribe the first dawn of botanical science in Greece. Their doctrines, however, were most confused and absurd. They supposed that vegetable substances had sentient souls, desires, and wishes, and were capable of experiencing pleasure and pain. They were followed by Pythagoras and his disciples, one of whom, Empedocles the Sicilian, even declared that he himself had been once a shrub, then a bird, then a fish, and lastly a man. But little progress was made until the increasing sufferings consequent upon the violation of the simple rules of our primitive forefathers induced many of the Greek philosophers to turn their attention to, and endeavour to increase and improve the means which had been handed down to them. A new era, however, commenced with Hippocrates, the Father of medicine, "the Homer of his profession." He first made experiments with different medicinal plants (of which he enumerates two hundred and thirty) on the human frame, which greatly tended to increase his knowledge, and by the observations deduced from them, he was supposed not only to have been able to prolong the lives of others, but his own; for he died at the age of one hundred and nine years, free from all disorders of mind and body.

To the Philosopher of Truth,* to him who killed himself rather than live when disappointed in his scientific investigations, we were first indebted to the introduction of botany as a philosophical science. His views and ideas were more fully followed out by his disciple Theophrastus, who gave a full account of all plants known in his time; in his work, περι Φυτων ιστοριας, he enumerates about five hundred species, all medicinal, but often applying the same name to plants totally dissimilar in their botanical and physiological characters. He paid great attention to the physiology of plants, and was aware of the difference of the exogenous and endogenous, or monocotyledons and dicotyledons of the moderns. He was also aware that nutrition was conveyed to plants by the leaves. We next come to Dioscorides the Cilician, who lived in the time of Nero; he enumerated about six hundred plants, and Pliny the elder increased the number to one thousand. He, however, acknowledged that there were many more undescribed, and which probably would be found useful for medicinal purposes. Then came the almost complete annihilation of the sciences by the barbarian inroads into civilized Europe.

* Aristotle, who drowned himself because he could not discover the cause of the flux and reflux of the waters in the Euripus.

All that remained sought refuge in Asia; and we find botanical writings, with others on natural history, in the works of Galen, Oribasius, Ætius, Paulus Ægineta, and, later, in those of the Arabian physicians, Aben Mesne, Serapion, Rhazes, Avicenna, etc.; they are, however, chiefly transcripts from the earlier writings of Hippocrates, Theophrastus, and Dioscorides.

"It is melancholy to look back upon the state of Europe during the period which has been justly denominated the dark ages. A dismal gloom enveloped the whole of the civilized world; ignorance, superstition, and barbarism tyrannized over learning and genius; knowledge of any kind was to be acquired only by searching among the rubbish of schools and monasteries; fabulous legends supplied the place of truth, and the deceptions of a crafty priesthood debased, at the same time they enslaved, the minds of men. During this long and melancholy course of years, the few scattered writings that appeared on natural history were the productions of the monks, and compiled from the old authors, but even these were cloaked in an almost unintelligible jargon, and it was not till the middle of the sixteenth century that the sun of science again burst this thick cloud, and shed its rays upon the north of Europe. At this period, botany, which was exactly in the same state as the ancients left it, could not be considered anything more than a catalogue or list of names of about one thousand plants; for although the ancients were great observers, they did not make much use of their observations. They looked at nature rather with the eye of the poet than the philosopher; and on giving the reins to imagination, were too powerfully charmed with her more striking beauty and sublimity, to descend to a calm and patient investigation of the causes of the effects which they observed."

It is, then, to Brunfels, a physician of Berne, in Switzerland, that we are indebted for the revival of botanical science, when the light of learning again shone forth upon the world after the period of the dark ages; he lived about the beginning of the sixteenth century, and was the first person who represented the figures of plants by means of woodcuts. About the same time lived Gesner, and soon after the celebrated naturalist Cæsalpinus; one of the professors of the University of Padua. He was born at Arezzo, in Tuscany, in 1519; his investigations threw great light upon vegetable structures, he was the first botanist who endeavoured to classify plants, and demonstrate their different sexes, although this latter fact had been hinted at by the ancients. He was followed by Jungius, who died in 1657; and then came Morison, and after him the celebrated John Ray, born in 1628, at Black Notley, in Essex, his father being the blacksmith of the village. His works show the most laborious research, and in his "Historia Plantarum generalis" is given all that was known of botanical learning at that time. Haller designated him as the greatest botanist in the memory of man. To him succeeded Grew in this country, and Malpighi on the Continent, whose splendid investigations and examinations of the structure of plants are almost unequalled. Then came Camerarius, to whom the honour is due of first discovering and proving by experiments the existence of the sexes of plants. He was followed by Tournefort, the celebrated

French botanist, the great leader of the French school, born at Aix, in Provence, in 1656, whose hardy frame and enterprising spirit made him despise the rigorous climate of the Alps and Pyrenees, and to whom we are indebted for the best botanical description of those regions. At this time, with the facilities and impetus given to all branches of science by the improvement in printing and engraving, shone forth the transcendent genius of the great Linnæus. His wonderful mind gave a new aspect to every branch of the study of natural history, and more particularly to botany. This great naturalist was born at Rashult, in the province of Smaland in Sweden, in the year 1707; his family name was Lindelius, supposed to have its origin from a famous linden tree which grew in the neighbourhood of the family residence. He was very early imbued with the love of botany, but the display of his extraordinary abilities, like those of many other illustrious men, depended upon accident, and but for the kind offices of a physician of the name of Rothman, those of Linnæus would have been for ever suppressed, his father having felt so much disappointment with his earlier studies, that he considered him only fit for a tradesman, and destined him to be a shoemaker. The poverty of Linnæus obliged him to struggle with great hardships in his earlier years, and when studying at Upsal he was glad to wear the cast-off clothes of his fellow-students, and mended his own shoes with the bark of trees, and it was owing to the kindness of the lady who afterwards became his wife that he could raise the money which enabled him to graduate at Leyden. Since the time of Linnæus, therefore, we may mark a rapid and progressive movement in the science of botany, until it has reached a position equal, if not superior, to almost all other branches of natural history. And when we find such names as Haller, Rumphius, Æder, Schreber, Jacquin, Bergius, Reinholdt, Forster who sailed with Captain Cook, Jussieu, Sir Joseph Banks, Miller, Dryander, Gærtner, Sir J. E. Smith, Withering, Wildenow, Humboldt, Roxburgh, Decandolle, Lindley, R. Brown, etc. etc., we may justly be proud of the science and study which includes such men as its votaries.

To the medical student and practitioner a knowledge of plants, more particularly those appertaining to medicine, is of the utmost importance. How often may he be placed in situations where such a knowledge may not only be of the greatest advantage to himself, but of the greatest benefit to his fellow-men. By this knowledge he can save whole armies from destruction; he is able to choose the most salubrious situations for towns and encampments; he can at once determine which plants are salutary and which are deleterious; that the natural families of the Cruciferæ, Rosaceæ, Malvaceæ, Labiatæ are innocuous, whilst the Solaneæ, Apocyneæ, Ranunculaceæ, and Papaveraceæ are almost all poisonous; which of the Umbelliferæ are edible, which are injurious; and by this knowledge he is enabled to distinguish the harmless weed from that which is a deadly poison.

CLASSIFICATION OF PLANTS.*

WHEN science was in its infancy, and when few plants were observed, they were described or treated without any particular arrangement; or if some method was adopted, it was merely empirical and of little use to others. Theophrastus, Dioscorides, and Pliny, who respectively treated of vegetables, may therefore be justly rejected as systematists; and we may place Gessner, born at Zurich in 1516, as the first who demonstrated that the characters drawn from the flowers and fruit were most to be depended upon. He also pointed out that certain groups possessed particular characters in common. To him succeeded Cæsalpinus: he distinguished vegetables into trees and herbs; with the former arranging shrubs, and with the latter suffruticose plants. He next divided each of these; the first into two classes, the last into thirteen, according to the fruit and situation of the embryo. In 1680 Monson offered a new system. His sections or secondary divisions are 108 in number, and are taken from the figure and substance of the fruit, the number of seeds, sepals, and petals, the figure of the root, the direction of the stem, the colour of the flower, the place of growth, and one from the medical virtues of some of the plants that compose it. In 1682 Ray proposed his method: he made thirty-five classes; the distinguishing marks of some of which were derived from the habit or external appearance; of others from a greater or less perfection of the plants, from their place of growth, the number of seeds, fruits, petals, or sepals of each flower, or from the nature of the fruit or inflorescence.

They were as follows:—I. *Herbs.*—1. Submarinæ or sea-plants, including Zoophytes and Corals. 2. Fungi. 3. Musci, including Hepaticæ and Lichens. 4. Capillares or Ferns. 5. Apetalous plants, comprehending, among other anomalies, the genus Equisetum. 6. Planipetalæ, or those with semi-flosculose, compound flowers, corresponding to the Cichoraceæ of Jussieu. 7. Discoideæ, containing such of the Corymbiferæ of Jussieu as have a pappus. 8. Capitatæ, corresponding principally to the Cynarocephalæ of Jussieu, but more extensive, and including all plants with tubular flowers that are collected into a scaly involucrum. 9. Corymbiferæ, similar to those of modern botanists, but limited to the species without a pappus. 10. Gymno-monospermæ, or such as were supposed to have one naked seed; to this belongs Valeriana and Armeria, and, by some unhappy chance, Thalictrum. 11. Umbelliferæ. 12. Stellatæ, corresponding to

* The following abridged account of the different natural and artificial systems is taken from *Arnott's Introduction to Botany* and *Lindley's Vegetable Kingdom.*

one of the sections of Rubiaceæ. 13. Asperifoliæ. 14. Verticillatæ, or the Labiatæ of Jussieu, and Didynamia angiospermia of Linnæus. 15. Polyspermæ, or those with many apparently naked seeds, as Ranunculus, Malva, Potentilla, and Alisma; a most unnatural assemblage. 16. Pomiferæ, the fruit of which resembled an apple, and among these the gourds and passion-flowers. 17. Bacciferæ, or every herb with a berry, whether a potato or asparagus. 18. Multisiliquæ, such as Aquilegia and Sedum, that had a fruit of apparently several pods. 19. Ditripetalæ, containing principally Tillandsia, but seemingly not understood by Ray himself. 21. Tetrapetalæ, with either a long or a short pod; not, however, confined to the Cruciferæ of Jussieu, but comprehending Veronica, Euphorbia, Plantago, etc. 22. Papilionaceæ or Leguminosæ, including Fumaria. 23. Pentapetalæ, as Dianthus, Cistus, Hypericum. 24. Pentapetaloideæ, or those with a monopetalous corolla, so divided as almost to resemble five petals, among which are enumerated Erythræa, Apocynum, Oxalis, etc.; but indeed the 19th, 23rd, and the present classes are much confused by the author. 25. Bulbosæ and their allies, including a great part of the monocotyledones, as Liliaceæ, Asphodeliæ, Orchideæ, or Irideæ. 26. Graminifoliæ, comprehending the Grasses, Cyperaceæ, and Junceæ. 27. Anomaleæ, or those herbs, as Nymphæa, Pipea, and Polygala, that were not reducible to any of these.

II. *Trees.*—28. Arundinaceæ, including the Palms. 29. Juliferæ, called also Apetalæ, containing those in which the fruit is separated from the staminiferous flower; under which Ray ranked the Amentaceæ and Coniferæ, the Elm, the Mulberry, etc. 30. Aggregatæ, or trees with the flower and fruit collected together in one mass, as the Fig. 31. Umbilicatæ, with an inferior, fleshy, or pulpy fruit; a heterogeneous set. 32. Non-umbilicatæ, or those where the flower adhered to the bottom of the fruit; these are again divided into Pruniferæ, Bacciferæ, and Pomiferæ. 33. Vasculiferæ, or trees with a dry fruit. 34. Siliquosæ, or trees or shrubs, bearing a legume, follicle, or any of such elongated fruits. 35. Anomalæ, or such as are not referrible to any of the above.

Most authors enumerate only thirty-three classes, omitting the 24th and 30th, but which, nevertheless, form part of his arrangement. Ray's principal division into herbs and trees is extremely faulty, and separates plants otherwise closely allied. His method, however, being a great approximation to a natural one, deserves much praise; and we believe it was the opinion of the late Sir J. E. Smith, who was well qualified to judge, that Ray as a botanist was eclipsed by few but Linnæus.

To pass over several of inferior note, we come now to Tournefort. This distinguished individual was born at Aix, in Provence, in 1656. He was Professor of Botany at the Jardin des Plantes of Paris, and in 1700 was sent by Louis XIV. to the Levant. He travelled through Greece, and surveyed the borders of the Black Sea and the islands of the Archipelago, and returned to Paris, where he published an interesting account of his expedition. But before his departure, he had made known his new system of the arrangement of plants in his "Institutiones Rei Herbariæ," illustrated by many plates, and containing a description of 688 genera and 10,146 species; and it is difficult to say whether he deserves most honour for his new classification, or for the attempt to characterise the genera and species.

The method of Tournefort is composed of twenty-two classes, of which the characters are derived—first, from the consistence and size of the stem—thus dividing vegetables into herbs or suffruticose plants and shrubs, or trees, in which respect his system is subject to the same fault as that of Ray, notwithstanding Rivinus, an intervening botanist, had demonstrated the absurdity of such a division; secondly, from the presence or absence of the corolla; thirdly, from the flower being simple or solitary, or compound, or united into a common involucrum; fourthly, from the corolla being of one (or gamopetalous) or of several petals; and, fifthly, from its regularity or irregularity. His classes are:—

HERBS OR UNDERSHRUBS.

§ 1. *Flowers Simple or Solitary.*

1. Flowers monopetalous, Campaniform.
2. Flowers monopetalous, Infundibuliform and Rotate.
3. Flowers monopetalous, Anomalous.
4. Flowers monopetalous, Labiate.
5. Flowers polypetalous, Cruciform.
6. Flowers polypetalous, Rosaceous.
7. Flowers polypetalous, Rosaceous Umbellate.
9. Flowers Liliaceous.
10. Flowers polypetalous, Caryophyllaceous.
11. Flowers polypetalous, Anomalous.

§ 2. *Flowers Compound.*

12. Flowers Flosculose.
13. Flowers Semi-flosculose.
14. Flowers Radiate.

§ 3. *Herbs without Petals.*

15. Flowers Apetalous or Staminiferous.
16. Flowers absent, Seed present.
17. Flowers and Fruit invisible.

TREES AND SHRUBS.

18. Flowers Apetalous.
19. Flowers Apetalous, Amentaceous.
20. Flowers Monopetalous.
21. Flowers Rosaceous.
22. Flowers Papilionaceous.

In the 3rd class, the term anomalous means irregular, but not labiate; in the 11th, irregular, but not papilionaceous. A liliaceous flower, as in the 9th class, he afterwards explains to be a regular corolla of six or three petals, or even a monopetalous one with six divisions, but always having a fruit of three cells. The 16th contains the Ferns; the 17th the other Cryptogamia, which, he says, were commonly destitute of both flower and fruit. Such were the twenty-two classes established by Tournefort. Each of them contains sections, of which there are in all 122; and though at first sight it may appear simple and easy of reference, it still presents considerable difficulties, from many of the characters being merely negative, and others by no means decisive.

The systems, whether of Cæsalpinus, Morison, Ray, or Tournefort, were all, more or less, attempts at a natural classification. We now come to the artificial system of Linnæus, the basis of which rests almost entirely on the male organs or stamens; and where no sexes could be distinguished, he termed the plants cryptogamous, and assigned to them the 24th class of his arrangement, Cryptogamia. His system is as follows:—

I. Stamens Definite and Equal.

1. Monandria; one stamen.
2. Diandria; two stamens.
3. Triandria; three stamens.
4. Tetrandria; four stamens.
5. Pentandria; five stamens.
6. Hexandria; six stamens.
7. Heptandria; seven stamens.
8. Octandria; eight stamens.
9. Enneandria; nine stamens.
10. Decandria; ten stamens.

II. Stamens Indefinite.

11. Dodecandria; stamens from eleven to nineteen.
12. Icosandria; stamens twenty and upwards, perigynous or inserted on the calyx.
13. Polyandria; stamens twenty and upwards, hypogenous or inserted on the receptacle.

III. Stamens Unequal.

14. Didynamia; stamens four, two longer than the others.
15. Tetradynamia; stamens six, four longer than the others.

IV. Filaments United.

16. Monadelphia; one bundle of stamens, or androphore.
17. Diadelphia; two bundles of stamens.
18. Polyadelphia; or several bundles of stamens.

V. Anthers United.

19. Syngenesia; stamens five, united by their anthers, flowers collected into a common involucre.

VI. Stamens united to the Pistil.

20. Gynandria.

VII. Flowers Unisexual.

21. Monœcia; stamens and pistils on the same individual.
22. Diœcia; stamens and pistils on different individuals.
23. Polygamia; hermaphrodite and unisexual flowers, either on the same or different individuals.

VIII. Flowers Invisible.

24. Cryptogamia; neither stamens nor pistils.

In the first thirteen classes the characters of the orders, or subdivisions of the classes, are derived from the number of the styles or female organs, the names Monogynia, Digynia, Trigynia, etc., indicating respectively one, two, three, etc., styles.

In the 14th class, or Didynamia, Linnæus took his ordinal characters from the structure of the fruit. When this is formed of four akenia, situated at the bottom of the calyx, so as to resemble naked seeds, he called the order Gymnospermia; and when the fruit was a capsule containing several seeds, he termed the group Angiospermia. Tetradynamia presents also two orders; the one with a silicule, the other with a siliqua; and hence they were called Siliculosæ and Siliquosæ. A third order has been added by Sprengel, for such as have an indehiscent fruit; and De Candolle has proposed to subdivide the class according to the relative position of the cotyledons and radicle. The 16th, 17th, and 18th classes being according to the union of the filaments, the number of stamens is made to serve as a character for the orders.

In Syngenesia, where the anthers are united, and there are almost always five stamens, other means were resorted to. Some florets were observed to be bisexual; others with stamens or pistils only. In reference, therefore, to the 23rd class, Linnæus gave to each of the orders the name Polygamia, with another epithet to mark their respective peculiarities. The first he terms Polygamia æqualis, all the florets being equally fertile and bisexual; the second, Polygamia superflua, where the florets of the disc are bisexual, but those of the circumference or ray female, both producing perfect seed; the third, Polygamia frustranea, have the florets of the disc bisexual and fertile, but those of the ray sterile and imperfect. In the second order the florets of the ray were only superfluous; here they are totally useless. The fourth, or Polygamia necessaria, has the florets of the disc bisexual, but sterile from the imperfection of the stigmas; those of the ray containing only pistils are fertilized by the pollen of the former.

The fifth, Polygamia segregata, has all the florets bisexual, but each of them contained an involucre peculiar to itself; the whole, as in the other orders, being collected within a common involucre. To these Linnæus added a sixth, Polygamia monogamia, wherein the flowers were not collected in a common involucrum; but this last has been transferred to Pentandria monogynia.

In Gynandria, the orders are taken from the number of the stamens. Monœcia and Diœcia, including plants that are monandrous, diandrous, monadelphous, or gynandrous, have the names of the orders, as Monandria, Decandria, Gynandria, taken from some of the preceding classes. The 23rd class, or Polygamia, containing plants with bisexual and unisexual flowers, mixed either on the same or distinct individuals, has in consequence been divided into three orders: Monœcia, in which the flowers are bisexual and unisexual on the same individual; Diœcia, where one bears the bisexual and another the unisexual blossoms of both kinds; and Trœcia, where one has the bisexual, another the male, and a third the female flowers.

Cryptogamia was originally divided by Linnæus into four orders: Ferns, Mosses, Algæ, and Fungi; but so little was then known about the structure and limits of these, that it is now generally agreed to adopt nearly the same divisions as are employed in the natural method.

The following is the natural distribution first proposed by Linnæus under the name of Fragments, in 1751. Many of his groups were taken from his predecessors; others were contrived by himself.

Natural Order.	*Examples.*
1. PIPERITÆ, as	Arum, Piper.
2. PALMÆ,	Corypha, Cycas.
3. SCITAMINA,	Canna, Amomum
4. ORCHIDEÆ.	
5. ENSATÆ,	Iris, etc.
6. TRIPETALOIDEÆ,	Butomus, etc.
7. DENUDATÆ,	Crocus.
8. SPATHACEÆ,	Amaryllis, etc.
9. CORONARIÆ,	Ornithogalum, Scilla.
10. LILIACEÆ,	Lilium, Tulipa, etc.
11. MURICATÆ,	Bromelia, etc.
12. COADUNATÆ,	Magnolia, etc.
13. CALIMARIÆ,	Juncus, etc.
14. GRAMINA,	as now.
15. CONIFERÆ,	Abies, Pinus.
16. AMENTACEÆ,	Pistacia, Populus. Quercus.
17. NUCAMENTACEÆ,	Xanthium, etc.
18. AGGREGATÆ,	Valerianum, etc.
19. DUMOSÆ,	Viburnum, Ilex, Rhus.
20. SCABRIDÆ,	Ficus, etc.
21. COMPOSITÆ,	as now.
22. UMBELLATÆ,	as now.
23. MULTISILIQUÆ,	Modern Crowfoots.
24. BICORNES,	Azalea, Myrsine, etc.
25. SEPIARIÆ,	Jasminum, Ligustrum.
26. CULMINIÆ,	Tilia, Bixa, China.
27. VAGINALES,	Polygonum, Laurus, etc.
28. CORYDALES,	Fumaria, etc.
29. CONTORTI,	Vinca, Asclepias, etc.
30. RHŒADES,	Papaver, etc.
31. PUTAMINEA,	Capparis, etc.
32. CAMPANACEI,	Convolvulus, Viola, Lobelia, etc.
33. LURIDÆ,	Solanum, Digitalis, etc.
34. COLUMNIFERÆ,	Camellia, the Mallowworts, etc.
35. SENTICOSÆ,	Roseworts exclusively.

Natural Order.	*Examples.*
36. CORNOSÆ,	Spiræa, Filipendula.
37. POMACEÆ,	Pyrus, Ribes, etc.
38. DRUPACEÆ,	as now.
39. ARBUSTIVA,	Philadelphus, and Myrtle blooms.
40. CALYCANTHEMÆ,	Œnothera, etc.
41. HESPERIDEÆ,	Citrus, Styrax.
42. CARYOPHYLLEI,	Cloveworts.
43. ASPERIFOLIÆ,	the Modern Borageworts.
44. STELLATÆ,	Galium, etc.
45. CUCURBITACEÆ,	Colocynthis, etc.
46. SUCCULENTÆ,	Cactus, Oxalis, Ledum, etc.
47. TRICOCCÆ,	Euphorbia, etc.
48. INUNDATÆ,	Hippuris, Elatine, etc.
49. SARMENTACEÆ.	Vitis, Hedera, Smilax, Menispermum, etc.
50. TRIHILATÆ,	Bigonia, Berberis, etc.
51. PRECIÆ,	Part of Modern Primworts.
52. ROTACEÆ,	Gentiana, Lysimachia, Anagallis, etc.
53. HOLERACEÆ,	Spinacia, etc.
54. VEPRECULÆ,	Rhamnus, Daphne, etc.
55. PAPILIONACEÆ,	as now.
56. LOMENTACEÆ,	Leguminous plants with pointed pods.
57. SILIQUOSÆ,	Crucifers.
58. VERTICILLATÆ,	Labiates, etc.
59. PERSONATÆ,	Figworts, etc.
60. PERFORATÆ,	Hypericum, Cistus.
61. STATUMINATÆ,	Ulmus, etc.
62. CANDELLARES,	Rhizophora, etc.
63. CYMOSÆ,	Lonicera, Cinchona, etc.
64. FILICES,	as now.
65. MUSCI,	as now.
66. ALGÆ,	nearly as now.
67. FUNGI,	as now.
68. VAGÆ,	all his doubtful genera.

At a later period, Nos. 7, 10, 11, 17, 26, 27, 36, 38, 39, 60, 61, 62, and 63 were cancelled, and four added:—

Natural Order.	*Examples.*	*Natural Order.*	*Examples.*
GRUINALES,	Cranesbills.	HEDERACEÆ,	Hedera, Vitis, etc.
CALYCIFLORÆ,	Osyris, Trophis, etc.	MISCELLANEÆ,	a curious mixture.

In 1789, Jussieu, Antoine Laurent de, adopting the views of Ray as to primary divisions, applied them to the system of Tournefort, which had been in common use in France from the year 1694. To this he added the position of the stamens with respect to the ovary, and thus constructed his fifteen classes in the following manner:—

					Class.
Acotyledones,					I.
Monocotyledones		Stamina,	hypogyna,		II.
		,,	perigyna,		III.
		,,	epigyna,		IV.
Dicotyledones	Apetalæ	Stamina,	epigyna,		V.
		,,	perigyna,		VI.
		,,	hypogyna,		VII.
	Monopetalæ	Corolla,	hypogyna,		VIII.
		,,	perigyna,		IX.
			epigyna	Antheris, connatis,	X.
				Antheris, distinctus,	XI.
	Polypetalæ	Stamina,	epigyna,		XII.
		,,	hypogyna,		XIII.
		,,	perigyna,		XIV.
	Diclines irregulares,				XV.

Under each of these classes he arranged his Natural Orders, as follows, usually deriving their name from some genus which he regarded as a good illustration of their structure:—

CLASS I.

1. Fungi.
2. Algæ.
3. Hepaticæ.
4. Musci.
5. Filices.
6. Naiades.

CLASS II.

7. Aroideæ.
8. Typhæ.
9. Cyperoïdeæ.
10. Gramineæ.

CLASS III.

11. Palmæ.
12. Asparagi.
13. Junci.
14. Liliæ.
15. Bromeliæ.
16. Asphodeli.
17. Narcissi.
18. Irides.

CLASS IV.

19. Musæ.
20. Cannæ.
21. Orchides.
22. Hydrocharides.

CLASS V.

23. Aristolochiæ.

CLASS VI.

24. Eleagni.
25. Thymeleæ.
26. Proteæ.
27. Lauri.
28. Polygoneæ.
29. Atriplice.

CLASS VII.

30. Amaranthi.
31. Plantagines.
32. Nyctagines.
33. Plumbagines.

CLASS VIII.

34. Lysimachiæ.
35. Pediculares.
36. Acanthi.
37. Jasmineæ.
38. Vitices.
39. Labiatæ.

40. Scrophulariæ.
41. Solaneæ.
42. Boragineæ.
43. Convolvuli.
44. Polemonia.
45. Bignoniæ.
46. Gentianeæ.
47. Apocyneæ.
48. Sapolæ.

CLASS IX.

49. Guaiacanæ.
50. Rhododendra.
51. Ericæ.
52. Campanulaceæ.

CLASS X.

53. Cichoraceæ.
54. Cinarocephalæ.
55. Corymbiferæ.

CLASS XI.

56. Dipsaceæ.
57. Rubiaceæ.
58. Caprifolia.

CLASS XII.

59. Araliæ.
60. Umbelliferæ.

CLASS XIII.

61. Ranunculaceæ.
62. Papaveraceæ.
63. Cruciferæ.
64. Capparides.
65. Sapindi.
66. Acera.
67. Malpighiæ.
68. Hyperica.
69. Guttiferæ.
70. Aurantiæ.
71. Meliæ.
72. Vitis.
73. Geraniæ.
74. Malvaceæ.
75. Magnoliæ.
76. Anonæ.
77. Menispermæ.
78. Berberides.
79. Tiliaceæ.
80. Cisti.
81. Rutaceæ.
82. Caryophylleæ.

CLASS XIV.

83. SemperviVæ.
84. Saxifragæ.
85. Cacti.
86. Portulaceæ.
87. Ficoideæ.
88. Onagræ.
89. Myrti.
90. Melastomæ.
91. Salicareæ.
92. Rosaceæ.
93. Leguminosæ.
94. Terebintaceæ.
95. Rhamni.

CLASS XV.

96. Euphorbiæ.
97. Cucurbitaceæ.
98. Urticeæ.
99. Amentaceæ.
100. Coniferæ.

In 1813, De Candolle, A.P., published his "Théorie Elémentaire de la Botanique, ou Exposition des Principes de la Classification Naturelle et de l'Art de décrire et d'étudier les Végétaux."

In this work is to be found the explanation of the principles which guided its clear-minded author to the construction of a method of arrangement, which has now almost superseded all others, chiefly because of its easiness and simplicity. He himself explains the course he has taken to the following effect: "I place Dicotyledons first, because they have the greatest number of distinct and separate organs. Then, as I find families where some of these organs become consolidated, and consequently seem to disappear, I refer them to a lower rank. The principle gives me the following series:—

1. Dicotyledons;	polypetalous and hypogynous.
2. „ „	„ „ and perigynous.
3. „ „	monopetalous and perigynous.
4. „ „	„ „ and hypogynous.
5. „ „	apetalous, or with a single perianth.
6. Monocotyledons;	phanærogamous.
7. „ „	cryptogamous.
8. Acotyledons;	leafy and sexual.
9. „ „	leafless and without any known sexes.

"I have adopted this series, partly because I think it that which is least removed from a natural sequence, and partly because it is convenient and easy for study. But let no one imagine that I attach the least importance to it. The true science of general natural history consists in the study of the symmetry peculiar to each family, and of the relation which these families bear to each other. All the rest is merely scaffolding, better or worse suited to accomplish that end" (p. 206, 1st edition).

At this time De Candolle made no attempt to combine the Natural Orders in Alliances; but at a later period (1819), in a second edition of the "Théorie," he proposed a few such groups, under the name of Cohorts, as will be seen by the following lists of his Orders, taken from the edition of 1819. In that of 1844, published by his son after his death, these Cohorts are all broken up, and considerable alteration is made in the sequence of the Natural Orders.

I. VASCULAR or COTYLEDONOUS PLANTS; *i. e.*, furnished with cellular tissue and vessels, and whose embryo is provided with one or more cotyledons.

1. Exogens or Dicotyledons; *i. e.*, where the vessels are arranged in concentric layers, of which the youngest are the outermost, and where the embryo has opposite or verticillate cotyledons.

A. Perianth double; *i. e.*, where the calyx and corolla are distinct.

THALAMIFLORÆ.

Petals distinct, inserted on the receptacle.

Cohort I.—Carpels numerous, or stamens opposite the petals.

1. Ranunculaceæ.
2. Dilleniaceæ.
3. Magnoliaceæ.
4. Anonaceæ.
5. Menispermeæ.
6. Berberidæ.
7. Podophyllæ.
8. Nymphæaceæ.

Cohort II.—Carpels solitary, or consolidated, placentæ parietal.

9. Papaveraceæ.
10. Fumariaceæ.
11. Cruciferæ.
12. Capparideæ.
13. Flacourtianeæ.
14. Passifloreæ.
15. Violaceæ.
16. Polygaleæ.
17. Resedaceæ.
18. Droseraceæ.
19. Frankencaceæ.
20. Cistineæ.

Cohort III.—Ovary solitary, placenta central.

21. Caryophylleæ.
22. Lineæ.
23. Malvaceæ.
24. Chlenaceæ.
25. Byttneriaceæ.
26. Sterculiaceæ.
27. Tiliaceæ.
28. Elæocarpeæ.
29. Sapindaceæ.
30. Hippocastaneæ.
31. Aceraceæ.
32. Malpighiaceæ.
33. Hippocratiaceæ.
34. Hypericineæ.
35. Guttiferæ.
36. Marcgraviaceæ.
37. Sarmentaceæ.
38. Geranieæ.
39. Cedreleæ.
40. Meliaceæ.
41. Hesperideæ.
42. Camellieæ.
43. Olacineæ.
44. Rutaceæ.

Cohort IV.—Fruit gynobasic.

45. Simaroubiaceæ.
46. Ochnaceæ.

CALYCIFLORÆ.

Petals free, more or less united, always perigynous, or inserted on the calyx.

47. Frangulaceæ.
48. Samydeæ.
49. Zanthoxyleæ.
50. Juglandeæ.
51. Terebinthaceæ.
52. Leguminosæ.
53. Rosaceæ.
54. Salicariæ.
55. Tamariscineæ.
56. Melastomeæ.
57. Myrtineæ.
58. Combretaceæ.
59. Cucurbitaceæ.

60. Loaceæ.
61. Onagrariceæ.
62. Ficoideæ.
63. Paronychieæ.
64. Portulaceæ.
65. Nopaleæ.
66. Grossulaceæ.
67. Crassulaceæ.
68. Saxifrageæ.
69. Cunoniaceæ.
70. Umbelliferæ.
71. Araliaceæ.
72. Caprifolieæ.
73. Loranthææ.
74. Rubiaceæ.
75. Opercularieæ.
76. Valerianeæ.
77. Dipsaceæ.
78. Calycereæ.
79. Compositæ.
80. Campanulaceæ.
81. Lobeliaceæ.
82. Gesnerieæ.
83. Vaccinieæ.
84. Ericineæ.

COROLLIFLORÆ.

Petals united into an hypogynous corolla, or not attached to the calyx.

85. Myrsineæ.
86. Sapoteæ.
87. Ternstromieæ.
88. Ebenaceæ.
89. Oleineæ.
90. Jasmineæ.
91. Strychneæ.
92. Apocyneæ.
93. Gentianeæ.
94. Bignoniaceæ.
95. Sesameæ.
96. Polemonideæ.
97. Convolvulaceæ.
98. Boragineæ.
99. Solaneæ.
100. Antirrhineæ.
101. Rhinanthaceæ.
102. Labiateæ.
103. Myroporineæ.
104. Pyrenaceæ.
105. Acanthaceæ.
106. Lentibularieæ.
107. Primulaceæ.
108. Globularieæ.

B. MONOCHLAMYDÆ.

Perianth simple, or whose calyx and corolla form only one envelope.

109. Plumbagineæ.
110. Plantagineæ.
111. Nyctagineæ.
112. Amaranthaceæ.
113. Chenopodeæ.
114. Begoniaceæ.
115. Polygoneæ.
116. Laurineæ.
117. Myristiceæ.
118. Proteaceæ.
119. Thymeleæ.
120. Santalaceæ.
121. Elæagneæ.
122. Aristolochiæ.
123. Euphorbiaceæ.
124. Monomieæ.
125. Urticeæ.
126. Piperiteæ.
127. Amentaceæ.
128. Coniferæ.

2. ENDOGENS, or MONOCOTYLEDONS; *i.e.*, plants whose vessels are arranged in bundles, the youngest being in the middle of the trunk, and whose embryo is furnished with solitary or alternate cotyledons.

A. PHANÆROGAMS.

Fructification visible, regular.

129. Cycadeæ.
130. Hydrocharideæ.
131. Alismaceæ.
132. Orchideæ.
133. Drymirrhizeæ.
134. Musaceæ.
135. Irideæ.
136. Hæmodoraceæ.
137. Amaryllideæ.
138. Hemerocallideæ.
139. Dioscoreæ.
140. Smilaceæ.
141. Liliaceæ.
142. Colchicaceæ.
143. Junceæ.
144. Commelineæ.
145. Palmæ.
146. Pandaneæ.
147. Typhaceæ.
148. Aroidiæ.
149. Cyperaceæ.
150. Gramineæ.

B. CRYPTOGAMS.

Fructification hidden, unknown, or irregular.

151. Naiades.
152. Equisetaceæ.
153. Marsileaceæ.
154. Lycopodineæ.
155. Filices.

II. CELLULAR OR ACOTYLEDONOUS PLANTS, *i. e.*, composed of cellular tissue only, not furnished with vessels, and whose embryo is without cotyledons.

A. FOLIACEÆ.

Having leaf-like expansions and known sexes.

156. Musci.
157. Hepaticæ.

B. APHYLLÆ.

Not having leaf-like expansions and no known sexes.

158. Lichenes.
159. Hypoxyla.
160. Fungi.
166. Algæ.

In 1845, Lindley, John, published "The Vegetable Kingdom," and the following is the arrangement adopted in his work.

CLASSES.

Asexual, or Flowerless Plants.

Stems and leaves undistinguishable - - -	I. THALLOGENS.
Stems and leaves distinguishable - - -	II. ACROGENS.

Sexual, or Flowering Plants.

Fructification springing from a thallus - -	III. RHIZOGENS.
Fructification springing from a stem; wood of stem youngest in the centre; cotyledon single; leaves parallel, veined, permanent; wood of the stem always confused - - - - - -	IV. ENDOGENS.
Leaves net-veined, deciduous; wood of the stem, when perennial, arranged in a circle of central pith	V. DICTYOGENS.
Wood of stem youngest at the circumference, always concentric; cotyledons two or more; seeds quite naked - - - - - - -	VI. GYMNOGENS.
Seeds enclosed in seed-vessels - - -	VII. EXOGENS.

CLASS I. THALLOGENS.—*Alliances of Thallogens.*

1. Algales.
2. Fungales.
3. Lichenales.

CLASS II. ACROGENS.—*Alliances of Acrogens.*

4. Muscales.
5. Lycopodales.
6. Filicales.

CLASS III. RHIZOGENS.—*Alliances the same as the Class.*

CLASS IV. ENDOGENS.

Flowers glumaceous; that is to say, composed of bracts not collected into true whorls, but consisting of imbricated, colourless, or herbaceous scales.

7. Glumales.
   Flowers petaloid, or furnished with a true calyx or corolla, or with both, or absolutely naked, ♂ ♀.
8. Arales.
9. Palmales.
10. Hydrales.
    Flowers furnished with a true calyx, and corolla adherent to the ovary, ☿.
11. Narcissales.
12. Amomales.
13. Orchidales.
    Flowers furnished with a true calyx, and corolla free from the ovary, ☿.
14. Xyridales.
15. Juncales.
16. Liliales.
17. Alismales.

CLASS V. DICTYOGENS.—*Alliance the same as the Class.*

CLASS VI. GYMNOGENS.—*Alliance the same as the Class.*

CLASS VII. EXOGENS.—*Alliances of Exogens.*

Sub-Class I. Declinous Exogens.

Flowers ♂ ♀, without any tendency to ⚥.

18. Amentales.
19. Urticales.
20. Euphorbiales.
21. Quernales.
22. Garryales.
23. Menispermales.
24. Cucurbitales.
25. Papayales.

Sub-Class II. Hypogynous Exogens.

Flowers ⚥, or ♂ ⚥ ♀; stamens entirely free from the calyx and corolla.

26. Violales.
27. Cistales.
28. Malvales.
29. Sapindales.
30. Guttiferales.
31. Nymphales.
32. Ranales.
33. Berberales.
34. Ericales.
35. Rutales.
36. Geraniales.
37. Silenales.
38. Chenopodales.
39. Piperales.

Sub-Class III. Perigynous Exogens.

Flowers ⚥, or ♂ ⚥ ♀; stamens growing to the side of either calyx or the corolla; ovary superior, or nearly so.

40. Ficoidales.
41. Daphnales.
42. Rosales.
43. Saxifragales.
44. Rhamnales.
45. Gentianales.
46. Solanales.
47. Cortusales.
48. Echiales.
49. Bignoniales.

Sub-Class IV. Epigynous Exogens.

Flowers ⚥, or ♂ ⚥ ♀; stamens growing to the side of either calyx or corolla; ovary inferior or nearly so.

50. Campanales.
51. Myrtales.
52. Cactales.
53. Grossales.
54. Cinchonales.
55. Umbellales.
56. Asarales.

GLOSSARY OF BOTANICAL TERMS.

A

ACEROSE, chaffy
Acicular, needle-shaped
Aciniform, scimitar-shaped
Aculeate, prickly
Adnate, adhering
Aggregate, many flowers included in one calyx
Alate, winged
Androgynous, bearing male and female flowers, distinct on the same root
Anther, summit of the stamen, containing the pollen
Apetalous, without petals
Apophysis, a swelling beneath the capsule of a moss
Appressed, squeezed close
Arborescent, becoming woody
Arboreous, woody
Arcuate, bowed
Articulate, jointed
Asci, small tubes in which the seeds of some cryptogamic plants are placed
Attenuated, growing slender
Auriculated, ear-shaped
Awn, a beard, sharp process, issuing from chaff in corn and seeds
Awnless, without beard
Axillary, flowers, etc., proceeding from an angle formed by a branch with a stem

B

Beaded, granulated
Beaked, like a bird's beak
Bearded, beset with parallel hairs, or tufts of hair
Bicapsular, having two capsules
Biennial, living two years
Bifid, two-cleft, cloven
Bifarious, pointing from opposite sides
Bilabiate, blossom with two lips
Bilocular, having two cells
Binate, in pairs
Bipartite, deeply divided into two parts
Bipinnate, double-winged
Biternate, doubly three-fold
Bivalved, two-valved
Border, the upper spreading part of a monopetalous flower
Bractea, floral leaf, may often be mistaken for the calyx, but is more permanent
Bulbiferous, flowers succeeded by bulbs instead of seeds

C

Calyptra, veil, covering the anther of mosses like a hood
Calyx, the outer covering of a flower
Campanulate, bell-shaped
Canaliculate, channelled
Cancellated, latticed
Capillary, hair-like
Capitate, growing in heads
Capsule, membranous hollow seed-vessel
Carinated, keeled
Carnose, fleshy
Catkin, flowers and chaff on a long, slender stalk, like a cat's tail
Caudate, tailed
Caulescent, having a stem
Cell, the hollow in a capsule for holding the seed
Central florets, which occupy the middle part of a flower
Chaff, dry calyx of corn and grasses
Ciliate, fringed
Cirrhi, tendrils
Cirrhose, terminating in a tendril
Clavated, club-shaped
Claw, the lower narrow part of the petal in flowers
Cleft, divided into parts
Club-shaped, thinner at the base than the termination
Coadunate, joined together at the base

Coated, composed of layers, as the bulb of the onion
Cochleated, snail-shaped
Column, the central pillar in a capsule
Columnar, like the shaft of a column
Compact, growing close, as it were pressed together
Complicate carinate, doubly keeled
Compound flowers, consisting of many florets or little flowers
Compressed, a stem having two opposite sides, plain or flat
Conduplicate, folded, or doubled together
Confluent, running one into another at the base
Congested, heaped together
Conjugated leaf, a pinnate leaf with only one pair of leaflets
Connate, united at the base
Connivent, converging
Converging, applied to the corolla, when the tips of the petals meet so close as to shut the flower
Convoluted, twisted spirally
Cordate, heart-shaped
Cordate-lanceolate, heart spear-shaped
Coriaceous, leather-like
Cornute, horn-shaped
Corolla, blossom
Corona, crown
Corymb, bunch of flowers supported on separate footstalks
Costated, ribbed
Cotyledones, seed-lobes
Crenate, scolloped
Crenato-serrulated, finely notched
Crested, having an appendage like a tuft or crest
Crinite, hairy
Cruciform, cross-shaped
Cucullate, cone-shaped
Culm, straw
Cuneiform, wedge-shaped
Curtain, the calyx of agarics
Cuspidate, prickly pointed
Cyathiform, cup-shaped
Cylindrical, round, without angles, like a walking-stick
Cyme, tuft
Cymose, tufted

D

Deciduous, falling off
Declining, bent like a bow, with the arch downwards
Decompound, doubly compound, or containing within a common calyx smaller calyxes common to several flowers
Decumbent, lying down
Decurrent leaf, having its base running down the stem
Decussated, crossed at right angles
Deflected, bowed or bent down
Dehiscent, gaping
Deltoid, trowel-shaped
Dentate, toothed
Denticulate, set with little teeth
Dichotomous, forked
Didymous, double
Digitate, finger-like
Dimidiate, divided in two parts
Diœcious, male and female flowers, growing on different plants
Dipetalous, of two petals
Diphyllous, two-leaved
Disk, the whole surface of a leaf or flower
Divaricating, straddling
Diverging, making a right angle
Drupe, a pulpy seed-vessel, containing a nut or stone
Duplicate, doubled

E

Echinate, set with prickles
Elliptic, oval
Elliptic-lanceolate, narrow oval
Emarginate, notched at the end
Ensiform, sword-shaped
Erose, gnawed
Exserted, protruded, opposed to inclosed
Extra-foliate, growing under the leaves

F

Farina, see Pollen
Fascicled, bundled
Fastigiate, flat-topped
Feathered, downy
Female flowers, containing pistils but no stamens
Fibres, woody strings or nerves
Filament, the thread-like part of a stamen, supporting the anther
Filiform, thread-shaped
Fistulous, hollow
Flexuose, zig-zag, winding
Floral leaf, the leaf next the flower, sometimes mistaken for the calyx

Floret, the separate little flower of an aggregate flower
Foliaceous, leafy
Frond, when the stem, root, and leaf are all in one
Fruit-stalk, a stalk bearing flowers but not leaves
Fruticose, shrub-like
Fuliginous, sooty
Furcated, forked
Fusiform, spindle-shaped

G

Geniculated, knee-jointed
Germen, seed-bud, the rudiment of fruit yet in embryo
Gibbous, bulging
Gills, the thin plates on the under side of a mushroom
Glands, secretory vessels
Glandular, formed of glands
Glaucous, grey, blueish-green
Glomerate, flowers growing close together in a globular form
Glume, husk
Granulated, headed

H

Hastate, halbert-shaped
Hastate-sinuated, jagged halbert-shaped
Herbaceous, succulent and tender, in opposition to woody
Hermaphrodite flowers, containing both stamens and pistils
Hirsute, roughed with strong hairs
Hispid, bristly
Husk, dry, semitransparent membranes, forming the calyx and blossoms of grasses
Hymenium, that part of a fungus which contains the reproductive organs

I

Inbricated, tiled
Imperfect flowers, such as want either anther or pistil, or both
Incise, serrated, gashed
Incrassated, thickened upwards
Incumbent, leaning or resting against
Incurved, bowing inwards
Indented, hollowed or deeply scolloped
Inflected, bent inwards
Infundibuliform, funnel-shaped
Internode, the space between the joints
Intrafoliaceous, within the leaves
Involucrum, the calyx of an umbel
Involucret, a partial involucrum
Involute, rolled inwards
Interrupted, divided by intervals of smaller flowers

K

Keeled, bent like the keel of a ship or boat

L

Labiated, having lips
Laciniated, jagged
Lactescent, milky
Lamellæ, the gills of a fungus
Laminated, the flat surface of leaves lying close upon each other
Lanceolate, spear-shaped
Lanceolate-ovate, spear egg-shaped
Leaflet, one of the single leaves of a compound leaf
Legumen, pod
Lenticular, spherically convex on both sides
Lid, a cover to the capsules of mosses
Lignose, woody
Limb, the upper flat, broad part of the petal is called the limb
Linear, strap-shaped
Linear-lanceolate, strap spear-shaped
Lineated, streaked
Lip, the upper or under division of a gaping blossom
Lobed, divided nearly half-way down into lobes
Lunated, crescent-shaped

M

Male flowers, containing stamens but no pistils
Marginate, bordered
Mid-rib, the principal nerve in the rib
Mitriform, mitre-formed
Moniliform, necklace-shaped, like beads strung together
Monopetalous, one-petalled
Monophyllous, one-leafed
Monospermous, one-seeded
Mucronated, sharppointed at the end

Multangular, many-cornered
Muricated, covered with sharp points

N

Navicular, boat-shaped
Nectary, honey-cup, part of flower designed to secrete and contain honey
Neutral, flowers without stamen or pistils, and producing no seeds
Node, knot
Nucule, a little nut

O

Obconic, inversely conic
Obcordate, inversely heart-shaped
Obovate, inversely egg-shaped, that is, with the small end downwards
Obsolete, indistinct
Octofid, eight-cleft
Olivaceous, having the quality of olives
Operculum, lid
Orbiculate, round and flat
Osseous, hard as bone
Ovate, egg-shaped
Ovate-lanceolate, egg spear-shaped

P

Palate, the inner part of the mouth of gaping blossoms
Paleaceous, chaffy
Palmate, hand-shaped
Panduriform, fiddle-shaped
Panicle, an assemblage of flowers growing upon subdivided fruit-stalks, as in oats and some grasses
Papilionaceous, butterfly-shaped
Papillose, pimpled
Parasitical, growing on some other plant, not on the ground
Partite, divided
Pectinated, comb-like
Pedate, bird-footed
Pedicle, a partial peduncle, or little fruit-stalk
Pedunculate, growing on a fruit-stalk
Peduncle, fruit-stalk
Peltate, when the stalk is fixed in the disk, instead of the margin
Pendulous, hanging down
Pentagonal, five-cornered
Pentapetalous, five petals
Pentaphyllous, five-leaved
Perennial, continuing for several years
Perfect flower, having both stamens and pistils
Perforated leaf, full of small holes, very apparent when held up to the light
Perfoliate, the stem passing through the leaf
Perianth, cup or calyx
Pericarp, seed-vessel
Perichætial leaves, surrounding the base of the fruit-stalk in mosses
Peristome, the rim surrounding the mouth of the capsule in mosses
Permanent, applied to calyxes, etc., remaining on the plant till the fruit is ripe
Personate blossom, gaping
Petaliform, resembling a petal
Petal, the coloured leaves which constitute the blossom
Petiolate, having leaf-stalks
Petiole, a leaf-stalk
Pileus, a cap of a fungus
Pilose, hairy
Pinnatifid, feather-cleft
Pinnated, winged, a compound leaf, formed of several little leaves fastened to each side of it
Pinnulate, when each pinna is subdivided
Pistil, part of the flower standing in the centre, and composed of germ, style, and summit
Plicate, plaited
Plumose, feathered
Pod, a seed-vessel
Pollen, the dust contained in the anther of flowers
Polypetalous, many-petalled
Procumbent, trailing
Proliferous, when one blossom grows out of another
Pubescent, covered with soft wool or hair
Punctated, dotted

Q

Quinate, growing in fives

R

Raceme, a cluster of flowers, attached by a pedicle to a common stalk; as in currants
Rachis, the common stalk, or recept.

to which the flowers of grasses, etc., are attached
Radiate, compound flowers in which the florets in the centre differ from those of the circumference
Radical, issuing immediately from the root
Radii, the outer florets of a radiate compound flower
Ramose, branched
Receptacle, the base upon which the other parts of a flower are placed
Reclining, bent downwards so that the point of the leaf is lower than the base
Recurved, curved downwards
Reflected, bent back
Reniform, kidney-shaped
Repens, creeping
Replicated, folded or plaited
Reticulated, veined like network
Revolute, rolled back
Retroflexed, distorted
Rhomboid-triangular, three-cornered, diamond-shaped
Rhomboid-ovate, egg-diamond-shaped
Ringent, gaping
Root-leaves, leaves proceeding immediately from the root, without a stem
Rostrate, beaked
Rotate, wheel-shaped
Rugose, wrinkled
Runcinate, notched, the notches pointing backwards

S

Sagittate, arrow-shaped
Salver-shaped, a blossom tubular at bottom, flat and expanding at top
Scaber, rough like a file
Scape, stalk
Scions, shoots
Scariose, skinny
Semibifid, half-cleft
Semicylindrical, half a cylinder divided lengthwise
Seminal leaves, arising immediately from the seed-lobes
Serrated, toothed like a saw
Serrulated, very minutely serrated
Sessile, sitting
Setaceous, bristle-shaped
Setose, bristly
Sexangular, six-sided
Shaggy, rough, with stiff hairs
Sheath, a membrane investing a stem or branch
Shield, a circular kind of fructification of some lichens
Shrubby, perennial with several woody stems
Silicle, a little pod
Silique, pod
Simple, undivided
Sitting, leaves having no leaf-stalk, or flowers without a fruit-stalk
Spadix, sheathed fruit-stalk
Spathe, sheath
Spatulate, battledore-shaped
Spike, sessile flowers placed alternately on each side of the fruit-stalk
Spikelet, a little spike
Spindle-shaped, gradually tapering
Spinose, thorny
Sporidia, small, transparent bodies containing seeds
Spur, shaped like the spur of a cock
Squamose, scaly
Stamens, long, slender bodies placed in the flower-cup round the pistil
Standard, the upright petal of a butterfly-shaped blossom
Stellate, starry, leaves surrounding the stem in a whorl
Stem-leaves, growing immediately upon the stem
Stigma, the summit of the pistil
Stipes, the stalk of a fungus
Stipitate, standing on a pedicle
Stipulæ, small leaves or scales at the base of the leaf-stalk
Stoloniferous, putting forth suckers
Strap-shaped, long and narrow
Striated, scored with slender lines
Style, the middle portion of the pistil, connecting the stigma with the germ
Subcymose, somewhat tufted
Subramose, a little branched
Subserrated, somewhat serrated
Subulate, awl-shaped
Succulent, juicy
Subsessile, almost sessile
Subfruticose, somewhat woody
Summit, the top of the pistil
Suture, seam
Sword-shaped, long, narrow, and pointed

T

Tendril, a spiral shoot
Terminal, ending in a branch or stem

Ternate, leaves, growing three together from the same point
Tesselate, chequered
Thallus, the part which bears the fructification in lichens
Theca, the seed-vessel in cryptogamic plants
Tiled, one leaf or scale partly covering another
Tomentose, cottony
Trifid, three-cleft
Trivalved, three-valved
Truncate, lopped
Tunicate, coated
Turbinate, top-shaped

U

Umbel, a composition of flowers, in which a number of slender fruit-stalks proceed from the same centre, like the spokes of an umbrella
Uncinate, hooked at the end
Undate, waved
Undulate, waved
Unequal florets, when those in the circumference of an umbel are larger than those in the centre.
Ungulate, hoof-shaped
Univalve, one-valved
Urceolate, pitcher-shaped

V

Vaginate, sheathed
Valves, the several pieces which compose a capsule, also the leaflets composing the calyx and corolla, in grasses
Veil, the calyx in mosses
Ventricose, distended
Verrucose, warty
Verticillate, growing in whorls
Vesicles, bladders
Villous, soft-haired
Volva, wrapper

W

Whorls, leaves or flowers surrounding the stem in a ring
Wings, the lateral petals of a butterfly-shaped blossom
Winged leaf, formed of many little leaves growing from each side of the stalk
Wing-cleft, a leaf cut deeply down the middle
Woolly, clothed with a pubescence resembling wool

CONTENTS OF VOL. I.

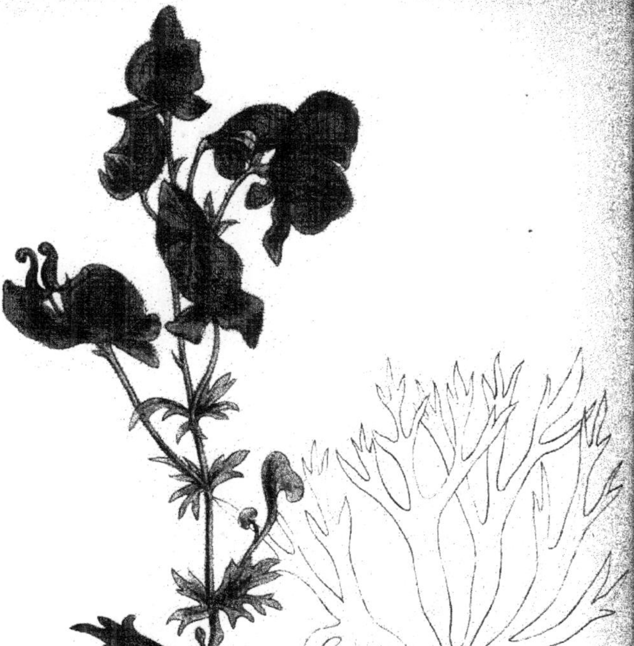

Aconitum Napellus.

FLORA HOMŒOPATHICA.

I.

ACONITUM NAPELLUS.

Monkshood, Wolfsbane, Helmet Flower, Friar's Cap.

SYNONYMS.—Aconitum cœruleum seu Napellus, *Bauh. Pin.;* Aconitum caule simplici, *n.* 1197. *Hall, Hist.* ii. 1235; Aconitum vulgare, *Decandolle.*

FOREIGN NAMES.—*Fr.:* Napel, Aconit. *Ger.:* Eisen-hut, Blauer Sturmhut. *Ital.:* Napello. *Span.:* Napelo. *Dut.:* Monnikskap. *Dan.:* Dreumunke. *Swed.:* Stormbat. *Russ.:* Borets.

Nat. Order, RANUNCULACEÆ.—POLYANDRIA, PENTAGYNIA.

DIAGNOSIS OF THE ORDER.—Ranal exogens, with distinct carpels; no separate stipules; an imbricated corolla; homogeneous albumen; and seeds without an awl. OF GENUS.—Calyx in æstivation imbricated. Fruit, many-seeded follicles.

GEN. CHAR.—*Calyx,* none. *Corolla* (calyx of Decandolle and others) inferior. *Petals* five, the upper arched or helmet-shaped. *Nectaries* (petals of Lindley) two, pedunculate, and recurved at the honey-bag behind, on long tubular stalks. *Filaments* numerous, some of the inner ones abortive. *Anthers* roundish. *Germens* spreading. *Styles* terminal, awl-shaped. *Stigmas* simple, acute. *Capsules* egg-shaped; one valve. *Seeds* numerous; angular, rugged at the edges of the capsule. *Root* tapering, placed perpendicularly in the earth, with numerous cylindrical fleshy fibres arising from it.

SPEC. CHAR.—Upper petal arched at the back. Spur of the nectary conical and bent down. Flowers densely spiked, or loosely panicled. Wings of the stamens cuspidate, or wanting. Lobes of the leaves cuneate, pinnatifid.

Fig. 1. exhibits a seed. 2. A capsule and follicle. 3. Germens, styles, and stigmas. 4. Nectaries and stamens (ap. Baxter).

The naked corolla of five petals, the upper one hooded, and the two recurved, stalked nectaries, concealed within the hollow of the uppermost petal or hood, will readily distinguish this from other genera in the same class and order (Baxter).

HISTORY.—The plant Ακόνιτον was known to the ancients, and mentioned by Nicander, Dioscorides, Theophrastus, Galen, Paulus Ægineta, and others. It is referred to as a virulent poison; but there have been many doubts as to whether the Aconite of the Greeks is the same as that used by us at the present day. Dioscorides described two species; Dodonæus, Sprengel, and Woodville agree that the second described by that author, viz. the λυκοτονον ("Aconitum alterum quod nonnulli Cycoctorum, alii Lycoctonum vocant, plurimum in Italia nascitur"), is the Aconitum napellus or Wolfsbane. The first species, the παρδαλιανχες ("Aconitum aliqui Pardalianches alii Cammarum), is supposed to be the Doronicum pardalianches, or Leopard's Bane. The Aconitum of Theophrastus has been referred, to the Ranunculus Thora, by Sprengel. *(Vide Supp. to Dunbar's Lex.)* Allalus, coeval with Cato, cultivated, in a garden, the Aconite, and other poisonous plants, and administered them for the purpose of experiment, so as to discover their antidotes. *(Plutarch, Demet.)*

Aconite is often referred to in mythological history; it was supposed to be the principal ingredient in the deadly draught given to the old men of Ceos, when they had become too infirm to be serviceable to their country. Medea was said to have used it in composing the poisonous drink she intended Theseus to quaff. It is also fabled as caused by Hecate to spring from the mouth of Cerberus: "Ut ab Hecate inventum aut ex Cerberi spuma enatum pronunciarent." Theophrastus relates that there was a mode of preparing the Aconite in his day, so that it should only destroy at the end of one or two years. It is asserted, that the huntsmen of the Alps dipped their arrows into the juice of this plant when hunting wolves; hence the name Wolfsbane. In later times it has been employed in the attempt to destroy whole armies, as the Indian poison Bihk or Bisch, with which the natives poisoned the tanks in the Burmese war, is supposed to have been a preparation of one of its species, the Aconitum ferox.

As a medicine, it was used by the ancients chiefly as an anodyne, and as an external application, to relieve pain in the eyes. It fell into disuse, until the time of Störck, who vaunted its powers as an antispasmodic, stimulant to the absorbents, diuretic and diaphoretic. From its very remarkable effects, as related by Störck, it was first introduced into the Pharmacopœias, but has been chiefly used since then as a topical remedy in neuralgic and rheumatic pains, and internally, in gout, rheumatism, some skin diseases, scrofula, phthisis, scirrhus and cancer, intermittents, dropsies, paralysis, epilepsy, amaurosis, uterine affections, and hypertrophy of the heart.

The name of this plant is derived, according to Theophrastus, from Aconis, a city of Bithynia, in the neighbourhood of which it grew in abundance. Pliny ascribes its etymology to Ακονη, a whetstone. Others, according to Burnett, derive its name from *ακονιγος*, *pulveris expers*, without dust, because the plant grows on rocks destitute of soil; but this applies more to the Aconitum neomontanum. Others, again, derive the word from *acon*, *acne*, a dart, because savage nations dipped their arrows into a poison made from this plant. The word Napellus is from *napus*, a turnip, from the similarity of its root to that vegetable.

Description. — Perennial, flowers May, June, and July. *Flowers* purple, glabrous. *Upper petal* helmet-shaped. *Leaves* palmated, in five wedge-shaped segments, deeply cut and toothed, standing alternately on channelled footstalks; the upper leaves not so deeply cut as the lower. *Stem* erect, from two to three feet high. Decandolle allows no less than twenty-nine varieties. That which is called by Miller Pyramidale, is most common in our gardens, being preferred on account of its long spike of blue flowers.

The following are the different species,* besides the Aconitum napellus, described in Martyn's edition of Miller's Dictionary.

1. *Acon. lycoctonum.* Great yellow Monkshood, or Wolfsbane, of which there are two varieties; viz. the bluish ash-coloured flower of Linnæus, and the Acon. altissimum of Miller. The common sort grows upwards of three feet high; both flower in the middle of June. In Sweden it is reckoned among the earliest spring flowers. First cultivated in this country by Gerarde, in 1596. Grows wild in the mountainous parts of Sweden, Austria, Carniola, and Siberia. A decoction of the powder of the root is used to destroy flies and other insects; but it is eaten in some parts of Sweden with impunity, being milder than some of the species. The ancients believed that it was fatal to those who slept under it.

2. *Acon. japonicum.* Native of Japan; there called Soo Huso.

3. *Acon. pyrenaicum.* Pyrenean, or fennel-leaved Monkshood. Grows wild in the Pyrenees, Tartary, and Siberia. First cultivated in England in 1739. Grows to the height of four feet, and the spike nods before flowering, which in this country is in July. It is poisonous.

4. *Acon. anthora.* Salutary Monkshood, as it has been erroneously called. Its root has two to four angular fleshy bulbs, and a stem from one foot to eighteen inches high. The flowers are of a *sulphur* colour. Grows wild in the Pyrenees, Alps, Austria, Siberia, etc. First cultivated in England in 1596. There is a variety of this with a white flower. Poisonous.

5. *Acon. variegatum.* Variegated or small blue Monkshood. Native of Italy and Bohemia. First cultivated in England in 1752. Flowers end of June. Two feet high. Spikes of flowers short; and the corollas change from variegated to plain. Poisonous.

* The Acon. napellus and cammarum are the most virulent European species. Horses will eat the napellus, when dried, without injury.

6. *Acon. album.* White Wolfsbane. Native of the Levant. Cultivated in England in 1739. Sometimes upwards of six feet high. Characterised by its tall stem, palmate leaves, and white flower. Poisonous.

7. *Acon. cammarum.* The paniculatum of the London Pharmacopœia. Purple Monkshood. Flowers of a pale blue. A much longer helmet and shorter raceme than Acon. napellus. Stem higher. Found wild in Switzerland, Austria, Styria, and Piedmont. First cultivated in England in 1748. Poisonous, but feeble compared to the napellus. A variety, with white and variegated flowers.

8. *Acon. uncinatum.* American Monkshood. Native of Pennsylvania. Leaves similar to the napellus; flowers resembling the cammarum. Cultivated in England in 1770. Highly poisonous.

9. *Acon. ferox.* Native of India. Highly poisonous.

10. *Acon. neomontanum.* 11. *Acon. volubile.* 12. *Acon. septentrionale.* 13. *Acon. tauricum.* 14. *Acon. cernuum.* All poisonous.

Geographical Distribution.—France, Sweden, Switzerland, Austria, Carniola, and other parts of Europe. One species Asiatic, one American, one British; although by some it is considered a doubtful native.

Localities.—In the mountainous districts of Carniola, Sweden, etc. *In England:* Watery places, by the side of streams. First discovered in a wild state by the Rev. Edward Whitehead, of Christchurch College, Oxford, in 1819. *Devonshire:* In some profusion on the margin of a limpid stream below Ogwell Mill; F. R., and Dr. Withering, 1827. *Herefordshire:* In a truly wild state by the side of the river Teme, and in great abundance on the banks of a brook running into that river; E. W., of Christchurch College, Oxon, 1819. Banks of a brook near Little Hereford; Dr. Lloyd. *Somersetshire:* In watery ground, on both sides of a brook at Ford, near Wiveliscombe and Milverton, where it grows in great abundance, and is collected for medicinal purposes.

PARTS USED IN MEDICINE.—The Roots, Flowers, and Leaves.

MODE OF PREPARATION.—The Homœopathic Pharmacopœia (Quin) orders the expressed juice of the recent plant to be mixed with equal quantity of spirits of wine, and after an interval of twenty-four hours, the clear liquid to be poured off. One drop of this is to be shaken twice with ninety-nine drops of spirits of wine, and marked with the sign (1). Afterwards, this is to be attenuated down to the 30th dilution, by adding one drop of the 1st dilution to ninety-nine drops of spirits of wine, and so on till the 30th is obtained. The qualities of the root and expressed juice vary much according to age, and if kept longer than a few months, become totally inert. Mr. Reuben Payne, of Milverton, finds the preparation made from the plant gathered in Somersetshire much more powerful than that procured from the best houses in London. This is probably owing to the above cause. The proper time of gathering the root for medicinal purposes is before the stem shoots; of the whole plant, in July and August.

POISONOUS EFFECTS. — The *poisonous* effects of medicinal substances on the animal economy, or the exhibition of over large doses of any medicine, are most interesting to the homœopathist; according to the law which governs them in their treatment of disease, these effects assist to indicate the general application of each medicinal substance, and from its baneful consequences its beneficial uses to mankind are made apparent.

The following are some of the most interesting cases which have occurred of poisoning by this plant, and which demonstrate its peculiar symptoms and actions.

A boy ate some of the leaves instead of parsley; in two hours, burning sensation in the mouth, throat, and stomach came on, followed by swooning and death. On inspection, the cerebral vessels were found enormously distended with a dark coloured fluid; a deep inflammatory blush extended over the whole mucous surface of the stomach, with dark coloured patches. (*Med. Chir. Review, July*, 1844.)

A dose (five grains) of the fresh extract was given to three patients, at the hospital of Bordeaux, by mistake. In a quarter of an hour, tremors of the muscles and a pricking sensation over the whole body came on, followed by vomiting, unconsciousness for a time, and afterwards confusion of sight, with intense headache, cold and clammy skin, pulse slow and irregular, respiration short and hurried; one died, the other two slowly recovered.

Dr. Geoghan (*Dub. Med. Jour.*, 1842) states a case of poisoning by the leaves of Aconite. *Two minutes* after eating, burning heat in the mouth, throat, gullet, and stomach ensued, with sensation of swelling of the face, general feeling of numbness and creeping of the skin; restlessness; dimness of sight; stupor, and partial insensibility; frothing at the nose and mouth; jaws and hands clenched; vomiting, purging; a sense of tenderness at the epigastrium; swooning and death.

A man boiled the fresh root and leaves, and half an hour after eating them, was found in bed rolling his arms about and foaming at the mouth; pupils widely dilated; lower extremities paralysed; surface cold and clammy; great nausea; pulse scarcely perceptible; followed by insensibility, and death.

The following are related by Dr. Pereira:—

A man, his wife, and child ate some roots at dinner, at two o'clock, by mistake for horse-radish. The greater part was eaten by the man. Three quarters of an hour after dinner the man complained of burning and numbness of the lips, mouth, and throat, which soon extended to the stomach, and was accompanied by vomiting of his dinner, and afterwards of a frothy mucus. His extremities were cold, but his chest warm; his head was bathed in a cold sweat; his eyes glaring; excessive trembling and violent pain in the head; lips blue; no cramp, spasm, or convulsion; his breathing was unaffected. He died apparently in a fainting state, about four hours after dinner.

The woman was affected in a similar way. She had the same burning and numbness of the lips, mouth, throat, and stomach, and violent vomiting. She experienced a curious sensation of numbness in the hands, arms, and legs, and she lost the power of articulating, her attempts to speak were attended with unintelligible sounds only; great muscular debility, unable to stand; some of the external senses were disordered; to use her own expression, though her eyes were wide open, her sight was very dim, and surrounding objects were seen indistinctly; the sensibility of the body was greatly impaired; her face and throat were almost insensible to the touch; she was very giddy, but neither delirious nor sleepy; her body and extremities were cold; she was frequently pulling her throat about, but she knew not why. Five or six hours afterwards she began to recover.

The child was similarly but slightly affected; like the others, she was constantly putting her hands to her throat. (*Pereira's Mat. Med., art. Aconite.*)

Mr. Sherwen mentions a case of a female poisoned by the alcoholic tincture of the root. The following were the chief symptoms. Five minutes after swallowing it, she was seized with prickling and tingling down the arms and fingers; painful numbness across the wrists; the tongue and mouth next felt the same; then the legs and feet; in less than ten minutes her face seemed to her to be swelling, and her throat getting tight; she felt sick, and made many efforts to vomit; her legs failed; she was almost blind, but was conscious of her state; the eyes were fixed and protruded, with contracted pupils; countenance livid; jaws and fauces rigid; arms and hands quite cold and pulseless; legs and trunk much in the same state; breathing short, imperfect, and laborious, with feeble fluttering of the heart. A strong convulsion occurred on attempting to give an emetic. Copious vomiting afterwards took place. Five hours after taking the poison, the pulse was becoming full, 58 per minute, and intermitting; there was less oppression at the præcordia, and the pupils were larger. She eventually recovered. (*Lancet, March* 25, 1837.)

The root of the Aconitum napellus was given to four brigands. Two of them, after having experienced most violent pains, were saved by appropriate means; the two others died. In one of these were the following symptoms. Some hours after the administration of the root he became imbecile; the face was covered by a cold sweat; asphyxia; spasms and syncope; involuntary alvine dejections; vomiting of bilious matter; swelling of the whole body; and he died apoplectic. (*Matthiolus in Dioscorid.*, p. 768.)

Willis reports a man dying maniacal, in a very short time after eating a salad containing some fresh leaves of the Aconite.

Linnæus relates, that an ignorant surgeon prescribed the leaves, which on his patient refusing to take, he swallowed them himself, and died in consequence.

A person having eaten some of the leaves became maniacal, and the surgeon who was called to his assistance, declared that the plant was not the cause of his disorder, and to convince the company that it was perfectly innocent, he ate freely of the leaves, and soon after died in great agony. (*Mord. in Kel. Acad.*, 1739.)

The juice of Aconite introduced into a small wound in the thumb excites pains in the fingers and arms; cardialgia; anxiety, with fear of suffocation; lipothymia (fainting); agitation; gangrene; abundant suppuration. (*Alberti, Junot. Med.*, vi. p. 724.)

Orfila relates that five persons partook of the leaves by mistake; three of them died two hours after. They all suffered from sensations of burning in the throat, œsophagus, and abdomen; desire to vomit; and when vomiting, violent colics, swelled face, and very tumid abdomen.

Some of the leaves of Aconite had been eaten by a man as a salad, and the following were the chief symptoms complained of. Sensation of tingling heat, which did not only affect the tongue but his jaws, so that the teeth seemed loose, and his cheeks were so much irritated, that he could scarce be persuaded but that his face was swelled to twice its proper size. This tingling sensation spread itself further and further, till it had taken hold of his whole body, especially the extremities. He had unsteadiness in the joints, especially of the knees and ankles, with twitching of the tendons, so that he could scarce walk across the room; he thought that in all his limbs he felt a sensible stop to the circulation of his blood, and that from the wrists to the finger-ends, and from the ankles to the toes, there was no circulation at all; giddiness of the head; eyes misty and wandering; humming and hissing noise in his ears, followed by syncope; strength and spirits exhausted; he must needs lie down (after vomiting produced by oil, etc., taken to eject the contents of the stomach); pulse interrupted and irregular, sometimes beating two or three strokes very quick together. (*Philos. Trans.*, vol. xxxviii. p. 287.)

"If the leaves or the root are chewed, a tingling sensation, with numbness, is produced; and if a rather larger quantity be taken, the palate and throat are affected. It appears as if the velum and soft palate were elongated, and rested on the dorsum of the tongue; to relieve this, frequent attempts are made to swallow." (*Pereira, art. Aconite.*) It has been affirmed, also, that the effluvium of the plant has produced fainting fits.

Dr. Fleming considers that the poison may cause death, "either by producing a powerful sedative impression on the nervous system (as in the case of Dr. Male, of Birmingham); by paralysing the muscles of respiration and causing asphyxia; or by producing syncope. A poisonous dose produces—1st, numbness and burning heat in the mouth, throat, and stomach; pain in the abdomen, with sickness and vomiting; diminished sensibility of the surface, with sensation of weight and fulness of different parts of the body, especially the face and ears: 2nd, vertigo; dimness of vision, or complete blindness; singing in the ears; deafness; frothing at the mouth; sense of constriction of the throat; great sense of debility; a trembling pulse, small, feeble, and irregular, and then imperceptible; extremities and surface cold and clammy; countenance blanched; bloodless lips; followed generally by sudden death. The common appearance on inspection is, general congestion of the venous system." (*Fleming on Ac. Nap.*, p. 134.)

Orfila remarks that, from the various experiments on animals, and effects on the human frame, it results that the different preparations of Aconite are absorbed, and transported in the current of the circulation; that they act specially on the nervous system, and particularly on the brain, where they produce a sort of mental alienation; that they exercise, besides, a local irritation, capable of developing an inflammation more or less intense; that they appear to act upon man as they do upon animals.

It will be seen, therefore, that every part of the fresh plant is strongly poisonous; but the root is particularly virulent, and many instances of its fatal effects are recorded both by ancient and modern writers; nevertheless, as frequently happens, "when *rightly understood*, qualities the most baneful may be converted into blessings."

MEDICAL USES (HOMŒOPATHIC).—The provings of Aconite, by Hahnemann, have given to the homœopathic practitioner a remedy which must ever hold a prominent, if not the first, place in our Pharmacopœia. The following are his observations upon this medicine, in his *Materia Medica Pura*. "Although the symptoms detailed do not fully express all the medicinal power of this precious plant, they afford the discerning homœopathist the means of judging how far it is useful in certain states of disease, in which the antiphlogistic treatment of the old practice has hitherto been applied. I refer to purely inflammatory fevers, in which a small dose of Aconite, taking the place of all antipathic remedies, produces a ready cure, without any subsequent affections.

"In measles, the purple miliary fever, inflammatory fever with pleurisy, etc., the efficacy of this plant is most powerful, provided the patient observes a cool diet, abstaining from everything medicinal, even from vegetable acids.

"Banishing from our system all idea of resemblance to that in ordinary usage, which is too often influenced by the names of imaginary diseases, it is necessary that the primary morbid conditions, under which Aconite is proposed, should present, in their principal symptoms, a strong analogy to those which are caused by this medicine. Its success is then most satisfactory.

"In acute inflammatory fevers, where it has been imagined that the patient can alone be relieved by copious and repeated bleedings, Homœopathy asserts its great superiority, in being, by the use of this medicine, able to overcome fevers and restore health in a shorter period of time than under the allopathic treatment, without being obliged to shed a single drop of blood, —that vital fluid which has been so often dangerously lavished under the old system.

"It is sometimes requisite, in acute disorders, to use another homœopathic medicine, to remove those morbid symptoms that still remain after those which the Aconite has subdued; but it is seldom needful to repeat the dose of Aconite.

"By giving Aconite with these precautions, in the diseases to which I refer, the circulation by degrees returns to its usual state.

"Although from the short duration of its action, which in small doses does not exceed thirty-six or forty-eight hours, Aconite would appear to be useful only in acute cases, yet it is not less so in the most obstinate chronic disorders, in which the condition of the body requires the modification of what is called *rigidity of fibre;* a subject upon which I cannot now enlarge. Its efficacy in such cases results from the development of the symptoms produced by it in the healthy subject.

"Aconite is also the chief and most powerful means of cure in the croup; in several species of angina, as well as in local acute inflammation in other parts of the body, especially when thirst and a quick pulse are connected with restless impatience, agitation that nothing can suppress, and a jactitation like that caused by Aconite. It produces, when given in health, all the morbid symptoms manifested by persons under the influence of fear, combined with anger; and it is also the most certain means of curing them rapidly.

"Whenever Aconite is chosen homœopathically, you must, above all, observe *moral* symptoms, and be careful that it closely resembles them.

"Aconite is found of great service in allaying all bad symptoms arising from suppression of secretions, alarm, agitation, or fear."

Clinical Observations.—*Noack and Trinks:* Aconite is especially suitable to individuals of a plethoric habit, lively character, bilio-nervous or sanguineous temperament, dark hair, bright complexion, and to old people. Congestion of blood in different organs; acute inflammation of all organs; violent hæmorrhages; attacks of violent general pain; effects of fright, anger, and chagrin; bilious affections; yellowness of skin, as in jaundice; congestion of blood to the head, when combined with vertigo; headache; catarrhal affections; great liability to catch cold; the exanthemata, in the first stages; erysipelas; nettle-rash; synochal fevers; acute rheumatism, especially of the joints; acute arthritis; gout; neuralgia; fainting fits; dementia, with apprehension of death, and great anxiety; ophthalmia; bleeding at the nose (epistaxis); catarrhal inflammation of the tonsils, palate, and pharynx; hæmatemesis; peritonitis; active metrorrhagia; croup; hæmoptysis; pleuritis; bronchitis and pneumonia (in first stage generally); organic affections of the left side of the heart; hypertrophy of the heart.

On comparing the homœopathic and allopathic uses of Aconite, it will be seen that both systems have given this medicine occasionally for the same diseases; but that the homœopathists have been led to the use of it in disease from the symptoms it produces, either in large or in repeated small doses, on persons in health; whilst, under the old school, it has been given empirically, chiefly because it is supposed to be a "*benumber*," and therefore useful in allaying increased pain and irritation of the nervous system; but whenever curative, it may be ascribed to its specific, *i. e.* homœopathic action.

It must also be remembered, that the homœopathic use of this and all other substances can never (owing to the mode of preparation) be attended with any possible degree of danger from their poisonous qualities, but that, under the old system, these medicines, often injurious from the manner of exhibiting them, may also become, either from inadvertence or ignorance, most fatal in their effects.

Antidotes.—Acids and wine; to its poisonous effects, vinegar.

Gerarde, in his Herbal, gives a curious antidote. He says, speaking of the Aconite, "It groweth on the mountains of Rhætia, and in sundry places of the Alps, where you shall find that the grass that groweth round it eaten up with cattle, but no part of the herb itself touched, except by certain flies, who in such abundant measure swarm about the same, that they cover the whole plant, and which is very strange, although these flies do with great delight feed hereupon, yet of them there is confected an antidote or most available medicine against the deadly bite of the spider called Tarantula, or any other venomous beast whatsoever; yea, an excellent remedie, not only against the Aconites, but all other poysons whatever." Also, Antoninus Geranaceus, of Pavia, a famous physician of his age, mentions a fly which eats very plentifully of Aconite leaves, as an antidote to its poisonous effects.

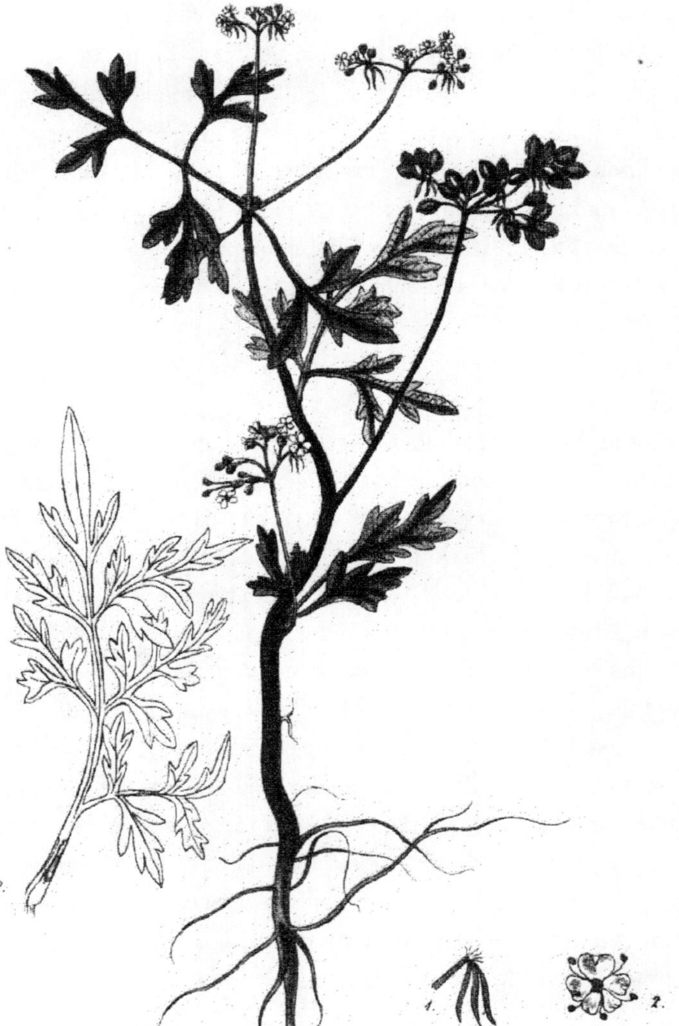

M.D. del. H. Sowerby lith.

Reeve & Nichols, imp.

Æthusa Cynapium..

II.

ÆTHUSA CYNAPIUM.

Lesser Hemlock, Fool's Parsley, Dog's Parsley.

SYNONYMS.—Cicutaria tenuifolia, *Raii Syn.* 215; Cicutaria apii folia, *Bauh. Hist.* v. 3; Cicutaria fatua, *Lob. Icon.* v. 2, 280; Cynapium, *Penlop;* Coriandrum Cynapium, *Crantz, Aust.;* Æthusa, *Hall, Hist.;* Æthusa Cynapium, *Linn. Wilden., Flor. Brit.*, etc., etc.; Cicuta minor, Petroselinus similis, *Tournefort.*

FOREIGN NAMES. — *Fr.:* La petite Cigue. *Ital.:* Cicuta minore. *Span.:* Cicuta menore. *Germ.:* Kleinen Scheiling, Hundspetersilie. *Dut.:* Tuin scheerling. *Russ.:* Medwjéscheis koren.

Nat. Order, UMBELLIFERÆ.—PENTANDRIA, DIGYNIA.

DIAGNOSIS OF THE ORDER.—Umbellal exogens, with didymous fruit, and a double epigynous disk.

GEN. CHAR.—*Calyx,* superior, minute. *Petals* five, inverse heart-shaped, with sharp, inflexed points. *Fruit* round, egg-shaped. *Carpels,* with five elevated, thick, sharply-keeled ridges. *Seeds* half globose. *General involucrum,* none. *Partial involucrum,* of three unilateral pendulous leaves.

SPEC. CHAR.—Leaves uniform. Leaflets wedge-shaped, decurrent, running down the leaf-stalk. Segments pear-shaped.

HISTORY.—According to Schulze (*De Toxicol. Veter.*), this plant was confounded by many early writers with the Conium maculatum, under the general term Cicuta. Hermolaus Barbarus first distinguished it under the name Cicuta terrestris minore. It is mentioned by Matthiolus, Jonston, Dodecampus, Jungius, Müller, and others, as producing extraordinary effects on those that eat of it. It is the Petroselinum vitium of Tragus. The Dauci inutilis genus of Gesner. Thalius calls it Apium

---

Fig. 1. Partial involucrum. 2. Corolla. 3. Carpellum. 4. Section of a seed-vessel. 5. Section of a carpellum. 6. Seed-vessel. 7. Germen, calyx, and style.

cicutarum. Lobel, Petroselinum canum; hence the name Dog Parsley. The name is derived from Αιθω, to burn, on account of its acrid qualities; another derivation is Αιθουσα, beggarly.

Description.—Annual, flowers July, August, and September. *Root* tapering, branched, and whitish. *Stem* from one to two feet high, upright branched, somewhat zig-zag, jointed, round, smooth, striated, sometimes purplish, but not spotted. *Leaves* bi-pinnated, smooth, dark lurid green; segments egg-spear-shaped, variously cut, lobed, and more or less decurrent; lower leaves sometimes tri-pinnate. *Umbels* terminal on long stalks, spreading and flattish; umbellules small, distant. *General involucrum* wanting. *Partial involucrum* of three long strap-shaped, unilateral, drooping leaves, by which it is readily distinguished. *Flowers* white. *Petals* somewhat radiating, inversely heart-shaped, with the summits bent in. *Anthers* purplish. *Fruit* egg-shaped, striated pale brown. Whole plant smooth, except the flower-stalks, which are angular, and the angles are furnished with a minute transparent, papillose membrane.

Geographical Distribution.—The British Islands, France, Germany, Italy, Russia, and other parts of Europe. One species, Æthusa meum (Spignel), grows wild in the mountains of Switzerland, Germany, Austria, Carniola, Italy, and Spain; and also in the high pastures of Westmoreland, Cumberland, Lancashire, and Merionethshire.

Localities.—A common weed in gardens and cultivated fields.

It is distinguished from garden parsley by the smell of the leaves, which is peculiar and disagreeable. The leaves themselves are finer, more acute, and decurrent, and of a darker green than the common parsley. The flower-stem is striated and grooved; and the plant is easily known by *the beard, or three long pendulous leaves under the flower.* Flowers are white, those of the common parsley pale yellow. Cows, horses, sheep, goats, and swine are said to eat it, but it is reported to be poisonous to geese.

PARTS USED IN MEDICINE, AND MODE OF PREPARATION.—The whole plant, prepared in the same manner as Aconite. (*Vide Quin, Pharm. Homœopath.*, p. 37.)

POISONOUS EFFECTS.—The following are the most interesting cases of poisoning by Æthusa, taken from Orfila and others.

A boy, six years of age, having eaten some of this herb by mistake for parsley, at four o'clock in the afternoon, commenced immediately after to cry out in great pain, and complained of great cramps in the stomach; whilst taking him home the whole body became excessively swollen, and of a livid hue; the respiration became difficult and short, and he died towards midnight. Another child was poisoned in the same manner, but he was fortunate enough to vomit up the herb; this, however, did not prevent many symptoms manifesting themselves; he talked wildly, and in his delirium he thought he saw numbers of dogs and cats. (*Orfila*, vol. ii. p. 324.)

Riviere reports a case of an individual who perished by this poison, and on a post-mortem examination, the tongue was found black. There was a brown serous fluid in the stomach; the liver was of a yellow colour; the spleen was livid; the body was not emphysematous.

Gmelin has related the case of a child who died in eight hours in consequence of having eaten the Æthusa. The symptoms were spasmodic pain in the stomach, swelling of the belly, lividity of the skin, and difficult breathing. (*Chris.*, p. 365.)

A woman gave two of her children some soup in which this herb had been boiled. They were both seized with severe pain in the abdomen, and next morning there was perfect unconsciousness; the lower jaw was spasmodically fixed; abdomen tumid; vomiting of a bloody mucus, and constant diarrhœa; cold extremities; convulsions; and death in twenty-four hours. Post-mortem appearance: redness of the lining membrane of œsophagus, and slight vascular congestion of stomach and duodenum. (*Medic. Jahrbuch.*)

Another child, who had eaten the bulbs by mistake for young

turnips, was suddenly seized with pain in the abdomen, followed by nausea, without vomiting; could not swallow; vacuity; inability to answer questions; lower jaw fixed; insensibility and death, an hour after the commencement of the symptoms. (*Med. Times, August* 23, 1845.)

Two ladies, of Castle Donnington, Leicestershire, partook of some salad in which the Æthusa had been put by mistake for common parsley. Serious symptoms soon followed. There was troublesome nausea, with vomiting; oppressive headache and giddiness; desire to sleep, with frequent startings and excessive agitations; pungent heat in the mouth, throat, and gullet, with great difficulty of swallowing; great thirst, with total loss of appetite for every kind of solid food; the extremities felt benumbed, and were affected with tremors; and all the vital and animal functions were performed with unusual activity. The ladies eventually recovered. (*Med. and Phys. Journal*, vol. xiv. p. 425.)

On Thursday, the 5th of June, W. Frekleton, a healthy, strong man, about thirty-five years of age, a publican, ate a handful of fool's parsley, with nearly the same quantity of young lettuce, about one o'clock at noon; in about ten minutes he was affected with a pain in the stomach and bowels, attended with a rumbling. He walked out in the fields, but was seized with such languor, weariness, and weakness, that he supported himself with difficulty. He was much troubled with giddiness in the head; his vision was confused, and sometimes objects appeared double. At seven o'clock he got an emetic, which brought up, he supposes, all the fool's parsley, but none of the lettuce; this relieved him of the unpleasant symptoms in the stomach, but the other sensations continued, and he passed a restless night. Next day he had much pain in his head and eyes, which last were inflamed and bloodshot. He had different circumscribed swellings in his face, which were painful and inflamed, but they were transient, and flew from place to place. On the Saturday his eyes were highly inflamed, painful, and entirely closed by the surrounding inflammation. He was bled, which gave him much relief in his face and eyes. From this time till the Monday he continued to get better, but had even then, pain, heat, and inflammation of the eyes, with œdematous swelling of the cheeks; his remaining symptoms went off gradually. (*Lowe.*)

Norembergus mentions two boys, whose bodies were much swollen after eating this plant.

Orfila gave seven ounces of the juice obtained from the leaves of Æthusa to a strong dog, and tied the œsophagus. Twenty minutes after giving it the dog became sick; in half an hour it did not appear to affect him much, when suddenly he stretched out his limbs and laid upon his stomach; in a few minutes he tried to rouse himself, but his efforts were vain. The muscles of his limbs, particularly of the posterior extremities, refused to obey the will, but the organs of sense exercised their functions; the pupils were scarcely dilated; the pulsations of the heart were slow and strong. This state lasted a quarter of an hour, and then the extremities were agitated by convulsive movements; the animal threw himself from one side to the other; the senses began to be enfeebled; and the œsophagus and the fauces were spasmodically contracted. This state of stupor increased, and the animal died an hour after taking the poison. On opening the body, the heart was contracted, and the left ventricle contained fluid and black blood. The lungs were a little less crepitant than natural. The stomach was found full of the poison; but there was no alteration in the digestive canal. (*Orfila*, vol. ii. p. 323.)

According to Schulze, Æthusa acts chiefly on the medulla spinalis.

On examining attentively the symptoms observed by many physicians in poisonings of this sort, we can reduce them to the following: heat in the throat; thirst; vomiting; sometimes diarrhœa; short, sighing respiration; small, frequent pulse; headache; vertigo; swellings of the extremities; delirium. (*Orfila*, l. c.)

Medical Uses (Homœopathic).—The chief symptoms in which Æthusa may be useful, are the following: great anguish; vertigo, with drowsiness; weight in the forehead, with ill-humour; rending tearing pain in the face and malar bones; continual thirst; violent vomiting of a frothy, milky substance; short, anxious respiration; in some kinds of tetanic convulsions; and also in hay fever.

Antidotes.—Vegetable acids. In treating the poisonous effects, produce, in the first place, vomiting, either by tickling the fauces with a feather, or by giving twenty grains of ipecacuanha; apply friction to the body, and mustard poultices to the feet; and give vinegar or citric acid after vomiting has been produced.

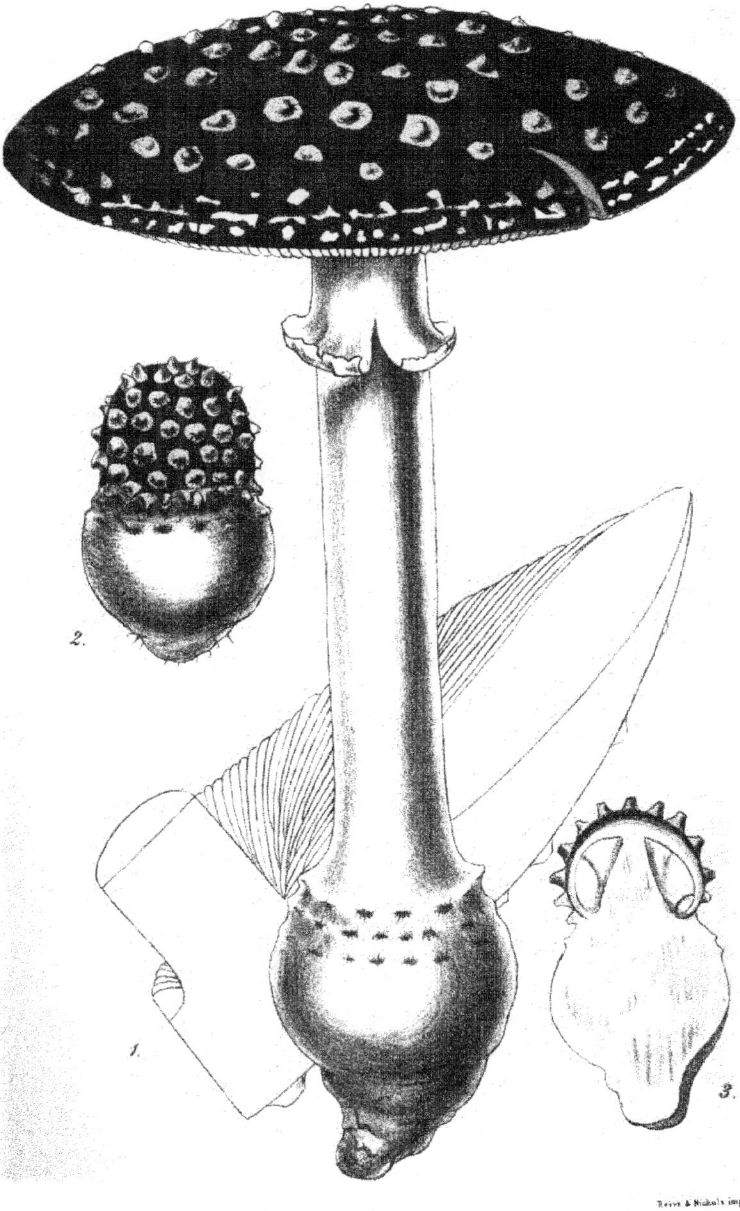

H. Sowerby lith.

Reeve & Nichols imp.

Agaricus muscarius.

III.

AGARICUS MUSCARIUS.

Fly Agaric, Bug Agaric.

SYNONYMS. — Amanita muscaria, Agaricus imperialis, *Batsch;* Amanita citrinus, *Schæffer;* Agaricus puella, *Bat.;* Agaricus plumbœus, *Id.;* Agaricus maculatus pustulatus, *Id.;* Agaricus verrucosus, *Id.;* Agaricus fulvus, *Id.*

These synonyms arise from its variety of colour, which it often assumes according to the locality in which it is found.

FOREIGN NAMES.—*Fr.:* Fausse Orange. *Ger.:* Fliegen-schwamm. *Ital.:* Amanita. *Russ.:* Moucho-more.

Class I. THALLOGENS.—CRYPTOGAMIA, FUNGI.

DIAGNOSIS OF THE ORDER.—Cellular flowerless plants, nourished through their thallus (spawn, or mycelinum), living in air; propagated by spores colourless or brown, and sometimes enclosed in asci; destitute of green gonidia (Lindley).

GEN. CHAR.—Margin of pileus striate. *Gills* white; stem subsolid, bulbous; vulva scaly. *Pileus* three to seven inches broad, convex at length, sometimes depressed; of a rich orange scarlet, but occasionally whitish, yellowish, or brown. *Sporules* white, rounded. *Stem* four to nine inches high, half to one inch thick. *Ring* deflexed.

HISTORY.—The Agaricus muscarius is supposed to be the black poisonous Agaric, described under the general name Μυκητον, by Theophrastus; and Αγαρικον, by Dioscorides, Paulus Ægineta, Galen, and Pliny. The Agaric of Serapion and the Arabian physicians is the Boletus ignarius.

Mr. Greville, in the fourth volume, Part II., of the "Transactions of the Wernerian Society," 1823, has the following remarks on this fungus:—"As the plant commonly known by the name of the fly agaric (from its property of destroying flies

---

Fig. 1. Represents a section and the under surface of the pileus. 2. A young plant. 3. Section of the same.

when steeped in milk) has made some noise of late on the Continent, I must warn those who might feel inclined to try it in this country, of the danger they would expose themselves to. It has not been clearly ascertained whether the species which grows in this country and in the south of Europe be indeed the same as that which is found in Kamtschatka, and called Amanita muscaria Kamtschatica. At any rate, our plant is known as highly poisonous, and the Kamtschatka variety may be another species, or having partly lost its virulence from inhabiting a more northern climate. The properties of this variety are exceedingly curious; and as they are contained in a German essay, "Annalen der Wetterauschen Gesellschaft für die Gesammte Naturkunde," by Dr. Langsdorf, I trust a concise account of them will not be unacceptable.

The variety of Amanita muscaria is used by the inhabitants of the north-eastern part of Asia in the same manner as wine, brandy, arrack, opium, etc., is by other nations.

These fungi are found most plentifully about Wischna, Kamtschatka and Milkowa Derewna, and are very abundant in some seasons, and scarce in others. They are collected in the hottest months, and hung up by a string in the air to dry; some dry of themselves on the ground, and are said to be far more narcotic than those artificially preserved. Small deep-coloured specimens, thickly covered with warts, are also said to be more powerful than those of a larger size and paler colour.

The usual mode of taking the fungus is to roll it up like a bolus, and swallow it without chewing, which the Kamtschadales say would disorder the stomach. It is sometimes eaten fresh, in soups and sauces, and then loses much of its intoxicating properties. When steeped in the juice of the berries of Vaccinium uliginosum, its effects are those of strong wine. One large or two small fungi is the common dose to produce a pleasant intoxication for a whole day, particularly if water be drank after it, which augments the narcotic principle. The desired effect comes on from one to two hours after taking the fungus; giddiness and drunkenness result in the same manner as wine and spirits; cheerful emotions of the mind are first produced; the countenance becomes flushed; involuntary words and actions follow, and sometimes at last an entire loss of consciousness. It renders some remarkably active, and proves highly stimulant to muscular exertion; with too large a dose violent spasmodic effects are produced. So very exciting to the nervous system in many individuals is this fungus, that the effects are often very ludicrous. If a person under its influence wishes to step over a straw or small stick, he takes a stride or a jump sufficient to clear the trunk of a tree; a talkative person cannot keep silence or secrets, and one fond of music is perpetually singing.

The most singular effect of the Amanita is the influence it possesses over the secretion of the kidneys. It is said, that from time immemorial, the inhabitants have known that the fungus imparts an intoxicating quality to this secretion, which continues for a considerable length of time after taking it.

This fungus is the Moucho-more of the Russians, Kamtschadales, and Koriacs, who use it for intoxication. It is often immersed in a liquid made from the Epilobium (Rosebay Willow herb); and when this liquor is drunk, the drinkers are seized with convulsions in all their limbs, followed with that kind of raving which attends a burning fever. They personify this mushroom; and if they are urged by its effects to suicide or other dreadful crime, they pretend to obey its commands. To fit themselves for premeditated assassination, they recur to the use of the Moucho-more.

It was recommended in early times as a remedy for *epilepsy*, and later employed externally to strumous, phagedenic, and fistulous ulcers.

Description.—This is one of the most splendid specimens of the order, and, as Mr. Greville remarks, "well may it be called imperial." The *pileus* varies occasionally in colour from blood red to orange, white, green, or brown; three to seven inches broad, fleshy, convex, at length nearly plane. *Lamellæ* white, broad. *Stipes* four to nine inches high, half to one inch thick, white or pinkish; solid, or with slight cavity, bulbous. *Keel* in the form of a deflexed collar.

Geographical Distribution.—Europe, Asia, and America. Not very common in England; but abundant in some parts of Scotland. In some parts of France and Germany. Common in Norway, Sweden, Russia, Lapland, etc.

Localities.—In dry places; sandy deserts in Asia; and in dry pine woods in Scotland and other parts of the north of Europe. "Its bright red colour contrasts beautifully with the sombre pines and white stems of the birch."

Parts used in Medicine, and mode of preparation.—The Stipes and Pileus can be used fresh, or carefully dried. If fresh, the stipes and pileus are to be well washed, and, the external part being removed, mashed up in a mortar, and to this add an equal part of spirits of wine; then put it aside for three days, and decant off the liquid from the remains; then attenuate to the 30th dilution, in the same manner as ordered for Aconite. If the dried fungus is taken, one grain is to be triturated with 100 grains of sugar of milk. (*Vide Quin, Pharm. Homœopath.*)

The time of collecting this fungus for medicinal purposes is in the autumn.

Poisonous Effects.—Haller relates, that six persons perished at one time from eating this mushroom; and that in others it causes delirium.

Orfila relates, that several French soldiers having eaten of this fungus, near Polosch, in Russia, were very shortly seized with anxiety, sense of suffocation, intense thirst, violent gripings, small, irregular pulse, universal cold sweat, altered expression of countenance, violet tint of the nose, general trembling, fetid evacuations, coldness and livid colour of limbs; violent delirium, and acute pains remaining to the last. On opening the bodies, large spots of inflammation and gangrene appeared in the stomach and alimentary canal, and putrefaction seemed advancing very rapidly.

M. Paulet reports many cases of poisoning by the Amanita. The sufferers experienced nausea, vomiting, faintings, anxiety, a state of stupor and insensibility, and a sensation of constriction of the throat; they neither had colic nor severe pains. Some grains of ipecacuanha were administered in hot water, and the Agaric was evacuated with sanguinolent matter. The patients slowly returned to health by the use of emollients; some of them experienced abdominal pains, and were treated by emollient fomentations and opiates.

M. Paulet gave to a dog some of the Agaric, mixed with parsley. Three hours after, the animal was seized with violent tremblings and weakness of the extremities. This state lasted about four hours, during which he moaned much; afterwards he fell into a state of stupor. The respiration was slow and deep, and he uttered, from time to time, plaintive cries; at one time he rolled upon the ground; at another, he turned over with sudden shivering, resembling electric shocks. Vinegar was given to him, which aggravated all the symptoms. Some oil of olives was afterwards given, which produced vomiting, and ejection of some of the poison, mixed with white mucus. He completely recovered in a few days, by giving him a little milk from time to time.

MEDICAL USES (HOMŒOPATHIC).—The Agaric was proved by Hahnemann and others, and the results recorded in his work on "Chronic Diseases," under the article Agaricus muscarius. This remedy has been successfully employed in convulsions and tremors, and some kinds of epilepsy. It is proposed for Paralysis of the upper and lower extremities, arising from incipient softening of the central portion of the spinal marrow. For the peculiar symptoms indicating its use, the reader is referred to Hahnemann's *Chronic Diseases*, Jahr's *Manual*, Noack and Trinks' *Homöop. Arzneimittellehre*, etc.

ANTIDOTES.—Camphor, Coffea, Pulsatilla,—Wine.

TREATMENT OF POISONING BY MUSHROOMS.—The following extract is from Orfila (*Toxicol. Gener.*, 3rd edit., p. 446): "I have tried the following experiments to ascertain the value of vinegar, common salt, ether, emetics, and volatile alkali, in cases of poisoning by mushrooms:—

"*Vinegar.*—1st. This vegetable acid has the property of dissolving the active parts of the Amanita and Agaricus bulbosus, so that one may with impunity swallow either of these kinds of mushrooms, cut in pieces, and cleansed in this acid, but the liquor is excessively poisonous." This agrees with the experience of M. Paulet.

"2nd. When these mushrooms are taken into the stomach with vinegar, in a quantity sufficient to produce death, it takes place sooner than without vinegar, provided the substance has not been vomited; which doubtless arises from the property of the vinegar to dissolve those parts which are most easily absorbed.

"3rd. Vinegar and water appears to be useful in this kind of poisoning, when the substance has been removed by evacuants.

"*Common salt* (muriate of soda) dissolved in water has the same property as vinegar in dissolving the active parts of the mushroom, and has of course the same advantages and disadvantages.

"*Sulphuric ether,* of late so much used in these cases, appears to be very useful after evacuants. In fact, we have restored dogs after giving them doses of Amanita sufficient to kill them, by making them swallow, after the poison was evacuated, alternately ether and etherated water, or the mineral anodyne liquor of Hoffmann.

"*Emetics and emeto-cathartics* are also eminent in treating these cases, for death almost always follows when the substance is not removed."

M. Paulet has found that volatile alkali (ammonia) is more injurious than otherwise, and that oil, butter, and milk are useless.

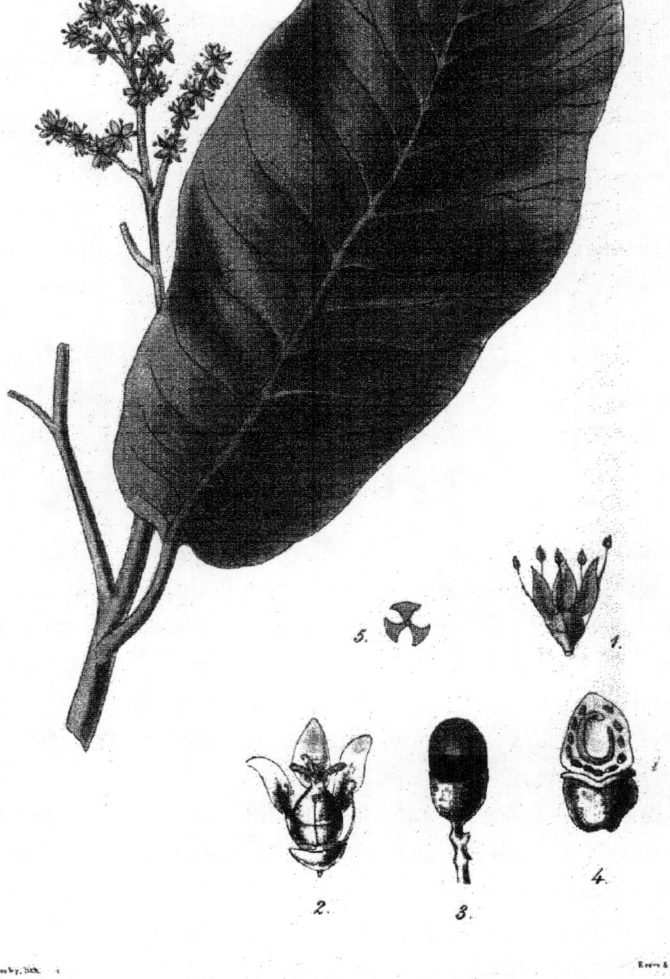

H. Sowerby, lith. Reeve & Nichols im

Anacardium semecarpus

IV.

ANACARDIUM.

(SEMECARPUS ANACARDIUM.)

Marking-nut Tree.

SYNONYMS.—Semecarpus Anacardium, *Linn. f. supp.*, 182; *Roxb. corom.*, i. t. 12; *Fl. Ind.*, ii. 83. Anacardium officinarum, *Gætn.* Anacardium latifolium, *Lam. Enc.* i. 139, t. 208. Anacard. orientale of *Mat. Med.*

FOREIGN NAMES.—*Fr.*: Anacardien, Anacarde à feuilles longues. *Ital.*: Anacardos. *Span.*: Anacard. *Germ.*: Elephantem Læusebaum, Anakardiem baum. *Dut.*: Anakardienboom, Hartjes. *Bengal*: Belaluhi. *Telinga:* Nellajiedy.

Nat. Order.—TEREBINTACEÆ.—POLYGAMIA, DIŒCIA.

GEN. CHAR.—*Calyx*, perianth inferior, of one leaf, bell-shaped, and cloven half-way down into five heart-shaped acute segments. *Petals* five, lanceolate, bordered, obtuse, larger than the segments of the calyx. *Stamens*, filaments five, awl-shaped, shorter than the corolla, inserted into the receptacle; anthers oblong, small. *Pistils*, germen superior, globular, flattened. *Styles* three, recurved, situated on the germen, and shorter than it. *Stigmas* club-shaped, retuse. *Pericarp*, none, except the receptacle, which is erect, fleshy, pear-shaped, smooth. *Seed*, a nut, resting on the receptacle, heart-shaped, flattened on both sides, smooth, and shining.

Roxburgh observed, that the flowers of the Anacardium were polygamous, diœcious; whereas nearly all those examined by Turpin were polygamous, which difference he ascribes to the character of the soil.

HISTORY.—The commentator of Paulus Ægineta (*Adams's Translation*, vol. iii. b. vii. p. 450) decides the Anacardium,

Fig. 1. The male flower. 2. The hermaphrodite flower. 3. The nut. 4. Section of the nut, showing the cells containing the juice.

mentioned by Serapion, Rhases, and Avicenna, to be the nut of the Semecarpus Anacardium, or the Marking-nut Tree; whilst others suppose that it is the seed of the Avicenna tomentosa, a didynamous plant. If the former is correct, this plant is mentioned by Galen (*De Comp. Med.*, sec. gen. viii.), under the name of χρυσο βαλανος, and by Myrepsus and Actuarius, under that of ξανθο βαλανος. Matthiolus (*Comment. in Dioscor.*, 189) supposes that the Greeks were entirely ignorant of this substance, but Adams (l. c.) comes to a different conclusion.

Hahnemann, in his account of this medicine (*Chronic Diseases, art. Anacardium*) confounds Avicenna with Semecarpus Anacardium; the two trees belong, in fact, to different natural orders, one to the Personatæ, and the other to the Terebintaceæ. The nut of the Avicenna or Malacca bean being kidney-shaped, that of the Semecarpus being heart-shaped.

The Indians, after depriving the nut of its external rind and juice, roast and eat it with much relish. The juice, which is in the cells under the rind, is of such acridity, that it is used by the natives to burn off warts, condylomata, and other excrescences, and to keep down excessive granulation in ulcers, both in man and beast; they used it also mixed with chalk for marking their linen. Hamel tells us that an excellent ink is made from this nut, with the addition of ash-lye and vinegar.

The ancient writers recommended it chiefly in mental diseases, particularly in loss of memory, paralysis, and spasms; and the Arabian physicians, who called the nut Balador, extolled its use in the same affections, and also as a prophylactic in those predisposed to paralysis. It was highly esteemed by the Telinga physicians as a remedy for nervous disorders. The natives give the kernel steeped in whey to those suffering from asthma; the Confectio Anacardium became celebrated under the name Confectio Sapientium, as a remedy against weakness of the mind; but Hoffman called it Confectio Stultorum, and condemns the internal use of it, as he says that "people have been made mad by it, and had lost their memory, and died miserably on account of using it too often." (*Hill, Mat. Med.*, p. 491.) Hence the abuse of this drug made it hurtful; applied homœopathically for the same diseases, it becomes a powerful and efficient remedy.

The name is derived from two Greek words, *ανα* without, and *καρδια* a heart, because the pulp of the fruit, instead of having the seed enclosed, has the nut growing out at the end of it.

Description.—As the nut mentioned by Hahnemann is without doubt the fruit of the Semecarpus, and not of the Avicenna or Malacca bean, by which name it is erroneously described in Gruhener's *Pharmacopœia* and *Materia Medica*, but correctly in Dr. Quin's *Pharmacopœia Homœop.;* a description of the three is subjoined; viz., the nut described by Hahnemann, the Semecarpus, and the Avicenna, by which it will be seen that Hahnemann's nut agrees with the former, and not with the Avicenna.

Hahnemann.

"Found in the forests of the East Indies:—between the external black, shining, heart-shaped, hard shell and the sweet kernel, which is covered with a brown, reddish, thin skin, there is a thick blackish juice, contained in a cellular tissue, with which the Indians mark their linen in an indelible manner. In the fruit which we receive here (Germany), this juice, which is commonly of the consistence of honey, is generally found dry."

Semecarpus.

Marking-nut Tree.

Linnæan Class and Order, Pentandria, Trigynia.

Nat. Ord.—Terebintaceæ.

A handsome, lofty tree, *whose bark is rough, ash-coloured*, and glutinous within. Branches numerous, spreading, rather hairy. Leaves alternate, on shortish foot-stalks, wedge-shaped, smooth above, rough beneath. Flowers in large terminal erect panicles of a dirty greenish yellow. Five petals, small, and deciduous. Branches numerous. Receptacle yellow. *Nut black, containing a corrosive, resinous juice*, at first of a pale milk colour, but turning black. Found in the mountainous dry forests of the East Indies. The seed is ripe in January and February.

Avicenna tomentosa.

Malacca Bean.

Linnæan Class and Order, Didynamia, Gymnospermia.

Nat. Ord.—Personatæ.

Leaves cordate, ovate, tomentose (cottony) underneath. This tree is like the mangrove, rising above sixteen feet high. Its trunk covered *with smooth, whitish green bark*, and the twigs from the stem propagate the tree like those of the mangrove. The leaves appear at the points of the branches, on very small petioles, *opposite*, having a large dark green rib; flowers, many, at the top of the branches, white, *four-petalled*. Capsule coriaceous, rhomboidal, compressed, one-celled, two-valved. Seed, one large, form of capsule, constructed of four fleshy folds; germinating in low lands along the coast of Malacca in the Indian Archipelago.

Geographical Distribution.—Asia, native of the East Indies, and found in mountainous dry forests.

Parts used in Medicine, and Mode of Preparation.—The Juice, contained in the cells under the external rind of the nut. Hahnemann gives the following directions: one grain of this juice is to be triturated with ninety-nine grains of sugar of milk to the 3rd attenuation; afterwards with alcohol to the 30th dilution. The juice is not soluble in water, and only diffusible in spirits of wine, it soon falls to the bottom unless the menstruum is previously alkalized.

Medical Uses (Homœopathic).—Noack and Trinks (*Handbuch der homöop. Arzneimittellehre, Leip.* 1842, *art. Anacardium*) offer the following remarks on Anacardium. It is adapted to nervous bilious constitutions; to the melancholic choleric temperament; and to irritable hypochondriacs. The following are the chief diseases in which it may be employed. *Weakness of mind, memory, and senses.* Imbecility. Loquacious dementia. Melancholia in all its forms. *Chronic deafness. Weakness of digestion and flatulence of hypochondriacs. Diseases of the liver. Asthma. Hysteric spasms of the chest,* which go off amid a flood of tears. (For the general symptoms produced by Anacardium, vide Hahnemann's *Chronic Diseases.*)

Antidotes.—Camphor, Coffee, Juglans. Camphor and spirits of nitre do not seem to act sufficiently as antidotes; smelling of coffea cruda is a powerful antidote against the anger and vehemence consequent on the use of Anacardium.

Plate V.

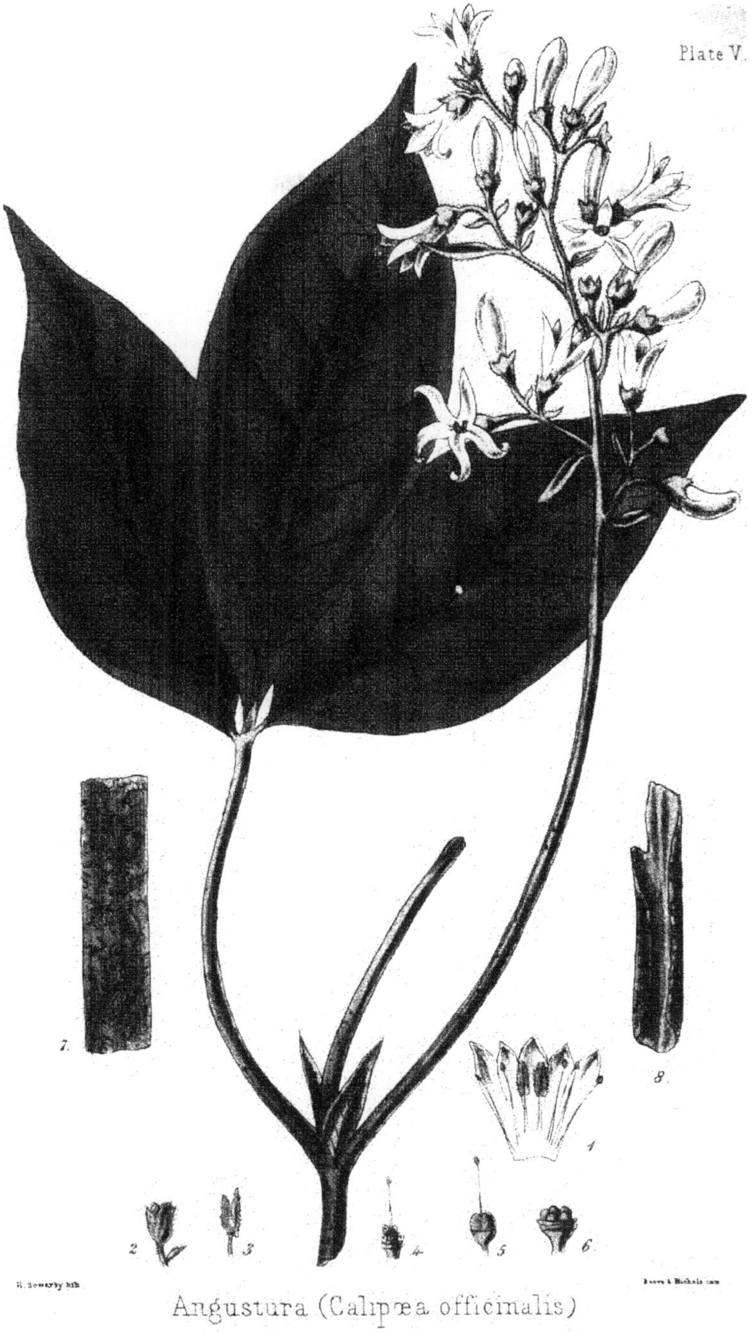

H. Sowerby lith

Reeve & Nichols imp

Angustura (Calipæa officinalis)

V.

ANGUSTURA.

(CORTEX ANGUSTURÆ.)

Bark of the Galipœa officinalis.

SYNONYMS.—Galipœa cusparia, *Decandolle.* Cusparia febrifuga, *Humboldt and Bonpland, Pl. Æquinoct.*, ii. 59, t. 57. Bonplandia trifoliata, *Willd.* Galipœa officinalis, *Hancock.*

FOREIGN NAMES.—*Fr.:* Ecorce d'Angusture. *Ital.:* Angustura. *Germ.:* Angustura rinde. *Dan. and Swed.:* Angusture. *Span.:* Quina de Carony. *Native name:* Orayuri.

Nat. Order, RUTACEÆ.—DIANDRIA, MONOGYNIA.

GEN. CHAR.—*Calyx* five-toothed. *Petals* five, unequal, two being one-ninth of an inch longer than the others, united at base, reflex, oblong, obtuse. *Stamens,* four to seven, somewhat adherent to the petals, unequal, generally two to five, sterile. *Nectary* cupuliform. *Styles* five, afterwards combining into one, and forming a four to five-grooved stigma. *Carpels* five, containing two ovules, sessile, with a separable endocarp. *Seeds,* two to a capsule, one often abortive. *Cotyledons* large, corrugated. *Leaves* alternate. *Peduncles* axillary, many-flowered.

SPEC. CHAR.—*Leaves* trifoliate. *Racemes* stalked, axillary, terminal, *Stamens* two. *Nectaries* (sterile stamens) five.

HISTORY.—Angustura was first made known in Europe in 1788, by Dr. Ewer, of Trinidad, and was called from the town of St. Thome d'Angustura, on the Orinoco. Its botanical source was long unknown, till Humboldt and Bonpland announced the discovery of the plant in their travels in tropical America; and it was for some time supposed that the medicinal bark was pro-

Fig. 1. The expanded corolla. 2. Calyx. 3. Stamens. 4. Pericarp. 5. Pistil. 6. Germen. 7. The bark, external appearance. 8. The bark, internal appearance.

duced from the Bonplandia trifoliata, and by which name it is called in Hahnemann's *Materia Medica Pura;* but Dr. Hancock, who resided in the district which yields the bark for some years, has shown that it is obtained from a different species of the same genus, which differs essentially from the plant described by Bonpland; the one being a magnificent, stately tree, sixty to eighty feet high, while that described by Hancock never exceeding twenty feet.

As a medicine it was in great request at the end of the last and beginning of this century; indeed, it had almost as great a reputation as Cinchona bark, and was used as a febrifuge in intermittent and remittent, in adynamic and continued fevers; in general relaxation and muscular debility, and in atonic conditions of the stomach. It was also given to check profuse mucous discharges, and was found efficacious in chronic dysentery and diarrhœa; but like very many of the remedies of the old school, owing to its indiscriminate use in diseases to which it was not specific, it fell into disuse, and is at present rarely employed in the allopathic prescriptions. The cause for this has been attributed by Christison and others to its dangerous adulterations with the bark of the Strychnos Nux Vomica.

Description.—The Galipœa officinalis is a beautiful shrub, seldom or ever exceeding the altitude of twenty feet, the usual medium being about twelve or fifteen feet, flowering in vast profusion during the months of August and September; the seeds ripening in October and November. Diameter of the trunk, which is tolerably erect, is from three to five inches. *Branches* scattered, slender, and bending nearly to the ground. *Bark* smooth, externally grey, and yellow within. *Leaves* placed, for the most part, alternately on branches composed of three folioles, supported on a common petiole of nearly the same length as the leaflets. *Leaflets* oblong, six to ten inches in length, two to four in breadth, centre one longer than the lateral, smooth and glossy, of a vivid green; when broken, yield a strong odour greatly resembling tobacco, from which the name Orayuri is derived, from *yuri*, tobacco. *Flowers* numerous, white, and having a peculiar odour, on longish spikes, which are both terminal and axillary. *Bracteæ* lanceolate, acute, in pairs.

Geographical Distribution.—South America, the neighbourhood of the Orinoco; Carony; Sumeremo; Uri; Alba Græcia; and Cupapui, in Columbian Guiana. It grows in abundance in the neighbourhood of St. Joaquin de Carony, between seven and eight degrees of North latitude. It delights in a rich soil, and flourishes at the height of 600 to 1000 feet above the level of the sea.

Parts used in Medicine, and Mode of Preparation.—The Bark. It is imported into this country in flat pieces or incomplete quills, from two to eight inches long, between half an inch and an inch and a half in breadth, from half a line to three lines in thickness, and composed of the epidermis and proper bark. Its external surface is dirty greyish yellow in colour, often speckled in the smaller pieces with lighter grey spots and elevations; the inner surface is dull brown, and the substance of the bark is yellowish brown. The transverse fracture is smooth and somewhat resinous in character. Powder greyish yellow, something like rhubarb; it has a peculiar odour, and a bitter, aromatic, hot taste; it imparts its properties to water, alcohol, and proof-spirit. It used to be adulterated abroad pretty considerably with what was supposed to be the bark of the Brucea ferruginea or antidysenterica, but which is now known to have been that of the Strychnos nux vomica, and many fatal accidents occurred from its use. The spurious bark, besides not being so speckled, is much thicker, more twisted, like dried horn, and arched backwards; the taste is much more bitter, without either aroma or pungency; the inner surface is not separable into laminæ, and the transverse fracture is rendered blood-red when touched by nitric acid. Hahnemann orders fifty grains of the powder of the Angustura bark to be mixed with

1000 drops of alcohol, at a low temperature, and the tincture so obtained to be applied to make the different attenuations as ordered in the preparation of other medicines. Dr. Quin (*Pharmacop. Homœop.*, p. 41) advises the tincture prepared after this manner to be left at rest for six days, and that the attenuations should only go as far as the ninth. Jahr (*Pharmacopœia and Posology*, American translation, p. 129) advises the three first attenuations to be prepared by trituration, rather than by digestion with twenty parts of alcohol, which should be done if we wish to preserve it under the form of tincture.*

Poisonous Effects.—Hahnemann has the following remarks upon the effects of an over dose of the medicine prepared from this bark. "The true bark, as described above, possesses also most powerful medicinal properties, so that when obtained fresh from the tree, as it now generally is, it may, like all other highly powerful drugs, cause serious consequences, when it has been administered inappropriately and in over large quantities. A child, six and a half years old, who had been given three teaspoonfuls of a decoction of Angustura, made of five ounces of bark, reduced by evaporation to five ounces of liquid, *i. e.* about an ounce and a half of the extract of Angustura, died in two hours under the following alarming symptoms, taken from the report of Emmert. Tremblings, becoming violent in about half an hour; tetanic convulsions on touching the arm; eyelids wide open; eyes fixed, starting, and immov-

* The mode of preparation by trituration is as follows: one grain of the medicinal substance, say the bark, is added to ninety-nine grains of sugar of milk, this is rubbed in a porcelain mortar for six minutes, and then is designated the first attenuation; to make the second, one grain of the first is mixed with ninety-nine grains of sugar of milk, and submitted to the same process; and the third attenuation is made in the same manner, by taking one grain of the second; to make the fourth, one grain of the third is dissolved in a bottle filled with 100 drops of water to two-thirds its capacity, and this mixture is shaken twice, as in the attenuations made with alcohol. The fourth attenuation is best made with water, or equal parts of water and alcohol, because the sugar of milk does not dissolve in pure alcohol, but all the following attenuations after the fourth are to be made with pure spirit.

able; the jaws fixed; the lips wide apart, showing the whole of the front teeth; tension of some of the muscles of the face; the limbs fully extended and stiff; the spine and head thrown violently back; the body from time to time was shaken and slightly raised by a violent shock, like an electric shock, along the back; the cheeks and lips became blue; the breathing interrupted. After an access of six minutes, the child breathed with much effort, the cheeks and lips becoming pale. There was frequent desire to drink coffee. Swallowing tepid water caused tetanic spasms. Pulse 200, spasmodic and irregular. The tetanus sometimes appeared of its own accord, at others, from noise or from contact with anything; and the child continually cried out from fear of being touched. After the tetanus the eyes were closed; the face and forehead covered with perspiration; cheeks and lips blue; moaning, apparently without pain. The whole body flexible and soft; the eyes glazed, with convulsive breathings at long intervals. Half an hour after death the body became stiff. After twenty-four hours, on opening the veins, the blood was found liquid and brownish; the right lung pale and emphysematous externally, full of blood internally. The left was blue externally, blackish at the division of the lobes, and very full of blood. Other facts also prove that too powerful doses of Angustura produce spasmodic convulsions, giddiness, anxiety, and loss of consciousness. Dr. Wuerzner informed me that four persons, each of whom took ten or twelve grains of the extract of Angustura in the form of pills, were seized with stiffness, somewhat analogous to tetanus, in all the muscles of the body, with tremors of the jaws, and fell suddenly to the ground without losing consciousness." Symptoms much resembling these, only much less powerful, are related in the provings of this medicine on persons in health; viz., Sensation of weakness and stiffness of the whole body. Stiffness and extension of the limbs. Tension in the muscles whilst walking. Sensation of paralysis of different parts. *Convulsive starts.* Attacks of spasms, excited mostly by the touch, while drinking and also by noise, terminating in blueness of the cheeks and of the lips. Difficult and panting respiration. Groaning, and closing of the eyelids. Cramp-like pains in the ears and cheekbones.

Noack and Trinks (*Handbuch der homöop. Arzneimitt., art. Angustura*) have the following clinical remarks. Angustura has a great action upon the motor and spinal nerves. It has been employed with success in Rheumatism, with paralytic conditions; in Lockjaw, with convulsions of the muscles of the back; in Irritation of the spine, and in Affections of the mucous membrane; Diarrhœa and Dysentery.

ANTIDOTE.—*Coffea.* Camphor is not an antidote to the powerful effects of Angustura.

Plate VI

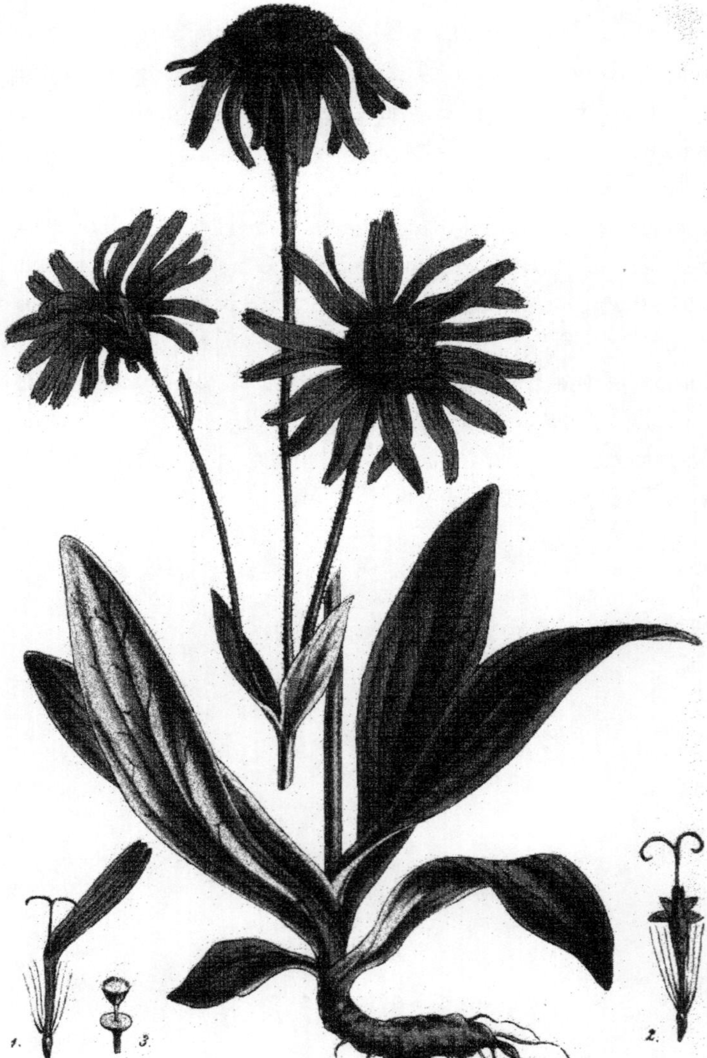

Arnica montana.

L.H. del. J. Sowerby lith. Reeve & Nichols imp.

VI.

ARNICA MONTANA.

Mountain Arnica, German Leopard's Bane, Mountain Tobacco.

SYNONYMS.—Arnica montana, *Lin. Sp. Pl.*, 1245; *Flor. Dan.*, t. 63; *Schhuhr, Handb.*, t. 248; *Villars, Dauph.*, iii., p. 257. Doronicum plantaginis folio alternum, *Bauhin*, πιναξ, lib. v., sect. 4; *Tournefort*, Class 14. Arnica montana foliis ovatis integris, caulinis geminis oppositis, *Linn.* Doronicum oppositifolium, *Lamar.*, *Dict.* ii., p. 312. Doronicum Austriacum quartum, *Clus. Pan.*, 522. Caltha alpina, *Tabern.* 336. Ptarmica montana, *Daleschamp.* Panacea lapsorum, *Fehr.* Chrysanthemum latifolium, *Dodonæus.* Nardus celtica altera, *Pena* and *Lobel.*

FOREIGN NAMES.—*Fr.:* Arnique, Arnica, Tabac des Vosges, Bétoine des Montagnes. *Ital.:* Arnica. *Span.:* Arnica, Tobaco de Montana. *Germ.:* Arnika, Wohl-verleih, Wolverley, Fallkraut, Luzianskraut. *Dut.:* Arnika, Val-kruid, Groot Luciaen-kruid. *Swed.:* Fibler.

Nat. Order, COMPOSITÆ, SENECIONIDÆ.—SYNGENESIA, POLYGAMIA SUPERFLUA.

GEN. CHAR.—*Calyx* common, shorter than the ray of the corolla; leaflets lanceolate, the length of the calyx, erect. *Corolla* compound, radiate; corollules hermaphrodite, in the disk very numerous; females in the ray about twenty; proper of the hermaphrodite, tubular, erect, five-cleft, equal; female lanceolate, very long, three-toothed, spreading. *Stamens* to the hermaphrodites: filaments very short, anthers cylindric; to the females: filaments subulate, erect; anthers none. *Pistil:* germen oblong; style simple, the length of the stamens; stigma bifid. *Perianth* none; calyx unchanged. *Seeds* solitary, oblong; down simple; in the hermaphrodites pubescent, long. *Receptacle* naked. *Corollules* of the disk often trifid, with the outer division twice as broad as the others.

SPEC. CHAR.—*Leaves* ovate, entire; two opposite cauline leaves.

Fig. 1. Hermaphrodite flower of the disk. 2. Floret of the ray. 3. The seed. The figure of the Arnica montana is taken from the specimen in the Herbarium of the Linnean Society, and coloured after Heyne.

History.—No notice is given in the earlier authors on medical botany, of the Arnica montana, although by some (*Chaumeton, Flore Médicale*) it is supposed that the Αλισμα of Dioscorides, commented on by Matthiolus (lib. iii., cxlvii.), is identical with this plant. However, Dr. Adams (*Supplement to Dunbar's Lexicon*, 3rd edit.), a good authority on these subjects, says, that Αλισμα is the same as Δαμασωνιον, as expressly stated by Galen (lib. iii. p. 154). R. Stephens calls it Plantago aquatica, and it is so acknowledged by Cordus, Sibthorp, and Sprengel; but the description given by Dioscorides is more like the Doronicum than the Plantain; Clusius (*Plant. Rariores*, p. xviii.) describes a plant under the name of Doronicum Pannonicum, which agrees in most respects with the Arnica montana. The same plant is mentioned by Gerarde (lib. ii. p. 742) as the German Marigold, or Chrysanthemum latifolium; by Gesner as Caltha alpina; by Dodonæus as Chrysanthemum latifolium; by Pena and Lobel as Nardus celtica altera; and as Ptarmica montana (*Daleschampii in Histor. Lugd.*, p. 1169). It was not brought into use till the beginning of the last century, when it was extolled by a German physician, of the name of Fehr, as the panacea for contusions and bruises; hence it obtained the name Panacea lapsorum. Dr. Collin, of Vienna, used it extensively in the Pazman Hospital in that city for four years, from 1771-74, with, as he relates, most unprecedented success, and through its agency hundreds of patients were snatched from the jaws of death. He used it extensively in intermittent and putrid fevers, supposing it to possess tonic and antiseptic qualities in the highest degree, and also in malignant dysentery. It was observed that on first giving this medicine, it frequently produced vomiting and uneasiness at the stomach; when given improperly, and in too large doses, it excites *great anxiety*, shooting and burning pains, and even dangerous hemorrhages, vomiting, vertigo, and coma.

It has also been recommended and given in paralytic disorders; chronic rheumatism; retention of urine from paralysis of the bladder; amaurosis; intermittent, putrid, and typhoid fevers, and, according to Haller, in epilepsy; it was also used much in France, at the end of the last century, in colliquative diarrhœa.

Althoff preferred Arnica to Peruvian bark, as an antiseptic to putrid fevers; and Stohl called it the Quinine of the poor, and declared it to be specific in dysentery.

Arnica was supposed to be contra-indicated by an inflammatory diathesis, a predisposition to hemorrhages, and internal congestions.

Besides Collin, as mentioned above, Stohl, Kausch, Crichton, and Gilbert advocated its use in mucous, adynamic, putrid, and petechial fevers. Müeller, Buechner, and La Marche, in peripneumonia, nephritis, rheumatism, and gout. Junker, Eschenbach, and Collin, in hemiplegia, epilepsy, and amaurosis.* It became what is termed a fashionable remedy about the latter part of the last century and commencement of the present one; but from its great abuse, or rather indiscriminate use, fell into disrepute, although, had it been discreetly administered in diseases for which it was appropriate, it would have become then, as it has now in homœopathic medicine, an invaluable remedy in many serious diseases.

Description.—Arnica montana is a perennial plant; flowers July and August. The *root* is woody, with numerous small

* The following are the chief essays which were written at that time on the virtues of the Arnica montana.—La Marche (George Auguste de), De Arnicæ veræ Usu. Diss. inaug Præs., 4to, *Halæ*, 1719; *id.* 1744. Meisner (L. F.), Panacea lapsorum seu Arnica, 4to, *Pragæ*, 1736. Buechner (André E.), De genuinis principiis et effectibus Arnicæ, 4to, *Erfordiæ*, 1741; *id. Lipsiæ*, 1749. Collin (Henry Joseph), Florum Arnicæ vires, etc., 8vo, *Viennæ*, 1773. Arnicæ in Febribus et aliis morbis putridis vires, 8vo, *Viennæ*, 1775. These observations fill about 800 pages. Schuelt (P. A.), De Viribus Arnicæ, 4to, *Gottingæ*, 1774. Döellinger (J. J.), Dissertatio inaugural. Observ. circa Arnica, 4to, *Bamberg*, 1776. Fried (Ignace), De Viribus et Usu Arnicæ, 8vo, *Viennæ*, 1780. Birhholz (A. M.), De Arnicæ virtute propriâ atque specificâ, 4to, *Lipsiæ*, 1785. Buchholz (G. H. S.), Versuche uëber die antiseptischen kroëfte des Wolferley, 4to, *Erford*, 1785.

radicles, and when macerated has a peculiar odour like apples, and an astringent taste. The *stem* is about a foot high, but in alpine situations very often not above six inches, simple, obscurely angular. The *leaves* are ovate, entire. The *stem-leaves* twin, and opposite, of a glossy green colour, veined, and lighter on the dorsal side. The *flowers* are bright yellow, having a deeper colour as they fade, about two inches in diameter, and placed on upright terminal peduncles. *Calyx* cylindrical, composed of rough, hairy scales. The *ligulate florets* are about sixteen to eighteen in number, three-toothed, and striated, twice as long as the calyx, hairy at the base. *Seeds* are oblong, blackish, and crowned with a straw-coloured down.

There are twelve different species of Arnica.

1. *Arnica montana*, as above.

2. *A. philoselloides*. Mouse-eared Arnica. "Leaves perfectly entire, elliptic, villose; scape one-flowered, woolly; calyx equalling the ray;" the stem and leaves covered with down; leaves two or three inches long, and about half this breadth, hairy, especially on the back, pointed; scape twice as long as the leaves, very woolly towards the top; flower large; calyx tomentose, of the length of the ray; florets of the ray very narrow, of a dark red or purple colour, and male. A native of the Cape of Good Hope.

3. *A. scorpioides*. Alternate-leaved Arnica (*Jacq. Flor. Aust.* ii. t. 349). Roots contorted, supposed to be like a scorpion; stems several, from six inches to a foot in height, terminated by a deep yellow flower of two inches diameter; root-leaves roundish, deeply serrated, on long foot-stalks. The whole plant has a strong, disagreeable smell. Native of Switzerland, Savoy, Dauphiné, etc.

4. *A. doronicum*. (*Jacq. Flor. Aust.*, i. t. 92; *Arn. clusii allion. ped.; Arn. Stiriaca; Villars Dauph.*, 210). Leaves hairy; stem four to eight inches in height, and never bears more than one flower. A native of the high Alps of the Grisons, Dauphiné, Piedmont, and Austria.

5. *A. maritima.* Sea Arnica. Aster Helenium maritimum (*Gmel.*, lib. ii. p. 175). Leaves lanceolate, lower ones serrate; stem leafy, many-flowered. Native of Kamtschatka and North America.

6. *A. crocea.* Saffron-flowered Arnica. A native of the Cape of Good Hope.

7. *A. ciliata.* Ciliate-leaved Arnica. The stem is erect, a foot high, angular, hispid, with white bristles; leaves alternate; flower terminating, red, the size of a small pear. A native of Japan.

8. *A. japonica.* Japonese Arnica (*Thunb.* 319). Flowers peduncled, red. A native of Japan.

9. *A. palmata.* Palmate-leaved Arnica (*Thunb.* l. c.) Leaves gashed, palmated, toothed; flowers panicled, terminating, small, yellow. Native of Japan.

10. *A. gerbera.* Leaves pinnatifid; one large flower, with a dark purple disk, and a yellow ray, purple underneath. Native of the Cape of Good Hope.

11. *A. coronopifolia.* Leaves pinnate; very much resembles the last, and is a native of the Cape of Good Hope.

12. *A. oporina* (*Forst. Pl. Aust.*, t. 299). Shrubby leaves, lanceolate, peduncles one-flowered, solitary, terminal, scaly. Native of New Zealand.

Geographical Distribution.—The Arnica montana is found in the mountainous districts of many parts of Europe, more particularly in Switzerland, the northern parts of Germany, and Siberia. There are five species European, but the A. montana is the only one supposed to have medicinal properties, and is that which Hahnemann proved. There is a peculiar parasitical insect which infests this plant, called Arnica, a species of Staphylinus.

Parts used in Medicine, and Mode of Preparation.—The Roots, Flowers, and Leaves. The powder of the root is prepared by making three attenuations by trituration; or else it is digested in twenty parts of alcohol to make the tincture. Should the fresh plant be procured, the expressed juice of the whole plant is mixed with equal parts of alcohol. For external use, as an application for contusions, etc., it is prepared as follows: the parts of the root selected should be about the size of a quill, the smaller fibrils being removed; this should be reduced to coarse powder and macerated in alcohol, and allowed to stand in a cool place eight or ten days, and then strained and decanted; great caution is necessary in the local application of this tincture, particularly in cases where there is abrasion of the skin, in such the tincture should be greatly diluted with water; in fact, in many cases it can hardly be applied weak enough.

Before making use of this plant, it is indispensable to clean the flowers, as they are often soiled by the eggs of the parasitical fly, previously mentioned, and it must be borne in mind that the root soon loses much of its medicinal virtue if exposed to the air, but if reduced to powder and dried in a sand-bath, and then placed into well-stopped bottles, it may be preserved for years.

From the very great demand for this drug for contusions, etc., a spurious root has been sent over from the Continent, and the author has seen bottles labelled "Tincture of Arnica Montana," which he has every reason to suppose did not contain one drop of the juice of that plant. It is therefore of the last importance that those interested either in the sale or the use of it, should be aware of its distinguishing characteristics.

The True Root.	The False Root.
Smell most peculiar, like that of apples or of an apple-room.	Smell faintish and very slight.
Taste biting, pungent, and astringent.	Taste insipid.
Colour dark brown.	Colour light, yellowish brown.
Structure woody, numerous small radicles proceeding from it in all directions, and generally from one and a half to two and a half inches in length, and a quarter of an inch in circumference.	Structure woody; no small radicle roots, but a mass of long fibres proceeding from a thick woody stem, tough and unyielding, and difficult to break.
Fracture sharp and brittle.	
When macerated in alcohol, it forms a brownish, yellowish green tincture, the characteristic odour prevailing over that of the alcohol.	When macerated in alcohol, gives a light yellowish tincture. Odour of alcohol pervading over that of the root.
Macerated in water, the peculiar apple odour is strongly perceptible.	Macerated in water, it has but little smell.

Medical Uses (Homœopathic).—Hahnemann, in his *Materia Medica Pura,* has the following observations upon

Arnica. "Notwithstanding all its carefully-constructed dogmas, its scholastic definitions, and subtle distinctions, the established system (*i. e.* allopathy) has never succeeded in discovering the specific properties of this plant, nor in finding any certain remedy for that general affection (often very serious) which results from severe falls, shocks, blows, contusions, etc., or from twisting or tearing the solid parts of the human frame. At length, after innumerable attempts and trials, the people discovered for themselves the desired remedy in Arnica. Two hundred years ago, a physician, named Fehr, communicated to his brethren, for the first time, the discovery of this domestic remedy; since when, Arnica has been called Panacea lapsorum. The case has been similar with regard to all other specifics; the art of medicine owes the knowledge of them to domestic practice, and has never made a single discovery for itself, because those who practise it, have not taken the trouble to try the pure effect of natural substances on persons in health."

Clinical Observations.—Noack and Trinks (*Handbuch der homöop. Arzneimittellehre*) offer the following remarks on the application of Arnica, according to the homœopathic principle. Arnica is suitable when the nervous system, the animal as well as the vegetative, is in a state of torpidity. *It is suitable for those stages of inflammation where the vital powers become extinct, where torpid fever or neurophlogosis sets in; under these circumstances, it is the contrary to Aconite, which corresponds to the purely inflammatory, especially the synochal character.* Arnica is especially useful in the so-called status gastricus nervosus stupidus; it appears to be suitable to nervous venous congestions; to plethoric young people with red face, or to persons of lymphatic temperament; to individuals weakened by disease, with pale, yellow, livid face.

As a remedy against the effects of blows, contusions, etc., Arnica rivals *Rhus toxicodendron, Conium maculatum, Acidum sulphuricum, Symphytum officinale, Calendula officinalis, Ruta, Ledum,* or *Ferrum muriaticum. Rhus,* however, corresponds more to the consequences attending an extension of membranous tissues, especially the ligaments of the joints. *Conium* is more suitable for contusions, which produce a condensation of the cellular tissue, and induration of glandular structures, accompanied by a sensation of numbness. *Symphytum* answers more to the pressure and contusions of bones. *Calendula* for sugillations, bloody and serous infiltrations of the cellular tissue in open wounds and ulcers. *Ruta* we know to be specific in cases of mechanical injury to the tarsal or carpal joints, and in rheumatic paralysis of these parts. *Ferrum muriaticum* is especially useful in a similar affection of the shoulder-joint; and *Ledum,* when the hip-joint is the seat of these affections.

Arnica montana has been serviceable, according to the homœopathic application, *in all cases arising from external injury, concussion of the brain, and the spinal marrow.* Soporous, apoplectic, and paralytic fits. Atonic hemorrhages. Nervous, gastric, and putrid fevers. Rheumatism and gout. Frozen limbs. Consequences of fright. Bad effects from the use of Cinchona. Poisoning by lead. Furunculus. *Stings of insects.* Hydrocephalus acutus, especially after Scarlatina miliaris. Epistaxis (bleeding from the nose). Swelling of one cheek. Hemorrhage from the mouth. Consequences of blows on the pit of the stomach. Cardialgia, consequent upon chronic gastritis or loss of animal fluids. Splenetic stitches. Serous and mucous enteritis. Proctitis. Dysentery. Retentio urinæ. Metrorrhagia. Pertussis. Spurious pleuritis. Pleurodynia. Pleuritis. Pneumonia, produced by mechanical causes.

Characteristic Peculiarities.—The pains increase by talking, moving about, blowing, and even by every sound. The pains quickly wander from one part to another. The violence of the pains almost drive him distracted.

Antidotes.—Camphor, Ignatia: it antidotes Ammoniacum, China, Cicuta, Ferrum, Ipecacuanha, Senega.

Wine increases the effects of Arnica, by aggravating the symptoms.

Plate VII

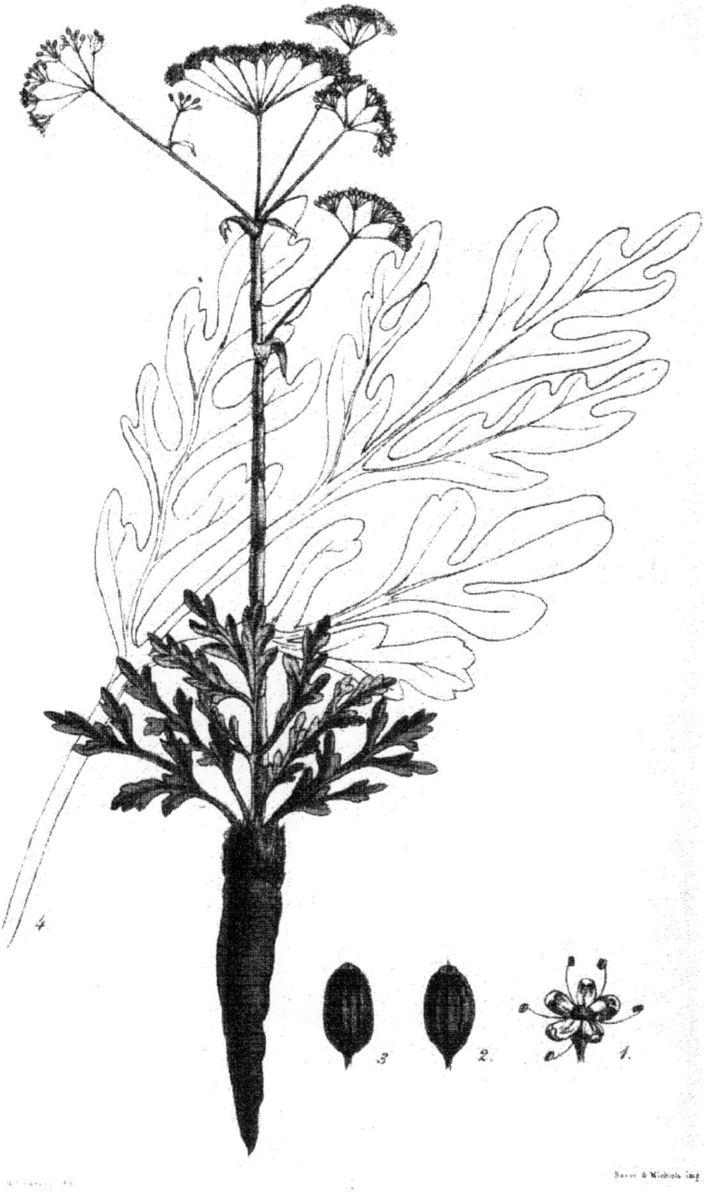

Asafœtida. (Ferula Asafœtida)

VII.

ASAFŒTIDA.

(GUM-RESIN FROM THE FERULA ASAFŒTIDA.)

Asafœtida.

SYNONYMS.—Asafœtida, *Bauhin*, Πιν., lib. xii. Ferula asafœtida, *Linn.* Ferula Persica, *Hope.* Asafœtida disgunensis, *Kæmpfer.* Narthex asafœtida, *Falconer.*

FOREIGN NAMES.—*Fr.:* Asafétida. *Ital.:* Assafetida, Zaffetica. *Span.:* Asa fetida. *Germ.:* Stinkasaut, Steckenkraut. *Dut.:* Duivels dreck. *Arab.:* Halsiit. *Pers.:* Ungooseh. *Hind.:* Hing. *Russ.:* Durnopathutschink.

Nat. Order, UMBELLIFERÆ.—PENTANDRIA, DIGYNIA.

GEN. CHAR.—*General umbel* of numerous rays, globose; *partial*, similar to it. *General involucrum* deciduous; *partial*, of numerous small linear leaves. *Perianth* scarcely discernible. Margin of the *calyx*, five-toothed. *Petals* ovate, entire, acuminate, with an ascending or incurved point. *Flowers* white, many rays, lateral, often opposite. *Fruit* oval, somewhat compressed, marked with three elevated lines on each side, separable into two parts. *Seeds* two, large, elliptical, flat on each side, marked with three distinct ribs.

SPEC. CHAR.—*Stem* terate, simple, clothed with leafless sheaths. *Leaves* radical, pinnatisect. The *segments*, one or two, pinnatifid, sinuate. *Lobes* oblong, obtuse. *Involucrum* none.

HISTORY.—The ancient history of Asafœtida is involved in mystery; it is supposed to be the Σιλφιον of Dioscorides, Herodotus, and Galen, and the Laserpitium of Pliny, which latter produced the Succus Cyrenaicus; but this plant becoming scarce, the ancients used another of the same genus, probably the Ferula communis, the Ναρθηξ of Dioscorides, in its place.

Fig. 1. The flower expanded. 2 and 3. The seed in different states. 4. The leaf.

Dioscorides, in describing the Σιλφιον, says that it grows in Syria, Armenia, Media, and Lybia; and Pliny—"For a long time past the only Laser (by which name this genus was called) brought to us, is that which is produced abundantly in Persia, Media, and Armenia, but it is far inferior to the Cyrenaic." It is probable that this Laser described by Pliny is the Asafœtida of modern times. Serapion also gives a long account of it under Assa, and likens it to Σιλφιον; and Avicenna records two kinds—the one fetid, the other odoriferous. Dioscorides (liber iii. cap. xciv.), in describing the Σιλφιον, vaunts its powers most highly; mixed with various ingredients, it prevents suffusion in inflammation of the eyes, cures toothaches, the bites of mad dogs, and wounds of scorpions. Mixed with ruta, it relieves carbuncles; and with other substances, cures sarcoma, polypus, tetanus, and opisthotonos; is an excellent gargle in sore throat; helps the catamenia, etc. He also describes another plant, Ναρθηξ, or Ferula (from *ferula*, a cane), which he recommends as most useful in hæmoptysis cœliacis, and, when given in wine, as a remedy against the bites of vipers.

Pliny (*Holland's Translation*, book xix.) says that "Laserpitium was discovered first in the province of Barbarie Cyrenaica. The juice or liquor drawn from this herb they call Laser; a drug so magnified, of such singularity and use in physicke especially, that it was sold by weight, and a drachm of which cost a Roman denier. For some years this plant is not to be found in Cyrenaica, owing to the farmers and publicans putting their cattle into the fields in which it grows, and is by them eaten greedily, and they grow fat and give much milk, whereby they gain more than by allowing it to stand for juice. If by chance a sheep or goat eat of the young plant, it may be known by the following sign, namely, the sheep, as soon as it hath tasted it, will drop asleep, and the goat begin sneezing. For many years the merchants have brought no other Laser than that which grows in Persia."

"It was so prized, that by great good fortune the consuls

C. Valerius and M. Herennius brought thirty pounds weight of it to Rome from Cyrenæ, and that it was set abroad to show to all comers; and that Cæsar, at the beginning of the civil war, took forth openly from the chamber of the city, with other treasure both of gold and silver, 111 pounds of the best Laser."

He also records the mode in which it originated in the following words:—"The most renowned Greek authors have left in writing, that seven years before the foundation of the city Cyrene, which was built 143 years after our city of Rome, this plant Laserpitium was engendered in one instant by occasion of a certain thick, gross, and black shower of rain, in manner of pitch, which suddenly fell and drenched the ground.

"That the herb will not choose to be cultivated, but dies if taken from barren soil.

"That cattle are first scoured by it, and then, after rid of humour, grow fat, and in flesh taste most delicate."

Geoffroy, Millar, and Fourcroy find a resemblance between the Cyrenaica and Asafœtida, and consider that it is without doubt the Σιλφιον of Dioscorides, the Laserpitium of Pliny, the Asafœtida disgunensis of Kæmpfer, and the Ferula Asafœtida of Linnæus. Captain Beechey, a modern traveller, found in the region of Cyrene a plant three feet high, resembling the hemlock, which he supposed the same as the ancient Σιλφιον. It has been a matter of uncertainty from what source the Asafœtida was procured, till within the last few years; the Ferula Persica having been given and figured as the plant from which the gum-resin proceeded, since Dr. Hope's cultivation of that plant in the Botanical Garden of Edinburgh. Dr. Hugh Falconer, however, in his late researches in Central Asia, has set the question at rest, and proves that the true Ferula is that which was described so accurately by Kæmpfer.

Asafœtida has been used extensively in allopathic medicine. In spasmodic and convulsive diseases. Hysteria. Infantine convulsions. Epilepsy. Pure spasmodic asthma. Hooping-cough. Flatulent colic of hysterical and dyspeptic individuals and of infants. As a stimulating expectorant and antispasmodic in chronic catarrh. In constipation, with flatulence; and as an emmenagogue in uterine obstructions (amenorrhœa and chlorosis), Asafœtida has been employed, from a notion that it acted specifically on the womb.

Description (From Dr. Falconer's account in Transactions of Linn. Soc., 1849).—A tall perennial plant, five to eight feet high. *Root* fusiform, simple or divided, a foot or more in length, about three inches in diameter at top, with a dark greyish, corrugated surface. The summit connected, above the soil, with dark hair-like, fibrous tegmenta, the persistent exuviæ of former years. *Leaves* collected into a fascicle above the roots, numerous, large, and spreading, about eighteen inches in length in the adult plant, of a light green colour, paler underneath, and of a dry leathery texture. *Stem* erect, striated, about two inches in diameter at the base, solid throughout. *General* as well as *partial involucra* wanting. *Umbels*, ten to twenty, rayed, emitted from the dilated spherical head of a common peduncle; the rays two to four inches in length. *Partial umbels*, with very short rays, aggregated into a round capitula, varying from ten to twenty rays in the fertile, and from twenty-five to thirty in the barren umbellæ. *Flowers* small, white, the barren generally mixed up with the fertile. *Styles* filiform, reflected in the ripe fruit, rather short and slender, attached by a broad base. *Fruit*, from seven to fifteen, ripening on the partial umbels, supported on short stalks.

"The plant above described, I believe to be the true Asafœtida disgunensis, or 'Hingesch' of Kæmpfer. It does not appear to have been met with by any other botanist since it was examined *in situ* by that excellent and careful observer, upwards of a century and a half ago."

The following is Kæmpfer's description of this plant:—"It has a long, generally undivided, root, black without, but internally white, fleshy, full of juice, and of an overpowering odour, something like garlic. This root, when about a year old, is the thickness of a man's thumb, and continues afterwards to increase until it shoots up a flowering stem, so that it sometimes reaches the size of a man's leg. It pushes out annually several large root-leaves, which resemble those of the pæony, and exhale a strong garlic odour like that of the root, but weaker. Rarely in its first year, generally, indeed, not till it is many years old, it produces a flowering stem, which is between six and nine feet tall, about two inches in diameter, and naked, except that it bears rudimentary leaves, in the form of the cylindrical bases of leaf-stalks. The whole plant dies after it has once flowered and ripened to seed." He describes the following process of procuring the gum-resin. "When the plant is at least four years old, and before it produces a flowering stem, the root-leaves are twisted off close to the root, in the beginning of April, and the soil is removed from the crown of the root. About forty days afterwards a slice is cut horizontally from its summit, upon which a milky juice, of an overpowering fetid odour, gradually exudes. In two days, when the exudation is somewhat hardened, it is scraped off, and at the same time a fresh slice is cut off the top of the root, from which the juice again flows, and is collected as before. This process may be repeated so often as twelve times in the course of six weeks, before the root is altogether exhausted. The roots are carefully kept from the sun, except after the last operation." The gum-resin, gathered from several plants at one time, is united into masses about one or two pounds in weight; and when farther hardened by keeping, is sent to the ports of Persia for exportation, or disposed of for consumption in the country as a condiment, many of the Asiatics being extremely fond of it; and from this cause some of the old writers have called it Cibus Deorum—food for the gods.

Asafœtida of commerce occurs in irregular pieces of variable size, externally yellowish or pinkish brown. The fracture is conchoidal, whitish or milk-white, translucent, pearly, with waxy lustre. By exposure to light and air, the recently-fractured surface acquires, in a few hours, a violet red or peach-blossom red colour, which, after some weeks, diminishes in intensity, and gradually passes into yellowish or pinkish brown. It is fusible and inflammable, burning in air with a white flame, and the evolution of much smoke. Its taste is acrid and bitter, and its odour strong, alliaceous, and peculiar. There are two different sorts generally found in the shops, Asafœtida in granis, or Asafœtida in tears; Asafœtida in massis, or lump Asafœtida: this latter is supposed to be the resin of the Ferula Asafœtida, the other being that of the Ferula Persica. Besides the gum-resin, the fruit of the Narthex Asafœtida is imported into India from Persia and Afghanistan, under the name of Anjoudan, being extensively employed by the native physicians.

GEOGRAPHICAL DISTRIBUTION. — Persia; Afghanistan; mountains of Chorassan and Laar. Dr. Falconer found it in the valley of Astore, one of the subordinate valleys of the Indus, behind Cashmeer. Sir Alexander Burnes also found it in the mountains of Hindoo Koosh, 7,000 feet above the level of the sea.

PARTS USED IN MEDICINE, AND MODE OF PREPARATION.— The Gum-resin, that which is known in commerce as the Lump Asafœtida, for the reason above stated. The tincture is prepared by infusing fifty grains of the powder in 1,000 drops of alcohol. The attenuations to be made as directed under Aconite.

MEDICAL USES (HOMŒOPATHIC).—Asafœtida was added to the *Hom. Materia Medica* by Stapf. According to Noack and Trinks (*Handbuch für Hom. Arzneimittell.*), Asafœtida acts principally upon that portion of the nervous system which regulates the vegetative functions, and is generally suitable when the sensibility of the organism is excessive, and accompanied by a corresponding excess of venous blood. Scrofulous or nervous individuals, with a venous and hemorrhoidal constitution and a phlegmatic temperament, are more particularly certain of the favourable action of Asafœtida. Hysteria and hypochondria. Globus hysterica. Ascites and anasarca, arising from disorganization of the abdominal organs. Chronic rheumatism and gout. Obesity. Swelling of the glands. Scrofulous affections and rachitis. Venereal mercurial ulcers of the bones. Hydrargyrosis. Rheumatic gastric fever, with menstrual colic. Amblyopia amaurotica. Ophthalmia scrofulosa. Ozœna scrofulosa. Otorrhœa scrofulosa, with discharge of bloody serum, having a putrid smell. Otorrhœa and deafness, from the abuse of mercury. Œsophagitis. Diaphragmitis. Chronic gastritis. Bilious and gastric conditions, particularly when the latter has arisen from eating too much fat. Weakness of digestion in hypochondriacal persons. Chronic affections of the liver. Pulsations of the abdomen. Obstruction and hardness of abdomen. Colic. Flatulent colic. Spasm of the bladder. Catamenia too scanty and too early, with labour-like pains. Asthmatic sufferings from exertion of any kind. Palpitation of the heart, particularly when arising from physical exertions, or the sudden suppression of some habitual discharge, or other secretions, and when accompanied with violent congestion of the lungs.

Characteristic Peculiarities.—Intermittent, pulsative, or oppressive darting; also, tearing pains from within outwards, transformed into different kinds of pains, or relieved by touching the parts, and sometimes accompanied by feeling of numbness; pains in the planes of the flexor muscles; the pains come on when sitting; they abate during a walk in the open air.

Professor Jorg (*Wibmer, Wirk d'Arzneim.*, ii. Gifte, bd. ii. 336) and his pupils (males and females) endeavoured to elucidate the effects of this medicine by experiments on themselves. Doses of Asafœtida, not exceeding a scruple, caused uneasiness and pain in the stomach, increased secretion of the gastro-intestinal membrane, and alvine evacuations. The pulse was increased in frequency; the animal heat augmented; the respiration quickened, and the excretion from the bronchial membranes increased. A very constant effect was headache and giddiness. The urino-genital organs appeared to be especially affected, and the catamenia appeared before the usual period.

A reference to the history of this plant will demonstrate how constantly it has been given for diseases, the symptoms of which it will produce when taken in over-large doses.

MM. Trousseau and Pidoux (*Traité de Thérap.*, pp. 12, 13) state that they felt no inconvenience from taking Asafœtida; the only effect it produced was altering the odour of the secretions, which was worse than the Asafœtida itself; and the perspiration of Asiatics who use Asafœtida daily, becomes extremely impregnated. Aristophanes (*Equites*, act ii. sc. 4) alludes to this circumstance.

In experiments made on animals, it was found that the odour of Asafœtida was discoverable in the veins of the stomach, the stomach itself, and the small intestines, but not in the arterial blood or the lymph. Hence it is concluded that the odorous principle of the gum-resin is but very slowly absorbed by the venous system.

Antidotes (to homœopathic doses).—China, Pulsatilla,—Electricity.

Plate VIII.

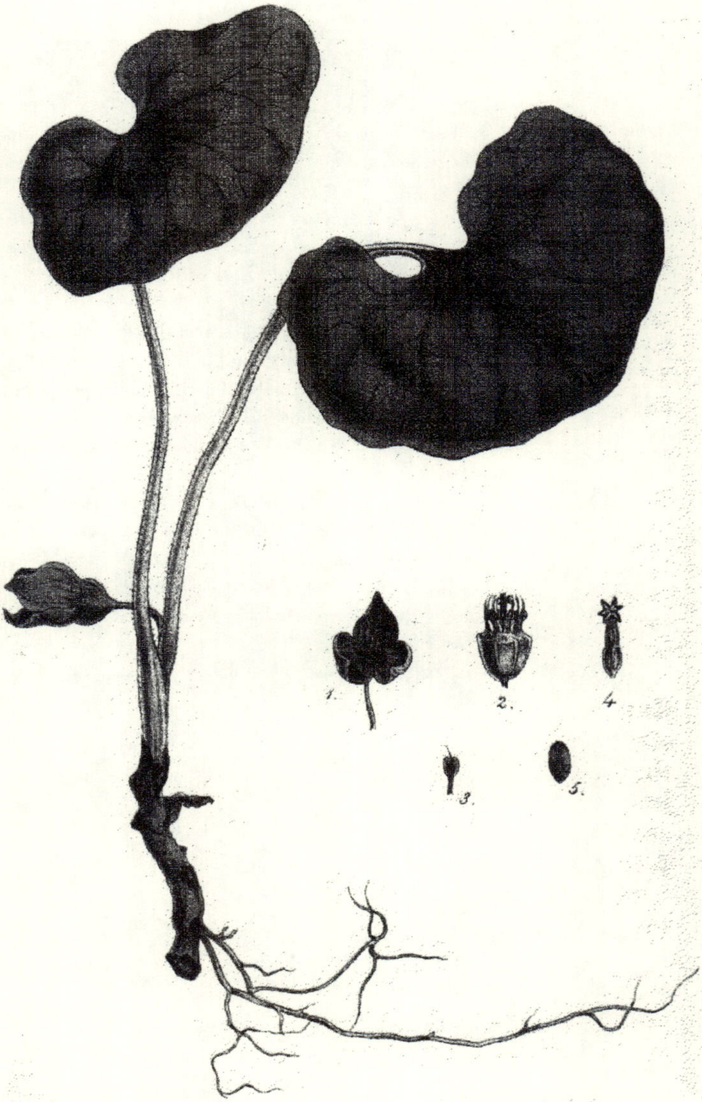

A. F. del. R. Sowerby lith. Reeve & Nichol, imp.

Asarum Europœum

VIII.

ASARUM EUROPÆUM.

Asarabacca, Fole's Foot, Hazelwort, Wild Nard.

SYNONYMS.—Asarum, *Bauhin*, Πιναξ, lib. v. sect. 6. Asarum vulgare. Asarum foliis reniformibus subhirsutis, *Linn.*

FOREIGN NAMES.—*Fr.:* Asaret, Cabaret, Bondelle, Oreille d'Homme, Narde sauvage. *Ital.:* Asaro. *Germ.:* Haselkraut, Hazelwurz. *Dut.:* Mansoor. *Swed.:* Hasselört. *Dan.:* Hasselurt. *Russ.:* Wodoler.

Nat. Order, ARISTOLOCHIÆ, *Juss.;* SARMENTACEÆ, *Linn.*—DODECANDRIA, MONOGYNIA.

GEN. CHAR.—*Calyx* campanulate, three-lobed, coriaceous, coloured; the points incurved. *Corolla* none. *Stamens* twelve, inserted in the ovary, awl-shaped, half the length of the calyx. *Anthers* adnate to the middle of the filaments, each of two round, separate cells. *Style* columnar, nearly as long as the stamens. *Stigma* stellate, six-lobed. *Capsule* six-celled.

SPEC. CHAR.—*Leaves* in pairs, kidney-shaped, obtuse.

HISTORY.—A substance which acts so perceptibly on the organs of smelling and of sight naturally soon attracted the attention of physicians, so we find the most ancient masters of our art celebrating the virtues of Asarum. Dioscorides (lib. i. cap. ix.) described it under the name of Ασαρον, and recommended its use in vomiting, dropsy, and inveterate ischias. Pliny asserts that it was often confounded with Nardus (Valerian) and Baccaris; but Sprengel maintains that the Baccaris of the ancients and

---

Fig. 1. A flower opened. 2. Unripe capsule, crowned with the stamens and pistils. 3. A separate stamen, showing its awl-shape. 4. A germen, style, and stigma. 5. A seed magnified.

the Asarabacca are identical, and he affirms that in the district of Verona, the Asarum is called Bacchera, and that the English name Asarabacca is a union of the two, Asarum and Baccaris; but it seems to have been a disputed point, even in the ancient times, as to what was the Baccaris. Galen says that it was a term applied both to a herb and a Lydian ointment; others have supposed it to be the Foxglove (Digitalis). Matthiolus and Bauhin think the Baccaris is the Conyza squamosa, to which it seems most identical, according to Adams. Pliny evidently did not confound the two plants; in lib. xxi. cap. vi. (*Holland's Trans.*), he says: "There is another plant which the Greeks call Ασαρον, very different from Baccaris. I do find that this plant is called Asarum, because it adorneth not garlands (from α, non; and σαιρω, to adorn)." Macer says that Asarum was called Vulgago. "Est Asaron, Græce, Vulgago dicta Latinè:—

> "This herbe *Asaron* do the Grecians name;
> Whereas the Latines *Vulgago* clepe the same."

It was also called by the great learned philosophers, according to Gerarde, Αιμα αρεως, *i. e.*, Martis sanguinis, or the blood of Mars; and Culpeper in his Herbal says it is under the dominion of Mars, and therefore inimical to nature. In giving an account of the virtues of the herb, this same physician deprecates the use of violent cathartics, etc., in the following words: "I shall desire ignorant people to forbear the use of the leaves. * * * * * The truth is, I fancy purging and vomiting medicines as little as any man breathing doth, for they weaken nature; nor shall ever advise them to be used unless upon urgent necessity. If a physician be Nature's servant, it is his duty to strengthen his mistress as much as he can, and weaken her as little as may be."

Dodonæus (*Lyte's Translation*, book iii.) gives the following account of the virtues of Asarabacca: "The root boiled in wine and drunken, is good against the strangury, the cough, shortness of breath, and difficulty of breathing, convulsions, cramps, and the shrinking together of members.

"The same, taken in like manner, is profitable against venom, and the biting and stinging of serpents.

"The same, in wine, is good for them that have the dropsy and sciatica.

"The leaves of the Asarabacca, stamped with wine and strained, and the juice thereof drunken, causeth vomiting, and purgeth, by vomiting, tough phlegm and choler.

"The same leaves, stamped, are good to be applied and laid to the ache and dolors of the head, to the inflammation of the eyes, and to women's breasts that are too full of milk when they list to dry the same, and it is good to be laid to the disease called the wildfire, especially at the beginning."

It was recommended by Coste and Willemet as a substitute for ipecacuanha, and indeed was used as an emetic previous to the introduction of that root into Europe. A few grains snuffed up the nose for several evenings will produce a considerable watery discharge, which sometimes continues for several days, by which headache, toothache, chronic ophthalmia, and some soporific and paralytic complaints have been relieved. It is supposed to be the chief ingredient in the cephalic snuffs. It was also used in arthritis, ascites, tertian and quartan agues, vertigo, hydrocephalus, amaurosis, deafness, bleeding from the nose, paralysis of the organs of deglutition, icterus, diseases of the kidneys, chronic bronchitis, and asthma. It was an ingredient in some of the nostrums used to procure abortions, and is used as a specific in dysentery by the Icelanders. It has been employed to cure malignant ulcers and other diseases in cattle. A comparison with the provings of this plant, will show how manifold are the homœopathic relations between the disorders produced by the Asarum and those which are cured by it. The following extract from Paulli (*Quadripartum Botanicum,* Argentorati, 1667, p. 23) is significant. "In super noto apud *Historiæ plantarum universalis autores,* tom. iii. pp. 550-6, hæc verba reperii subdit *Tragus Asari,* foliis carpo admotis uti mulierculas Argentoratenses ad febris ardorem depellendum, cum tamen tota planta aromatica sit et gustu mordax, quod insignis calidatis indicium est. Cæterum cum folia adstringendi naturam habeant, calorem ipsum febrilem, sic admota ad interiorem retrudunt, atque ita morbum adangent." And Zorn also says in his *Botanologia Medica* (Berlin, 1714, s. 96), "That the pounded leaves, placed upon the pulse, will remove the fever; but we also know by manifold experience, that Asarum will produce ebullition of the blood and feverish excitement."

Description.—The Asarabacca is a perennial plant; flowering in May and June; with a short, simple stem, round and pubescent, from which come two kidney-shaped leaves of a glossy green colour, and from the axils of the two leaves springs a solitary drooping flower, upon a short footstalk, of a greenish colour, streaked, and tipped with chocolate outside, and purplish brown within. The leaves darken as they fade, and emit a peculiar pungent odour.

There are two species besides the As. Europæum, viz.: 1. As. Canadensis, Canadian Asarabacca. 2. As. Virginicum, sweet-scented Asarabacca; a native of Virginia and Carolina, in North America; China, and Japan.

Geographical Distribution.—A native of most parts of Europe; found in the mountainous woods, in all climates, in Pontus, Phrygia, Illyria, Italy, and in many parts of the north of Germany, Poland, France, both in Provence and in the neighbourhood of Paris. It is indigenous in this country.

Localities.—In dark mountainous woods, in the most shady places; rare; found in the mountainous woods in Yorkshire, Lancashire, Cumberland, Westmoreland, and Northumberland; rather plentiful in the neighbourhood of Halifax, Yorkshire; and has occasionally been found between Henley and Maidenhead, in Berkshire. In Scotland, it was found by Miss Liston, at West Binny, near Linlithgow.

Parts used in Medicine, and Mode of Preparation.—The Leaves and Root. The expressed juice of the whole plant, mixed with equal parts of alcohol, and then attenuated to the 30th dilution, as directed under Aconite.

MEDICAL USES (HOMŒOPATHIC). — This medicine was described by Hahnemann and others, and the symptoms recorded in the *Materia Medica Pura.* The following are his observations: "If any proof were wanting to show the negligence with which the old school of medicine has attempted to study the effects of simple medicinal substances, it would be supplied by the labours of Coste and Willemet, who, in their chief work (*Essais sur quelques Plantes indigènes*, Nancy, 1778), have treated of Asarum. What results have they obtained from their examination? Not one of those remarkable symptoms hereafter enumerated, excepting that a dose, from twenty-eight to forty grains, caused vomiting five or six times. But of what nature? They say not a word. They add that a porter having taken forty-eight grains of Asarum, experienced severe colic, with purgation and vomiting, which was allayed by a lavement of milk; from which they inferred that the root of this plant acts similarly to ipecacuanha. But did it produce no other effects? and was this all the benefit to be expected from it? With what negligence must the observations have been made, in a matter of so much importance, when they profess to have seen nothing more; to have noticed no other effects; to have discovered no other cases in which Asarum might be more beneficial.

"No, Asarum is not better adapted as an emetic, to take the place of ipecacuanha, than many other substances which, when given in too powerful doses, are also expelled by nature, by means of violent vomiting, such as arsenic, sulphate of zinc, sulphate of copper, white hellebore, etc.

"Then, do all these substances which, when taken in excess, excite dangerous vomiting, exist to be used only as emetics? How short-sighted, how contented with superficial notions, and therefore dangerous ones, must one be to admit such opinions!

What I say applies not only to Coste and Willemet, the same reproaches are due to all our common observers. *Mutato nomine, de te fabula narratur.* In their view, almost all medicinal substances produce no other effect than to evacuate by perspiration, etc., etc., because they are always preoccupied with the idea of removing morbid matters, which very seldom exist, but which they fancy could not be cured otherwise.

"By connecting what Coste and Willemet have stated, with regard to the porter (an insignificant fact, because the unfortunate man did not die on the spot), with what we find written subsequently, it seems highly probable that in doses large enough to produce that upward evacuation which the partisans of saburres are so fond of, the root of Asarum places men in manifest danger of dying, and sometimes really kills them, as Wedel has seen. That is truly an admirable method, that can only expel these supposed saburres from the stomach by endangering the life of the patient. Are we permitted to act so barbarous a part towards our sick brethren? No, the Sovereign Preserver of life has bestowed this plant with a far nobler design. To put a stop to natural and morbid vomiting, accompanied by important symptoms analogous to those it produces, by means of the minutest dose of the tincture highly diluted; such is the true use to be made of this root, a use diametrically opposed to its mischievous abuse by those who recommend it in a large dose as an emetic.

"But its symptoms show also what other homœopathic resources are to be found in Asarum. It is enough to hint them to the physician capable of reflection, without naming expressly the diseases that may be cured by their aid.

"The homœopathic physician who acts exactly contrary to what the common school has hitherto done, knows how to take advantage of this powerful gift, and never abuses it to excite those shocks, those pernicious changes in the human frame. It is our duty also to spare the domestic animals those cruel potions called horse-medicines.

"The Creator has ordained that we should learn to heal severe diseases by minute, and therefore safe, doses of those valuable remedies that call out symptoms analogous to their own. He has not given medicines in abundance that we should use them lavishly to the injury of our species, as in ordinary allopathic treatment. These substances are intended by Nature for other purposes, with which we are not yet acquainted, and for which they have been created in such large quantities. Nature does nothing with one mere view, and each of its productions has more than one mode of usefulness. Although we employ them under the name of medicines, there is no reason because the earth yields them abundantly that we should administer them in large doses. For instance, arsenic certainly answers other important ends in the economy of Nature, since out of many hundred quintals supplied by the mines of Saxony alone, a most insignificant portion is required as medicine, if we would use it to a good purpose. One drop, or rather a very small part of a drop of the quadrillionth of a grain of the tincture, or the quintillionth dilution of the mixture of the fresh juice with equal parts of alcohol, appears to be the best dose for use in homœopathy."

According to Noack and Trinks (*Handbuch für Hom. Arzneimittell.*), Asarum is especially suitable to chilly individuals and to literary men; also in cases of great irritability of the nervous system, and after operations on the eye, when the patient suffers from darting pains. Helminthiasis, when ascarides are present. Intermittent fevers, accompanied with partial chilliness and partial heat of single parts, with external heat and internal chilliness, or with alternate heat and chills. Megrim. Periodical headache. Ophthalmia. Amblyopia. Amaurosis. Excessive vomiting. Colic and vomiting.

ANTIDOTES.—Vinegar. Camphor has the power also to calm any injurious effects of Asarum, either when given in large or in minute doses.

IX.

ATROPA BELLADONNA.

Common Dwale, Deadly Nightshade.

Synonyms.—Belladonna, *Raii Syn.* Solanum maniacum; Sol. furiosum, *Olim.* Sol. lethale, *Ger. Em.* 340; *Park.* 346; *Clus. Hist.*, pp. 86, 166. Sol. melanoceros, *Bauhin*, Πιν. Sol. somniferum, *Buch. Hist. Scot.; Lobel.* Bell. trichotoma, Atropa lethalis, *Salisb. Prodr.* Sol. sylvaticum, *Gesner. Scop. Carn.* Sol. Hortense, *Tragus.* Sol. magus, *Matthiolus.* Sol. lethale, *Gerarde.* Atropa Belladonna, *Lin.*, *Sp. Plant.*, 260, etc.

Foreign Names.—*Fr.:* Belladone. *Ital.:* Belladonna. *Span. and Port.:* Belladona. *Germ.:* Tollkirsche. *Dut.:* Besiedraagend doodkruit; Doodelyke naghtschade. *Swed.:* Wargbär. *Dan.:* Natskade. *Russ.:* Krasavitsa, Odurnik. *Arab.:* Inubas saleb. *Pers.:* Rorbah turbuc. *Hind.:* Sug-unggor.

Nat. Order, Solaneæ.—Pentandria, Monogynia.

Gen. Char.—*Calyx* five, partite. *Corolla* campanulate, twice the length of calyx; the lobes equal. *Stamens* distinct. *Berry* of two cells.

Spec. Char.—*Stem* herbaceous. *Leaves* ovate, undivided. *Flowers* axillary, on short peduncles, solitary.

History.—Like most of the medicinal substances known to the ancient physicians, the early history of Belladonna is involved in uncertainty. Dodonæus supposed that this plant is synonymous with the Mandragora described by Theophrastus. Dioscorides also (lib. vii. cap. 71), under the name Solanum Hortense, describes a plant which, both in its botanical as well as medicinal character, is very similar to the Atropa. "The seed is round, at first green, then turning black, and is pecu-

---

Fig. 1. The corolla and stamens. 2. Calyx and pistil. 3. Section of the pericarp.

Plate IX.

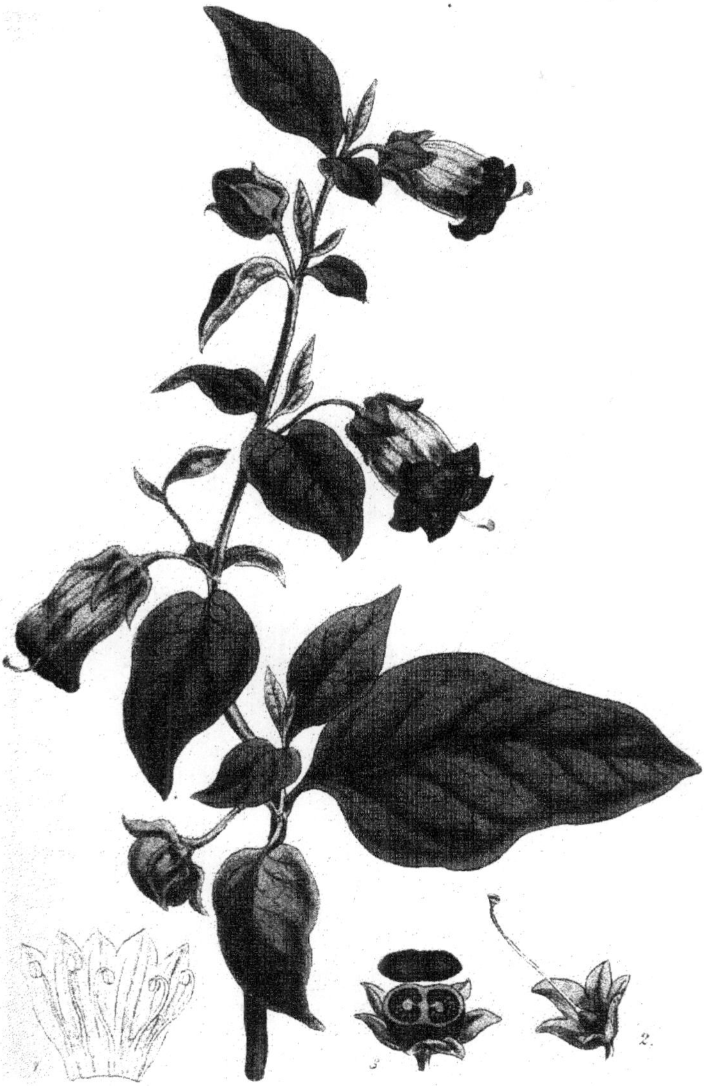

Atropa Belladonna

liarly efficacious in erysipelas, herpes, parotitis, and disperses swellings of the glands," etc. etc.

Pliny (*Nat. Hist.*, lib. xxi., *Holland's Trans.*) also describes a Solanum, "which hath leaves like to basil; for certes this hearbe is so dangerous, that a very little of the juice thereof is enough to trouble a man's brain, and put him besides his right wits."

The Greeks knew of three varieties of Nightshade. The Garden, which they deemed innocent; the Somniferous, which caused sleep; and the Furious, which caused madness and death; but none of them precisely agree with our Atropa.

Matthiolus, however, seems to have considered that Atropa Belladonna was unknown to the Greek physicians. Pereira mentions that the earliest undoubted notice of Belladonna occurs in the work of Tragus, A. D. 1532, who calls it Solanum Hortense nigrum. Joannes Bodæus says it is the same as the Solanum maniacum of Dioscorides. Among the Arabians, the juice of the recent leaves was applied in burns, in that disease common to them, called Buhe. Paulus Ægineta mentions, that an over-dose will produce madness and death. Klinger tried many experiments with it, and gave it at the time of Alberti in cancer.

Bergius, Evers, and Greding used the remedy, particularly in obstinate jaundice, from infarction of the liver; in epilepsy, chorea, and other convulsive disorders, as well as in palsy; in mania, and in hydrophobia. Buckhave instituted a variety of experiments in diseases of the class neuroses, particularly in tussis convulsiva. He employed the root only, and notes as follows: "That adults had dryness of the fauces and nose for three or four hours, impeded deglutition, indistinct articulation, and that acids held only in the mouth were sufficient to remove these unpleasant sensations; that all kinds of drinks were useless; the pulse full and quick, vertigo, congestion of the vessels of the head, flushings, dulness of the eyes, drunkenness, dilated pupils, etc., were the consequences. But that children had but few of these symptoms, and they were always more slight, showing the effect only by increased heat and swelling of the cheeks." Yet he says: "If the child be over-dosed, uncommon loquacity, staring of the eyes, similar to that of epileptics, deep sleep, with profuse perspiration, would take place; and the patient would then awake quite free from the above-mentioned symptoms."

The Danes were accustomed to employ the berries, mixed with wine or beer, in dysentery and gout.

Limberger, who was the cause of Belladonna being first used in this country, applied it in cancer. He tried it on himself, in proportion of a scruple of the leaves or root to ten cups of water, infused for a night, taking a cupful for a dose. It produced slight vertigo and unusual thirst, with increased arterial action.

Cullen, Graham, and Münch employed it in cancerous affections. Münch advises it in melancholia, epilepsy, and mania, and effected many cures. He says, however, "that even small doses have produced mania where none existed."

Münch, Ritcher, Mayerne, Bucholz, and Neimeche, have all witnessed the good effects of the Belladonna in rabies canina; in patients when they have become morose, vitiated in their minds, shuddered at food and drink, excessively convulsed, and yet they have been successful enough to have witnessed them recovered after a short time, to perfect health.

Cullen mentions a case of a person using the infusion of Belladonna, at a distance, and without communicating with him, in cancer of the lip, and that dryness and stricture of the œsophagus came on, and he suddenly died by a very copious throwing up of blood.

In hydrophobia, the old physicians used it with great success. It would be well if its application in such cases were renewed, or at least minutely investigated. A German journal states, that in a case of hydrophobia, when the female patient was unable to swallow, it was determined to inject Belladonna into the veins; the injection acted promptly, and the patient fell into a stupor, the convulsions, anxiety, and oppression entirely ceasing. She began to be able to swallow liquids, though with difficulty; some slight hopes of recovery were entertained, but the symptoms soon became severe, and terminated in death. (*Blackett on Effect of Atropa*, p. 32.)

Mr. Green, of Wenlock, in Shropshire, often found, in using Belladonna as an embrocation, that he was obliged to discontinue it, from its producing vertigo and great irritation of the nervous system.

Van Swieten relates a case where a lady applied a Belladonna leaf to an ulcer beneath the eye, suspected to be cancerous. In a few hours the pupil was dilated even when exposed to a strong light. The nightshade was removed and the vision returned. The experiment was repeated several times, and Ray was a witness to it.

Belladonna has been employed to allay pain and nervous irritation, as in neuralgia, prosopalgia, and tic-douloureux. As an antispasmodic, to relieve rigidity and spasmodic contraction of muscular fibres. As a topical remedy, in a case of angina pectoris, unconnected with organic disease, the application of Belladonna plaster to the chest (before the ulceration caused by tartar emetic had healed) produced alarming poisonous symptoms, which, when subsided, the symptoms of angina had quite disappeared. (*Davies' Lecture on Diseases of Lungs and Heart.*) In hooping-cough, with great relief. In maladies of the eyes, dilatation of pupil, iritis, and other inflammatory diseases of that organ, and to diminish the morbid sensibility of this organ to the influence of light. As a resolvent and discutient in enlargement of the lymphatic glands, scirrhus, and cancer.

Description.—The Atropa Belladonna is a perennial plant; flowering in June. The *root* is branched and spreading; a fleshy, pulpy, and juicy white when fresh internally, greyish when dry; of a mawkish, slightly bitter taste, and faint peculiar odour. The whole plant is fetid when bruised, of a dark and lurid aspect, indicative of its deadly narcotic quality. The *stem* is herbaceous, upright, round, somewhat hairy, and reddish, three feet high. The *leaves*, which it is particularly important to distinguish accurately, are sometimes alternate, more commonly in pairs, in which case, one leaf of each pair is for the most part less than the other. They are ovate and acuminated, between four and six inches long, or even larger, thin, and soft, entire on the edge, without any hair, except on the *nerves behind*, and supported on a short leaf-stalk; and when dry they have a brownish-green or greyish-green colour; scarcely any odour; of a faint, bitterish taste. The *flowers* are nearly an inch in length, solitary, axillary, bell-shaped; greenish towards the flower-stalk externally, dingy purple towards the rim and internally. The *fruit* is a dark black, shining berry, resting on a widely-extended calyx, roundish, but flattened appearance, and size of a black cherry; bilocular, and containing many kidney-shaped seeds, in a mucilaginous, mawkish, rather sweet, but not pleasantly-tasted pulp.

The leaves have been sometimes confounded with those of the Solanum Dulcamara and Solanum nigrum.

Those of the Dulcamara are considerably smaller, are supported on a leaf-stalk, often half as long nearly as themselves, and generally present a pair of small pinnæ at a short distance from their base.

Those of the Solanum nigrum are small, not acuminated, and their edges coarsely serrated.

The name is derived from Atropos, one of the Fates, and Belladonna, because it was employed by Leucota, a famous poisoner of Italy, to destroy the beautiful women.

The following are the different species:

1. *Atropa Belladonna*, as described above.

2. *Atropa Mandragora* or *Mandrake*. A native of the south of Europe. Stemless; scapes one-flowered; root perennial, large, and tapering; three or four feet long; externally brown, internally whitish; from the crown of the root arise a circle

of leaves, and from amongst these are three or four slender scapes, each supporting a single flower of an herbaceous, white colour; the fruit is a globular, soft berry, of a yellowish colour, about the size of a nutmeg. It was the subject of most ridiculous superstitions, from the supposed likeness of the root to the human form; it was certain death to dig it up.

3. *Atropa Physaloides*. Peruvian Deadly Nightshade. The flower bell-shaped slightly; five-lobed, and blue with a white edge, having blue spots. Berry the size of a cherry, with fine sharp angles.

4. *Atropa Solanaceæ*. A native of the Cape of Good Hope. Six feet high; peduncles axillary; one-flowered.

5. *Atropa arborescens*. Tree Atropa. A native of South America and Jamaica. A small tree or shrub; leaves alternate, and tufted towards the end of the branches; flowers white, fragrant, and nodding. This species is often tetrandrous.

6. *Atropa frutescens*. A native of Spain. Six or eight feet high; leaves alternate, roundish; flowers come out between the leaves on short peduncles, resembling those of the Belladonna, but much smaller, and of a dirty yellow colour.

7. *Atropa herbacea*. Two feet high; flowers white. Native of Campeachy.

8. *Atropa procumbens*. Wheel-flowered Atropa. A native of Mexico. Corolla herbaceous; yellow, wheel-shaped, which sufficiently distinguishes it from all its compeers.

GEOGRAPHICAL DISTRIBUTION.—Atropa Belladonna is a native of nearly the whole of Europe, more especially in the south. It is indigenous in Great Britain.

LOCALITIES.—In waste grounds, more particularly on a calcareous soil; not common. In this country it may be found in Whichwood Forest, near Witney; between Nettlebed and Henley, Oxon; Woodstock Park, near the Monument; Tilehurst Common and Englefield, Berks; near the ruins of Dudley Castle, Worcestershire; Cottenham, Triplow, Fulbourn, and Wisbeach, Cambridgeshire; roadside, near Peterborough;

Blathewick Park, at Kingscliff, Northamptonshire; Furness Abbey, among the ruins, which is called Vale of Nightshade; Cuxstone, near Rochester, Kent; Reigate, Surrey; about Box-hill, near Dorking, Surrey; on Inchcolm, and near the ruins of Borthwick Castle, Scotland.

Gerarde found it growing "without Highgate, near unto a pond or penfold on the left hand." Ray mentions it as growing in a ditch at the end of Goswell-street, on the road to Islington; and in the Annual Register of 1762, there is an account of the death of two persons by this plant, with the following caution by Dr. Hill: "This plant is now a quarter of a yard high, and has an aspect so inviting, that one almost wonders how Nature gave to it a poison. It has invited many to boil it, and death was always in the pot. Ray mentions it growing there; it has been thought lost in that place, but I fear those unhappy persons have found it."

The specimen from which the drawing is made was found near Reigate, in Surrey.

From its very poisonous character, it should never be cultivated, either for ornamental or medicinal purposes, where children or ignorant persons have access.

Parts used in Medicine, and Mode of Preparation.—The Leaves, Stem, and Flowers. The leaves readily yield their virtues to alcohol. In Quin's *Pharmacopœia Homœopathica*, it is ordered to be prepared as follows: the expressed juice of the recently-gathered leaves and stem is to be mixed with equal parts of spirits of wine, and after twenty-four hours the liquid is to be decanted clear and limpid. One drop of this is to be agitated twice with ninety-nine drops of spirits of wine, and the sign (I) inscribed; afterwards attenuate to the thirtieth dilution. It should likewise be known that the extract of Belladonna, if kept for a length of time, becomes chemically changed, decomposition takes place, a new combination is formed, and a greater portion becomes insoluble in water. The leaves may be preserved in hermetically-sealed glass jars for a considerable time without losing their virtue.

Poisonous Effects.—The symptoms produced by taking an over or poisonous dose are most interesting to all homœopathists. It is one of the most energetic of the indigenous poisons. Every part of the plant is injurious, but we are best acquainted with the effect of the berries, as from their tempting and luscious appearance they are often eaten by children and ignorant people. The usual effects are, dryness of the mouth, and heat attended with thirst. If the dose has been large, besides these, there are difficulty of deglutition and articulation, feeling of constriction about the throat; nausea; sometimes vomiting, and at times swelling and redness of the face; dilatation of the pupils; obscurity of vision, or absolute blindness; visual illusions; suffused eyes; singing in the ears; numbness of the face; confusion of the head; giddiness; delirium simulating intoxication, which may be combined with or followed by sopor; and, if the dose has been very large, complete coma, and death.

The berry of this plant is supposed to be that which poisoned Marc Antony's troops in the Parthian war, for being much distressed for food, they ate berries, etc.; and Plutarch gives the following description: "Those who sought for herbs and pot-herbs, and they found but few, and tasting unknown herbs, they found one which brought on madness and death. He that had eaten it immediately lost all memory and knowledge, but at the same time would busy himself in turning and moving every stone he met with, as if he were upon some very important pursuit. The camp was full of unhappy men bending to the ground, and thus digging up or removing stones, till at last they were carried off by bilious vomiting, when wine, the only remedy, was not to be found."

Its poisonous properties were also known to the Scots. The Danes, under Sweno, were defeated by Macbeth, and many destroyed by the Scots sending bread to their enemies, and a mixture of wine and ale poisoned by this plant, during a truce. (Vide *Rer. Scotic. Hist.*, lib. vi. cap. vi.)

Above 150 soldiers were poisoned by the berries of Belladonna, which they gathered at Pirna, near Dresden. And Orfila (*Toxicol. Génér.*, 3rd edit., tom. ii. p. 265) gives an account of the symptoms: dilatation and immobility of the pupil; insensibility, almost complete, of the eye to the presence of external objects, or at least confused vision; injection of the conjunctiva with bluish blood; protrusion of the eye, which in some appeared as if it were dull, and in others ardent and furious; dryness of the lips, tongue, palate, and throat; difficult deglutition, or total incapacity to swallow; nausea, attended with vomiting; sense of weakness; lipothymia, syncope; frequent bending forward of the trunk; continual motion of the hands and fingers; gay delirium, with vacant smile; aphonia.

Muller, of Vienna, gives an interesting description of five persons (one family) who had eaten of the berries of Belladonna. Two of the children (boys), having eaten plentifully, had the following symptoms. They attempted to get from their beds, and were with difficulty restrained; continual motion of their hands and fingers, and desire to lay hold of the coverlets or other objects within reach; thrusting the fingers up the nostrils; acute delirium; vision nearly gone, but both patients at the same time fancied they saw a number of objects; great dilatation and insensibility of the pupil; eyeballs alternately fixed and rolling; spasmodic action of the muscles of the face; grinding of the teeth; yawning, etc.; voice hoarse and weak; slight swelling of the left side of the throat, and burning sensation in the œsophagus; *decided aversion to all liquids in both; and spasmodic attacks whenever they were forced to swallow anything.*

The following cases are extracted from Orfila (l. c.) A child, of four years of age, of a feeble constitution, but otherwise well, ate at eleven o'clock a quantity of the berries of Belladonna.

The following symptoms soon set in: want of appetite; nausea; vomiting, and symptoms of drunkenness; slight delirium, and inextinguishable thirst; afterwards tumefaction, and redness of the face and lips; elevation of the eyelids; dilatation of the pupil; insensibility of the eye to light, etc.; convulsive contraction of the jaw and muscles of the face and extremities; delirium; very feeble pulse and irregular respiration. The next day there was increase of convulsive movements, with redness of the face, and great perspiration; the pupil remained dilated; there was great rigidity down the spine; tumefaction of the abdomen, which was very tender to the touch; constipation, and weak pulse. The next day these symptoms continued, but in a less degree, but he complained of great pain in his teeth. On the 31st all the symptoms had disappeared. It seems that, after an emetic, vinegar and honey had the best antidotal effects.

Some children ate in a garden some of the fruit of the Belladonna. They soon suffered from violent fever, accompanied by convulsions and strong palpitation of the heart; they lost consciousness, and were very delirious. One died the next day. One of the children ate four, the other six berries of Belladonna; an hour after, both of them were so extravagant in their manners, that they astonished their mother. Their pupils were dilated; their vision was altered; and a gay delirium, accompanied with fever, set in. The physician who was called in found them in a state of great agitation; talking here and there; running; leaping; laughing sardonically; with purple face and rapid pulse. After some tartar emetic, as an emetic, and some Glauber salts, the berries were got rid of, and the symptoms gradually disappeared.

Mappi (*Plant. Alsat.*, p. 36) says that the wine of Belladonna occasions a universal gangrene, followed by death.

It has also been observed, that the berries of the Belladonna have been taken without producing any sensible effect, viz.: two children, after dinner, ate each two berries of the Belladonna, without being incommoded. Also, an idiot of twenty years, swallowed upwards of thirty of the berries, and, with the exception of a few slight symptoms, he was not affected; but these observations only prove that a small quantity of the poison did not affect after a copious meal, and that an idiot, whose nervous system was but slightly impressionable, was not violently acted upon by this poison.

It appears that the berries of Belladonna possess a purely narcotic power, while the leaves and the root contain more acrid and exciting properties. From the effect of *the berries* on the organs of deglutition, and from the similarity of the symptoms to hydrophobia, it would perhaps be better that a homœopathic preparation be made solely from *the berries*, and tried in this disease.

Effect.—On animals generally. Belladonna proves poisonous to mammals and birds, but much less so to herbivorous than to carnivorous animals. Given to dogs, Belladonna causes dilatation of the pupils; plaintive cries; efforts to vomit; weakness of the posterior extremities; staggering; frequent pulse; a state like intoxication and death. (*Orfila, Toxicol. Génér.*, 3rd edit., p. 269.)

On vegetables.—An aqueous solution of extract of Belladonna is poisonous to plants. (*Marcet, Ann. Chim. et Physiol.*)

MEDICAL USES (HOMŒOPATHIC).—It has been truly observed by Hahnemann that Belladonna corresponds with a number of the morbid conditions often met with in the human frame, and that consequently there is frequent occasion to administer it homœopathically. " What remedy may not prove most prejudicial in the hands of ignorant people? Certainly every active medicine may become so if given injudiciously, and in too large doses; but then it is only prejudicial through the fault of him who calls himself a physician. On the other hand, the most powerful and violent medicines become as mild as they are beneficial by proper attenuation, even when taken by the most feeble and sensitive persons, while diminishing the doses as far as possible; they are given only in cases where the disease is composed of symptoms strictly analogous to those they excite in a healthy subject.

"Guided by numerous trials made upon sick persons, I am at length resolved to use only the decillionth dilution, of which I find the smallest part of a drop sufficient to include all the indications that can apply to this medicine.

"In this dose (when it is homœopathic), Belladonna cures the most violent maladies, its action being exerted with a rapidity that harmonizes with the nature of the disease."

Belladonna has become remarkable in homœopathic therapeutics as a PROPHYLACTIC IN SCARLET FEVER. The following are Hahnemann's remarks on this subject: "The property I have discovered in Belladonna, given in a small dose every six or seven days, of being a preservative against scarlatina, as Sydenham, Plenciz, and others, have described, was for nineteen years brought into contempt by physicians, who, ignorant that this disease belongs only to children, have confounded it with the *purple miliary* introduced from Belgium in 1801, and have applied to the latter my method, which, of course, failed. I rejoice, however, that of late years other physicians have distinguished the ancient and true scarlatina, establishing the preservative property of Belladonna in that disease, and have thus rendered justice to my labours so long misunderstood."

The following are the practical observations of Dr. Fleischmann, described in *Hufeland's Journal*, June and July, 1835, on the preservative effect of Belladonna against scarlatina:

Some experiments with this medicine were made on fifty-two children during an epidemy of scarlatina, and though not on a sufficiently extensive scale to have much weight, deserve to be added to the number of those instituted for a similar purpose.

The extract of Belladonna, two grains to an ounce of distilled water, was administered to fifty-two children, from six months to fourteen years of age; the remedy was administered according to the formula, for five weeks, the duration of the epidemic. Of the fifty-two, forty-eight remained free from the attack, and four were affected. In two families, where the children commenced taking the remedy immediately on the disease attacking one of the family, all the children remained free from contagion, although in constant communication with the affected person.

In several cases (twenty-three) the author remarked symptoms of the action of Belladonna, a few days after its use, such as disturbed nights, slight inflammation about the throat, salivation, thirst, torpor, dilated pupils, pain in the head, vomiting; and one girl, six years old, was seized on the tenth day after the first dose with fever, pain in the throat, restlessness, and delirium; on the following day the whole of the body, except the face, became red, and was covered with miliary vesicles. This continued two days, and then disappeared.

A boy, four years of age, who had taken Belladonna for three weeks, became very uneasy and disturbed on the 5th of March; on the 6th, this had passed off; on the 9th, the child, enjoying perfect health, was covered on all parts of the body, except the face, with a red eruption, which remained till the 11th; on the 12th, it diminished; and had completely disappeared on the 13th.

A child, eighteen months old, who had taken Belladonna six days, was seized with difficult deglutition, slight tumour of the cervical glands, salivation, fever, with excessive thirst, and general redness of the skin. The eruption was much diminished on the second day; and the child was well on the fifth.

From the above-mentioned experiments the author concludes—

1. That Belladonna seems to have an influence in counteracting the contagiousness of scarlatina.

2. That in some cases it diminishes the susceptibility for the contraction of the disease, though it does not altogether remove it.

3. That when the disease does occur during the use of Bel-

ladonna, its character is much more mild than in ordinary cases."

The following is from the *Edinburgh Philosophical Journal and Monthly Archives of Medical Science*: "In 1829, scarlatina raged both among our troops and the inhabitants of the towns and villages where we were quartered. The Grand Vizier, who had expended much time and money on the discipline of this his favourite *corps d'armée*, gladly accepted the proposal of Dr. Oppenheim to try the effects of Belladonna. As the troops were generally very young men and totally unaccustomed to narcotics, the dose he gave was comparatively small: thirty-six grains of the extract of Belladonna were mixed up with one pound of liquorice, and ten grains of this were given morning and evening to each soldier. The success of the experiment far exceeded his most sanguine expectations, for not more than twelve men out of 1,200 sickened after this plan was adopted; of these twelve, six died; and it is to be remarked that the disease continued *unabated* among the inhabitants where the soldiers were quartered, after it had ceased among the latter, although they lived in the same house."

In the *London Medical Gazette*, July 1829, the following letter from Messrs. Jander and Williams, of Bromley, Kent, concerning Belladonna as a preservative of scarlatina, addressed to the editor, is particularly interesting. "During the months of April and May, scarlet fever was very prevalent in this town and neighbourhood, and in many cases it proved fatal. Our attention was called by a friend to a notice in the *Lancet* of May, 'On the prophylactic powers of Belladonna against scarlet fever, by M. Hufeland.' We were at that time attending in a boarding-school, where the disease had attacked twelve of the boys, many of whom had been most dangerously ill, but none died. There still remained several boys, perhaps twenty, who had not taken the infection; also four young children of the master's, and several servants. We immediately commenced the use of the Belladonna, in the exact manner and doses advised by Hufeland. *Only* six or seven persons in the house took the disease *afterwards*, and in every instance it assumed the mildest form. In another small school we were called to visit a child about two years old, who had been attacked the evening before; the disease was of the most malignant character, and the child died on the following morning, the third day of the attack. The house is a very small one. There were in it three other children and five boarders, and a servant girl. The Belladonna was faithfully administered, and not *one* individual took the disease.

"We will not offer any conjecture on the *modus operandi* of the Belladonna, or whether it did or did not prevent the other members of these families from taking the disease. The facts are stated exactly as they occurred, and we entreat our medical brethren to make trial of Belladonna whenever a favourable opportunity offers. The following was the manner of giving the medicine: three grains of the extract of Belladonna, dissolved in three ounces of proof spirit; of this solution as many drops are to be taken as the patient is years old."

The *Medical Gazette* then goes on: "As our readers may not be fully aware of the circumstances alluded to in the above paper, we subjoin some observations on this subject made by Professor Koreff, in a letter to the late M. Laennec, published in the *Bulletin des Sciences Médicales*. 'Observation clearly proves,' says he, 'that the Belladonna taken for some time, either in powder or in extract, produces, especially in infants, a redness of the skin, which is sometimes transient, but at others more durable; dryness of the mouth, with a sense of heat in the throat; dilatation of the pupil; anxiety; occasional swelling of the submaxillary glands; symptoms having a great resemblance to those which accompany the eruption of scarlatina.

"'The effect of the Belladonna has also this, in common with scarlatina, that neither of them produce the redness of the skin invariably, whilst the symptoms about the throat are always present. I confess to you, however, that all these analogies did not appear to me sufficiently strong to persuade me, that in this plant was really to be found a preservative of scarlatina, similar to that which the cowpock affords against variola. It was not till I had received the authority of the celebrated Soemmering, who informed me that he had obtained the most satisfactory results with it, when the disease raged epidemically, that I determined to employ it. This malady, accompanied by the most unfavourable symptoms, and having entirely changed its usual character, was at that time producing ravages almost as fatal as contagious typhus. I then, for the first time, had the happiness to protect from this dreadful contagion almost all those who took the Belladonna with a little perseverance (and of these there *were many thousands*); since that time I have never lost sight of the discovery, which becomes the more valuable, as the scarlatina has increased during the last thirty years, both in violence and extent, in many countries, and I have always found the same effects in different climates and in epidemics of opposite characters. Many other physicians have equally confirmed the preventive powers of this plant; and the German journals are daily filled with proofs of a benefit which, with respect to some countries, equals that of vaccination. In France, the capital and provinces of which appear less subject to these fatal epidemics than Germany, Switzerland, the Tyrol, Poland, and the north in general, less attention has been given to this discovery, and it has been rejected, it must be said too lightly, and without sufficient examination, as may be seen in the article Belladonna, in the *Dict. des Sciences Médicales*. I only remember a single observation on this important subject by Dr. Meglin, who gives an account of a trial which he gave to this preservative during an epidemic of scarlatina at Colmar, and which confirms all the assertions of the German physicians. The absence of present danger is perhaps the cause of this indifference towards a discovery which, important in itself, might also be fruitful in results applicable to other diseases. At present, however, I shall confine myself to an account of the results which have been ascertained (by repeated observations, and by a great number of individuals placed in very different circumstances), without incurring the reproach of having proceeded in a manner not sufficiently vigorous. * * * *

"'The powder mixed with sugar, or the extract made very carefully from the juice of the recent plant, are employed after the following manner: Extract of Belladonna, three grains dissolved in an ounce of cinnamon-water; powder or root of Belladonna mixed with drachms *(sic)* of white sugar, divided into sixty doses. From half a dose to a whole one is given to a child from six months to two years old, four times a day; to children from three to six years old, from a dose to one and a half; to those from six to nine, two to two and a half; to those from ten to twelve, three to four and a half; of the solution, a drop is given for every year of the child's age, once a day, fasting. Observation has shown that when the epidemic is very fatal, or the intercourse with the patients very frequent and intimate, it is prudent to increase the dose a little. It has not yet been possible to determine the length of time which is necessary to eradicate by this remedy the susceptibility of contagion. Everything leads us to believe that the remedy, if used during a time too short to ward off contagion, moderates very much the malignity of the disease. We know for certain that the remedy does not permanently overcome the disposition to scarlatina, and it is necessary to resume its use on every occurrence of the epidemic. We have always observed that the most intimate communication with the sick does not produce the disease, provided the medicine has been employed eight or nine times previous to being exposed to the contagion, and continued up to the period of desquamation, a circumstance very important to nurses.

"'It appears more certain to begin with rather strong doses, in order to guard against the first impression of the contagion, and to diminish the quantity after a few days. No sensible effect has been observed to follow the continued use of this small quantity of Belladonna. Up to the present time, neither season nor locality, nor any other circumstance has appeared to diminish the preservative effect of this plant. * * * * Do not believe, my learned colleague, that these results have been too lightly deduced, or from a small number of individuals, or from epidemics of little violence. *It is from entire provinces*, from cities affected with this terrible scourge—from epidemics the most fatal in all seasons, and in localities the most diversified—on individuals of every age and of every condition, that observations have been made with the greatest accuracy, and have led to the above results.'" (*London Medical Gazette*, vol. iv. p. 293.)

The following are the remarks from the *Lancet*, which drew attention in the letter quoted above:—

"*On the Prophylactic Powers of Belladonna against Scarlet Fever.* By C. W. Hufeland.—The author has been led, both by his own experience and that of a great many other practitioners, to form such a favourable opinion with respect to the powers of this medicine, that he is convinced that in epidemics of scarlet fever it ought universally to be resorted to, as the best means of preventing the disease altogether, or mitigating its violence. The following are his general conclusions:—

"1. The proper use of Belladonna has, in most cases, prevented infection, even in those instances where, by the continual intercourse with patients labouring under scarlet fever, the predisposition towards it was greatly increased.

"2. Numerous observations have shown that, by the general use of Belladonna, epidemics of scarlet fever have actually been arrested.

"3. In those few instances where the use of Belladonna was insufficient to prevent infection, the disease has been invariably slight.

"4. There are exceptions to the above three points, but their number is extremely small.

"It seems that in some epidemics Belladonna has no protective powers at all; the individual disposition, the method of using the remedy, and the quality of it will of course have considerable influence on the result of the experiment. Three grains of extract, which must have been *recently* prepared, are dissolved in three ounces of dilute alcohol, of this solution the individual takes twice a day as many drops as he is years old; its use must be continued as long as contagion is possible. The dose, it appears, is so very small, that even if it should fail in its effects, it will at all events not be injurious.

"In consequence of Hufeland's communication on the above subject, the Prussian Government has issued an official decree, ordering the general use of Belladonna as a prophylactic, in all instances when scarlet fever prevails as an epidemic." (*Liter. Ann. der Ges. Heilk.*, extracted from *Lancet,* vol. ii. p. 135, 1838—9).

The following account of Hahnemann's discovery of the prophylactic effect of Belladonna in scarlet fever will be read with interest.*

"I shall now relate the mode in which I made the discovery of this specific preservative remedy.

"The mother of a large family, at the commencement of July, 1799, when the scarlet fever was most prevalent and fatal, had got a new counterpane made up by a sempstress, who (without the knowledge of the former) had in her small chamber a boy just recovering from scarlet fever. The first-mentioned woman, on receiving it, examined and smelt it, to ascertain whether it might require airing, but as she could detect no smell, she placed it beside her on a sofa, on which some hours later she laid down to sleep. In this way *alone* she imbibed this miasm. A week subsequently she was suddenly attacked with quinsy, and its characteristic shooting pains in the throat, which was subdued after four days. Several days afterwards, her daughter, ten years of age, was attacked in the evening by severe pressive pain in the abdomen, itching of the head and body,

* From Hahnemann's Lesser Writings. Translated by Dr. Dudgeon. Headland, 1851.

rigor over the head and arms, and paralytic stiffness of the joints. Her sleep was restless during the night, with frightful dreams and general perspiration, excepting the head. I found her in the morning with pressive headache, dimness of vision, slimy tongue, some ptyalism, the submaxillary glands hard, swollen, and painful to the touch, and shooting pains in the throat when attempting to swallow. She was free from thirst; pulse quick and small; breathing hurried and anxious; very pale, though feeling hot; horripilation; leaning forward to lessen the pain; she complained of stiffness, with an air of much dejection, and shunned conversation, feeling that she could only speak in a whisper. Her look was dull, yet staring; her eyelids widely stretched, face pale, and features sunk.

"Knowing too well the ineffectual nature of the ordinary favourite remedies, I resolved in this case of incipient scarlet fever not to act with reference to individual symptoms, but (agreeably to my new synthetical principle) to obtain, if possible, a remedy calculated to produce in a healthy person most of the morbid symptoms I now observed; and my memory and written remarks suggested no remedy so appropriate as Belladonna, which I had observed to produce precisely the above-mentioned symptoms.

"I therefore gave the girl, who was already affected by the first indications of scarlet fever, a dose of Belladonna (1) 432,000th part of a grain of the extract, which, according to my subsequent experience, is too large a dose. She remained quietly seated all day, without lying down; the heat of her body diminished; she drank but little; none of her symptoms increased, and no new ones appeared. She slept quietly, and the following morning, twenty hours after taking the medicine, most of the symptoms had disappeared without any crisis; the sore throat only continued, but in a less degree, till the evening, when it went off. The following day she was lively, and ate and played as usual. I gave her a second dose, and she remained perfectly well; while two other children of the family fell ill of the scarlet fever, without my knowledge, whom I could only treat according to my general plan detailed above. I gave my convalescent a smaller dose of Belladonna every three or four days, and she remained in perfect health.

"I now earnestly desired to preserve the other five children from infection, their removal being impossible; and I thus reasoned: a remedy capable of quickly checking a disease in its first onset, must be its best preventive, and the following occurrence strengthened my opinion. Some weeks previously, three children of another family were ill of severe scarlet fever; the eldest daughter alone, who had been taking Belladonna internally for an external affection of the joints of her fingers, to my great astonishment escaped the infection, although in other cases of epidemics she had readily taken them.

"This decided me to administer to the other five children very small doses of this excellent remedy, as a preservative, and as its action lasts only three days, I repeated the dose every seventy-two hours, and they all remained in perfect health, though surrounded with infection.

"In the meantime I was called in to attend another family, where the eldest son was ill of scarlet fever. I found him in the height of the fever, with the eruption on the chest and arms. He was seriously ill, and it was too late to give the specific prophylactic remedy. But wishing to preserve the other three children, of four and two years of age, and nine months, I directed the parents to give the requisite dose of Belladonna, every three days, and had the happiness of seeing them entirely escape the disease, in spite of constant intercourse with their sick brother.

"Also, a number of other occasions presented themselves, in which this specific preventive remedy never failed.

"To prepare this remedy for preventing the infection of scarlet fever, we take a handful of the fresh leaves of the wild Atropa Belladonna, at the season when the flowers are not yet blown; these we bruise in a mortar to a pulp, and press the juice through linen, and immediately spread it, about as thick as the back of a knife, on flat porcelain plates, and expose it to a draught of dry air, and the moisture will evaporate in a few hours. We stir it and spread it out again with the spatula, so that it may harden uniformly, until dry enough to be pulverized. The powder is to be kept in a warmed and well-stopped bottle.

"To prepare from this the prophylactic remedy, we dissolve a grain of this powder in 100 drops of common distilled water, by rubbing it up in a small mortar; we pour the thick solution into a one-ounce bottle, and rinse the mortar and the pestle with 300 drops of diluted alcohol (five parts of water to one of alcohol), and add this to the solution, and render the union perfect by diligently shaking the liquid. We label the bottle *Strong Solution of Belladonna.* One drop of this is intimately mixed with 200 drops of the diluted alcohol, by shaking it for a minute, and marked *Weak Solution of Belladonna;* and this is our prophylactic remedy for scarlet fever, each drop containing the 24,000,000th part of a grain of the dry Belladonna juice.

"Of this weak solution we give, to prevent liability to infection, to an infant, one drop; to a child of a year old, two drops; two years old, three; three years old, four; to a child of four years old, according to the strength of his constitution, from five to six; at five years, six to seven; at six years, from seven to eight; at seven years, from nine to ten; eight years, from eleven to thirteen; nine years, from fourteen to sixteen; and with each successive year up to the twentieth, two additional drops; from twenty to thirty, not above forty drops, a dose every seventy-two hours, well stirred in any kind of drink, as long as the epidemic lasts, and for four or five weeks afterwards.

"Should the epidemic be very violent, it would be safer, if the children could bear it, to give the second dose twenty-four hours after the first; the third, thirty-six hours after the second; the fourth, forty-eight hours after the third; and thenceforth every seventy-two hours.

"This course does not disturb the health of the children. They should follow their usual manner of life in all respects, both in food, air, and exercise, but avoiding all excess.

"The only thing I prohibit is, the use of too much vegetable acid, as sour fruits, vinegar, etc., which tend to increase enormously the action of Belladonna, as my experience has taught me."

Dr. Sigmond, a strong opponent to homœopathy, in his lecture on Belladonna, when quoting the supposed effects of this medicine as a prophylactic in scarlet fever, thus speaks of Hahnemann: "I have to speak to you of a man of high intellectual attainments, of great sagacity, of inflexible courage, of unwearied industry, who, amid difficulties of no common kind, has laid the foundation of a system which, whilst it cannot but create a few smiles at its singularity, is the work of great erudition, much toil, and striking ingenuity; we must not confound Hahnemann with those despicable charlatans who would sacrifice at the altar of avarice the lives and the happiness of thousands, who prey upon their deluded victims by the most daring and insolent effrontery, who have neither the education nor the feelings of men of principle, and whose success in their vile occupations is a reflection upon the state of society. The great acquirements of Hahnemann, the boldness with which he has promulgated his doctrine, the skill and fierceness with which he has carried on his arduous controversies, mark him as a man of no ordinary stamp. It is a disgrace to the character of our humane and liberal science, that her votaries should so often, in their zeal for their cause, forget that which is due even to the mistaken labourer in the arduous paths we have to pursue" (*Lancet*, 1836—7, vol. iii.)

Pereira (*Elem. of Materia Medica*, vol. ii. p. 859) endeavours to prove that the prophylactic powers of Belladonna are useless, and that the evidence brought forward in its favour is only negative, whilst that which is adduced against it is positive; for he conceives that twenty cases of failing to prevent the disease are more conclusive than one thousand cases of its non-occurrence. He quotes the following in its favour. Bayle (*Bibl. Thérap.*, tom. ii. p. 504) has collected from various sources 2,027 cases of persons who took this medicine, of these 1,948 escaped. Oppenheim (*Lond. Med. Gazette*, vol. xiii. p. 814) gave it to 1,200 soldiers, and only twelve became affected. Also Hufeland and Koreff, who admit, from their own personal observations, the efficacy of the remedy. Against it, he mentions Lehman, Bach, Wendel, Muhrbeck, and Hoffman, who say that it has failed in their hands, but he does not mention the particulars; and he quotes the remarkable failure mentioned by Dr. Sigmond (*Lancet*, 1836—7, vol. ii. p. 78), of a family of eleven persons who took the supposed specific, yet every individual contracted the disease.*

Clinical Observations.—According to Noack and Trinks (l. c.), Belladonna produces phenomena similar to those of Aconite, not directly, however, by exciting the central points of the nervous system into a more expansive activity, which, by a process of reaction, produces phenomena of inflammation in the peripheral tissues. Belladonna is especially suitable to plethoric, scrofulous, irritable individuals; persons disposed to affections of the head and brain, congestions, and spasms, in whom the nervous system is highly susceptible of impressions, and the circulatory system is easily excited; to the sanguine choleric temperament; to the organism of the child and the female, and such constitutions as are analogous to those organisms.

* On referring to the cases mentioned by Dr. Sigmond, he says: "In one family in which I had occasion to know that it was administered under the auspices of an eminent physician"—*i. e.*, he knew a physician who said he had given it. Not very good evidence upon which to reject any assertion, however absurd. Besides, independent of the knowledge that the medicinal action of Belladonna very materially alters by keeping, we may just as well reason that it is useless to vaccinate, because it is not a complete preventive of the smallpox.

Belladonna is, therefore, suitable especially for diseases of women and children, and all those diseases in which the whole nervous system is in a state of erethism. What Aconite is to inflammatory fevers, or the feverish reaction excited in the arterial system, Belladonna is to the inflammation itself, or the inflammatory action of the capillaries. If, after inflammatory action has been subdued by Aconite, the other symptoms of the nervous stage of inflammation continue, and sensation and irritability be alternately affected, Belladonna is then of the greatest use, if otherwise indicated.

The chief affections in which Belladonna is indicated are the following. Phlegmonous and erysipelatous inflammations, *the more delicate the inflamed organ or tissue the more suitable is Belladonna.* Catarrhal affections. Affections consequent upon fear, fright, and chagrin. Nervous affections. Spasms of every kind. Epilepsy. St. Vitus's dance. Ergotism. Tarantism. *Hydrophobia.* Congestions of the head, especially the eyes, chest, abdomen, uterus, and hemorrhoidal vessels. Sanguineous apoplexy. Erratic rheumatic pains. (Belladonna is said to be powerless against fixed pains.) Scrofulosis. Scrofulosis mucosa et ossea, when the periosteum and bones are inflamed. Scrofulous ulcers. Scirrhus and carcinoma. Measles, when combined with great intolerance of light. Miliaria alba et rubra, et herpetica. Pseudo-erysipelas. Erysipelas læve, fugas, et bulbosum. Erysipelas of the head, with delirium. Erysipelas of the face. Erysipelas neonatorum. Erysipelatous inflammations of the face, consequent upon the stings of insects. Impetigo erysipelatodes. Scarlatina lævigata et miliaris, especially with subsequent hydrocephalus, or with swelling of the parotid glands. Variola, when accompanied with severe headache. Varicella coniformis. *Metastases of acute exanthemata to the membranes of the brain.* Rubeola. Pemphigus. Acne. Eczema mercuriale. Porrigo larvalis in children of a plethoric habit. Sleeplessness, with congestion of the head. Lethargy, when combined with redness of the face. Fevers, where the symptoms indicate a more or less distinctly marked inflammatory action of the brain in nervous and typhoid fevers. Typhus versatilis et cerebralis. Febris lactea. Intermittent fevers. Derangements of the mind. Weakness of the memory. Hallucinations of the senses. Exaltation of the mind. Depression of spirits. Melancholia. Mania furens. Vertigo consequent on an irritable state of the cerebrum. Headache from congestion of the blood to the head. Violent neuralgia of the head (with Hyos. and Ign.) Paraphrenitis metastica. Inflammation of the brain and its membranes (after Aconite). *Hydrocephalus acutus*, in first stage. Meningitis. Arachnitis. Encephalitis vera. Delirium tremens. Inflammation of the eye. Scrofulous inflammation of the eye, with photophobia (followed by Sulphur). Fungus medullaris oculi. Contraction and distortion of the pupil. *Iritis*. Retinitis. Hemeralopia gravidum. Paropsis invertens. Strabismus. Amblyopia amaurotica. Amaurosis. Phlegmonous inflammation of the nose. Ozæna. Parotitis. Prosopalgia nervosa. Difficult dentition of children. Toothache in pregnant women. Inflammatory or congestive toothache. Ptyalism. Angina tonsillaris, uvularis, et pharyngea. Angina faucium phlegmonodes. Singultus spasticus. Pyrosis potatorum. Vomiting, when accompanied by congestion of the head; also during and after acute exanthemata. Chronic cardialgia. Acute and chronic gastritis. Peritonitis, especially puerperal. Enteritis. Chronic hepatitis. Colica spasmodica, flatulenta, et calculosa. Colica nephritica. Nephritis. Inflammation of the urinary organs. Enuresis. Dysuria. Metritis. Oophoritis. Intumescentia uteri benigna. Prolopsus uteri. Scirrhus and carcinoma uteri. Dysmenorrhœa. Too profuse menses. Abortus. Bad consequences of weaning. Mastodynia nervosa. Erysipelas of the mammæ. Mastitis. Galactorrhœa. Scirrhus and carcinoma of the mammæ. Aphonia. Aphonia catarrhalis. Catarrhal inflammation of the air-passages. Grippe. Whooping cough. Dry cough. Nightly attacks of dry cough. Rheumatism of the chest. Asthma thymicum. Asthma spasticum, hystericum, congesticum. Asthma Millari. Pneumonia, especially when nervous, or when occurring at the period of epidemics. Scarlet fever. Rheumatic stiffness of the neck. Inflammation of the spinal marrow. Phlegmasia alba dolens.

The effects of poisonous or large doses of Belladonna on the healthy subject have, in conjunction with other experiments, plainly pointed out its uses to the homœopathic physician, and it is remarkable to perceive how often the same disease has been treated by both schools with this medicine. By the homœopathist, from the symptoms it will produce on the healthy subject; by the allopathist, from the effect of this medicine on disease. In such cases as scirrhus and cancer, one must bear in mind that the homœopathist uses Belladonna, not because it produces such symptoms on the healthy body, but because, when Belladonna has been given for another disease, and in which patient this affection has existed, the scirrhus has been seen to yield under its influence.

Antidotes.—Large doses of Belladonna are counteracted by black coffee; but as the berries are often the cause of the poisoning, the stomach-pump must be put in requisition, and also some emetic.

Almost all authors have recommended vinegar as an antidote against Belladonna. (One man at Dresden was relieved on drinking acids.) Abundant experience, however, shows that vinegar increases the pain produced by Belladonna. Stapf has also observed that applications of vinegar to the forehead increased the headache caused by Belladonna, so as to make it insupportable. Fits of paralysis and colic produced by Belladonna may be assuaged by Opium, although it acts only as a palliative. Stupor, insanity, and frenzy produced by Belladonna are homœopathically relieved in the speediest and most certain manner by a few doses of Hyoscyamus. The intoxication of Belladonna is relieved by wine. Adequate help is most necessary when a large quantity of the berries have been swallowed; in this case relief may be obtained by large potions of strong coffee, which restores the irritability of the muscular fibre, puts a stop to the tetanic convulsions, although acting as a mere palliative, and secures the vomiting of the berries; this may, moreover, be facilitated by tickling the pharynx with a long feather. Camphor is an antidote against some of the symptoms of Belladonna; and Hepar Sulphuris, if Belladonna causes erysipelatous swellings.

X.

BERBERIS VULGARIS.

Common Barberry, Pipperidge Bush.

Synonyms.—Berberis dumetorum, *Raii Syn*, 465. Spina acida, or Oxyacantha, *Ger. Em.* 1325.

Foreign Names.—*Fr.:* L'Epine vinette. *Germ.:* Sauerdorn. *Ital.:* Crespino. *Span.:* Berberis. *Dut.:* Berberis. *Russ.:* Barbariss.

Gen. Char.—*Calyx* inferior, of six spreading, concave, coloured, deciduous sepals; the three outer ones the smallest. *Corolla* of six roundish, egg-shaped, concave, spreading petals, opposite to the sepals, each with two oblong, more deeply coloured, probably nectariferous glands at the base (fig. 2). *Filaments* six, strap-shaped, flattened, blunt, opposite to the petals, but shorter, attached to the base of each. *Anthers* of two separate lobes, on the opposite edges of the summit of the filament, each opening by a valve from the bottom upwards. *Germen* superior, cylindrical, as long as the stamens. *Style* none. *Stigma* single, round, and flat, broader than the germen, acutely bordered, permanent. *Berry* oblong, blunt, of one cell, pulpy, opening at the top. *Seeds* two or three, oblong, cylindrical, upright; attached by short stalks to the lower part of the cell.

The calyx of six sepals, the inferior corolla of six petals, and the two or three-seeded berry, will distinguish this from other genera in the same class and order.

Spec. Char.—*Thorns* three-cleft. *Clusters* pendulous. *Leaves* inversely egg-shaped, oblong, with bristly serratures. *Petals* entire.

History.—This is one of the medicinal plants of the ancient physicians, and, according to Gerarde, is described by Galen as Oxycantha, or Acuta spina, and differing from the Oxy-

---

Fig. 1. A petal. 2. Ditto, showing the nectariferous glands. 3. Stamens, germen, and stigma. 4. Stigma and germen. 5. A single stamen.

Plate X.

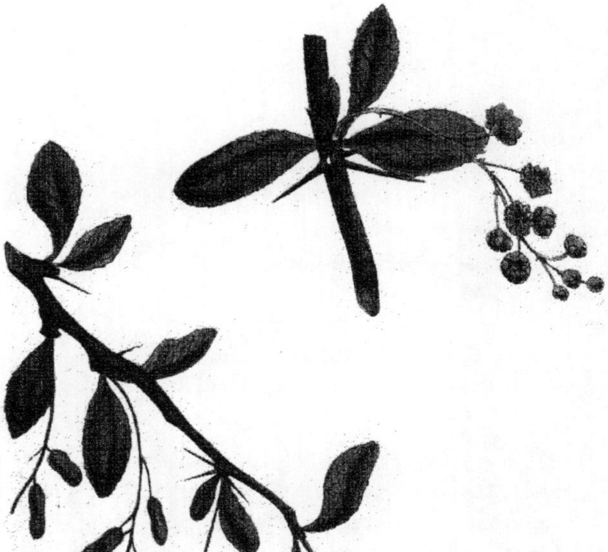

J. W. del. H. Sowerby, lith.

Reeve & Nichols imp.

Berberis vulgaris.

canthus of Dioscorides, or the Hawthorn. "The fruit," he says, "being most like that of the myrtle;" but J. Bodæus remarks, that the fruit of the Barberry is not at all similar to the myrtle, and he therefore concludes that the plants described by Dioscorides and Galen are identical.

Galen (*De Nutrimentis*) reckons the tender sprigs of the Barberries among the tender shoots that are to be eaten, such as Oxycanthus, or the Hawthorn, bringeth not forth. He evidently, therefore, considers them two distinct plants. It was called Καλμωριος by the Greeks, according to Rhases. The Arabian physicians, Avicenna and Serapion, make no distinction between this and the Hawthorn, and call both Amyrberis. Dr. Royle supposes the Lycium Indicum of Dioscorides to be the Barberry; but the commentator of Paulus Ægineta (vol. iii. p. 435) thinks it more probable that the Barberry was but the succedaneum of the Lycium. According to Leroux, it was much used by the old Egyptians.

Gerarde, in giving a description of the uses of this plant, says, that the leaves and berries of this thorn are cold and dry in the second degree; and as Galen also affirmeth, they are of thin parts, and have "a certaine cuttinge qualitie."

Under the head of the "Vertues," he divides them into the following:—

"A. The leaves are used of divers to season meat with, and instead of a sallad, as be those of sorrell.

"B. The decoction thereof is good against hot burnings and cholericke agues; it allayeth the heat of the blood, and tempereth the overmuch heat of the liver.

"C. The fruit or berries are good for the same things, and be also profitable for hot laskes and for the 'bloudy flixe,' and they stay all manner of superfluous bleedings.

"D. The greene leaves of the Barberry bush, stamped and made into sauce, as that made of sorrell, called greene sauce, doth cool hot stomachs, and those that are vexed with hot burnings, agues, and procureth appetite.

"E. The conserve made of the fruit and sugar performeth all those things before remembered, but with better force and success.

"F. The roots of the tree, steeped for certain days together in strong lie, made with ashes of the ash-tree, and the hair often moistened therewith, makes it yellow.

"G. The bark of the root is also used in medicine for the jaundice, and that with good success" (*Gerarde*, p. 1326).

In Quincey's *Pharmacopœia Officinalis*, 1742, p. 147, he says, the fruit of the Barberry is useful in diarrhœas and dysentery, and the bark for jaundice and other distempers, from foulness and obstruction of the viscera. It is likewise, for the same purposes, an ingredient in many of the medicated ales which are publicly sold.

The inner bark of the stem, infused in beer, has the reputation of curing the jaundice.

With the assistance of alum, it dyes linen a beautiful yellow. The roots boiled in lye, dye wool yellow. In Poland it is used, from its astringent qualities, to tan leather, and at the same time dyes it a most beautiful yellow.

The acid present in the Barberry is the oxalic, and it renders the berries so sour that birds, swine, and horses will refuse it, but kine, sheep, and goats will eat of it.

The Barberry has been said to mildew corn growing in its neighbourhood; this, however, has been proved to be fallacious. There is a parasite often on the leaves of this shrub, the Lysiphe berberides, frequently covering the whole surface of the leaves with a thin, white substance, which *perhaps* may have a pernicious influence on corn growing in the neighbourhood, but it is not at all certain.

Berberis, is a corruption of Amerberys, the Arabic name of the fruit.

It was used as a lithontriptic, styptic, and alexipharmic, according to Badigorius, Oribasius, Mesne, and others. Serapion (*De Simpl.* 229) recommends it as cooling and incisive, and of benefit in all fluxes; and later, according to Paulli, Bauhin, etc., in inflammations of the throat and other affections of the mucous membranes. According to Ray (*Hist. Plant.*, vol. ii. p. 1605), in diseases of the liver, jaundice, etc. According to Koch (*Buchner's Rep.*, vol. viii. fas. 1), in choleraic diarrhœa, when the secretion of the bile continues to be irregular and wanting, the Berberis has been given with great success. There are so many different opinions relating to the effects of the Berberis, as to make its classification difficult. If medical men had better distinguished between its positive and its medical effects, there would have been fewer contradictions. Its effects are noted as tonic and refrigerant, quenching the thirst, weakening, attenuating; dispelling fever and inflammation; desiccant and dissolving; purgative and antiseptic; astringent and styptic; anodyne, sudorific, and diuretical; expelling worms and causing abortion.

It was a popular remedy for feverish diseases and inflammations; but it gradually passed from the hands of the people into those of the physicians, who, for a time, extensively used it in these affections, but always, it is to be remarked, with that disunion and dissension which runs through the Materia Medica, and which arises either from faulty and incomplete observation, erroneous explanation of the facts, ignorance, or thoughtless echoing the opinions of others. While the Berberis was formerly employed for asthenic fevers, and recommended as a restorative remedy, it has also a so-called antiphlogistic effect. It is rejected by modern physicians in the first point, and recommended only in the others. Schœne (*Pract. Arzneim.*, vol. i. p. 83) considers it useful only in sthenic fevers, and forbids it in the asthenic form. Korn (*Arzneimittel.*, 2nd edit., p. 190) advises it only in hypersthenic fevers, etc. Herberger and Koch recommended the Berberis in inflammation of the bowels, diseases of the liver, cholera, and dysentery, in total opposition to Hesse, who considers that this medicine creates congestion of blood in the head, chest, and abdomen, bleeding from the nose and gums, and turgescence of the hemorrhoidal vessels.

Description.—A bushy shrub, from three to six feet high; in a cultivated state, often much higher; flowers May and June. *Branches* alternate, flexible, angular, with a yellowish-brown bark. Leaves in tufts, from lateral buds, deciduous, stalked, somewhat inversely egg-shaped, more or less pointed, between serrated and fringed. *Thorns* at the base of each leaf-bud, three-cleft, spreading, sharp, channelled underneath. *Clusters* solitary, from the centre of each bud, stalked, simple, many-flowered, drooping longer than the leaves. *Flowers* of a bright yellow colour, with red glands. *Berries* red, oblong, a little curved, very acid. The irritability of the stamens of this plant is very remarkable; if the inside of the filaments be touched near the base by any extraneous body, they immediately spring up and strike the anthers against the stigma. This may be repeated several times, as after each irritation the stamens return to their original position. Dr. Smith observes, that the spring of the stamens is owing to a high degree of irritability in the side of the filament next the germ (the outside of the filament and the anther having none), by which, when touched, it contracts, that side becoming shorter than the other, and consequently, the filament being bent towards the germ. The purpose which this curious contrivance in nature is designed to answer is evident; when the stamina stand in their original position, their anthers are effectually sheltered from rain by the concavity of the petals, thus they probably remain till some insect, in order to abstract honey from the base of the flower, thrusts itself between the filaments, and almost unavoidably touches them in their most irritable parts, and in this way the impregnation of the germens is performed; and as it is chiefly in sunny weather that insects are on the wing, so it is only in fine weather that the pollen is fit for the purpose of germination.

Geographical Distribution.—The Berberis vulgaris is indigenous in Great Britain and other parts of Europe. The genera, in Europe, Asia, and America. Rare in South America.

LOCALITIES IN BRITAIN.—In woods and hedges, and on bushy calcareous hills; in hedges by the roadside between Middleton Stones and Ardley; in Berks, Bedfordshire, Cambridgeshire, Devon, Essex, Norfolk, Suffolk, Somersetshire, Warwickshire, etc.

PARTS USED IN MEDICINE, AND MODE OF PREPARATION.—The small branches of the roots, or the bark of the branches of the roots of moderate size (the large roots being too fibrous). The tincture is prepared with alcohol.

PHYSIOLOGICAL EFFECTS.—Hesse discovered by his experiments that Berberis produces a remarkable feverish condition. One grain given to a perfectly healthy girl three times a day, for four days (altogether twelve grains), produced general relaxation; slight shivering along the back in the morning; heat in the face towards night; inflammation of the conjunctiva; great thirst; anorexia; slight griping in the abdomen, and pains before micturition. After giving an infusion of the root, he observed still more remarkable symptoms, and a fully-developed inflammation of the tonsils, uvula, and pharynx, accompanied by much redness and swelling; it is also remarkable that Paulli (*Quadripart. Bot.*, Argent. 1667, p. 103) praises the antiphlogistic effect of Berberis in fevers and inflammations, particularly in those of the tonsils and uvula, thus proving its homœopathic action. The same remarks apply to the cases of inflammations of the liver and lining membranes of the intestines, dysentery, and inflammations and congestion of the uterus. The experiments of Herberger, Wibmer, Whür, Buchner, and Hesse (vide *Wibmer and Hesse*, a. a. O. p. 26) give many significant proofs of the exciting effects of Berberis on the digestive organs, and this was shown also by Clusius (*Hist. Rar. Plant.*, 1661, p. 121), and others. Dioscorides recommends it as a medicine to produce abortion.

MEDICAL USES (HOMŒOPATHIC). — This medicine was not

proved by Hahnemann, and is not in the *Materia Medica Pura*, but is described and proved in the *Journal für Arzneimittellehre*. According to Noack and Trinks, Berberis is principally suited to gastric, bilious, and venous hemorrhoidal constitutions, and to the choleric or choleric-sanguine temperament. It seems to act upon the venous system and mucous membranes, particularly the eyes and digestive organs. Berberis deserves particular attention when disease of a bilious character prevails as an epidemic; also in acne; erythema intertrigo; urticaria; warts on the fingers; panaritia; chilblains; rheumatic fever; bilious gastric fever; arthritic fever; yellow fever; febrile conditions characterised by internal heat and external coldness, or partial chilliness; headache, particularly of the venous congestive kind, occasioned by derangements of the digestive functions, and accompanied by rheumatic and arthritic affections; catarrhal, rheumatic, and arthritic ophthalmia. Erysipelatous angina faucium, particularly when accompanied with striking bilious affections; affections of the liver; hepatitis, when occasioned by irritation from biliary calculi and from suppression of hemorrhoids; jaundice; diseases of the kidneys and urinary organs; hemorrhoidal affections; dysmenorrhœa; lumbago; arthritic and rheumatic affections of the extremities; arthritis nodosa.

Antidotes.—Camphor. Buchner says that Berberis antidotes Aconite.

Plate XI.

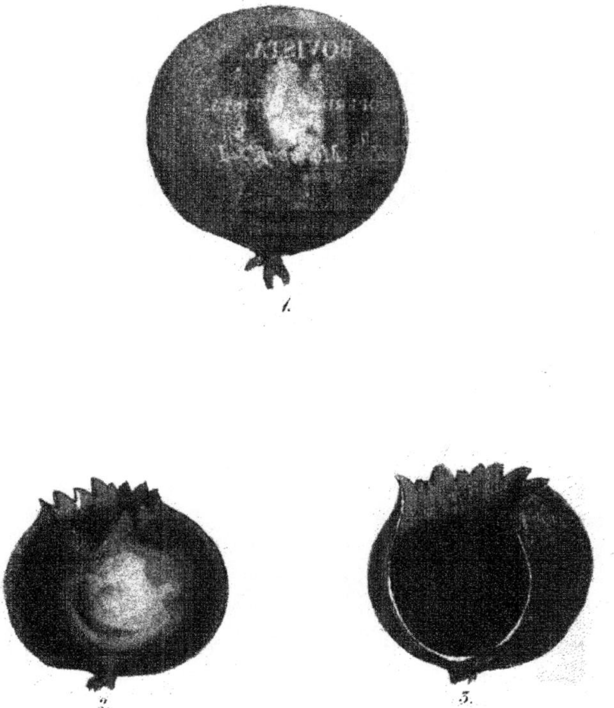

1. 2. 3.

E Sowerby, lith. Reeve & Nichols, imp.

Bovista (Lycoperdon Bovista)

XI.

BOVISTA.

(LYCOPERDON BOVISTA.*)

Puff-ball. Mollypuf. Puff-fist.

SYNONYMS.—Lycoperdon bovista, *Linn.* Lycop. cælatum, *Fries.* Lycop. globosum, *Bolton, Fung. Hal.* Bovista nigrescens, *Pers. Synop. Fungi.* Crepitus lupi, *Matthiol.* Fungus ovatus.

FOREIGN NAMES.—*Fr.:* Boviste, Vesse loup, Vesse de loup des bouviers. *Germ.:* Wolfsrauch, Kugelschwamm, Rauchpitz, Der Staubschwamm. *Dut.:* Stuifzwamm. *Ital.:* Licoperdo. *Span.:* Licoperdo. *Dan.:* Storsvam. *Swed.:* Klotsvamp.

Nat. Order, FUNGI (MYCETES), *Tribus* GASTERONYCETES, CRYPTOGAMIA—FUNGI.

GEN. CHAR.—*Fungus* roundish, fleshy, opening at the top, full of powdery, impalpable seeds.

SPEC. CHAR.—Stemless, white, changing to black; a regular globe, with only two coats.

HISTORY.—There is no notice of this fungus being used as a medicine by the old physicians, although it is mentioned by Pliny (*Nat. Hist.*, c. xix., *Holland's Trans.*) "In these toad-stools of the mushroom kind, are those flat tuffes or puffes to be reckoned which the Greeks name Perzitœ, as they have no root at all, so they be altogether without either stele or taste." It had an early reputation, and became a popular remedy for all

---

Figs. 1, 2, and 3. The fungus in different stages of its growth.

* The name is derived from λυκος, a wolf; and περδω, to explode backwards. Bovista, from the German Bofist.

kinds of hemorrhages, and was used extensively as an external application for this purpose by the common people, particularly in epistaxis. Linnæus mentions this in his account of it in the *Flor. Sued.*, p. 460; and that there is a general belief in Sweden, and also in Germany, that it promotes blindness. There can be no doubt that the fine powdery, spun-like contents may cause inflammation when introduced into the eye, and a fatal contraction when inhaled into the lungs. (Vide Loséke, *Mat. Med.*, 6th edit., p. 419.) It was not, therefore, attempted to administer it as an internal remedy. The Bovista does not enter into the allopathic Pharmacopœia; but Linnæus (*Mat. Med.*, 5th edit., 1787, p. 280) writes of a vis adstringens, obstipans, absorbens, incrassans, ophthalmica, gastrica.

The styptic properties of the Bovista, however, do not rest only on its mechanical action, but in reality on the physiological effects on the human organism, as indicated by the homœopathic provings of this fungus on persons in health. By reference to Noack and Trinks's *Handbuch für Hom. Arzneimittellehre*, art. Bovista, it will be seen that it produces the very symptom it has been given to cure, as a popular remedy, viz., bleeding from the nose.

Description.—It may be generally known by its globose structure, smoothish surface, and light colour, the whole forming a simple covering to the white cottony substance within, which substance, in an advanced age, becomes a mass of firmly-entangled fibres of a dark colour, holding an immense quantity of extremely fine sable powder—we presume the seeds. The covering, too, becomes dark, more or less of a brownish slate-colour, of a silky lustre, and stiff satiny texture. Small plants of this slate-colour have been called Lycoperdon ardosiaceum. It has been confounded with the Lycoperdon proteus, but is less common, and has the same number of skins, but the outer one is never so rough, which will help to distinguish it, as well as its being destitute of the cellular part at the base (*Sowerb. Fungi*).

According to Withering, it is snow-white when young, and white within; black in decay; opens with a very large aperture, the diameter being about two inches.

According to Buchner, when growing, it is white when young.

GEOGRAPHICAL DISTRIBUTION.—Most parts of Europe, Great Britain, Germany, France, Sweden, Norway, Russia, and Asia Minor.

LOCALITIES.—In dry meadows and on downs. (In Kensington Gardens, from the size of a pea to twenty or thirty inches in circumference. *Sowerby*).

PARTS USED IN MEDICINE, AND MODE OF PREPARATION.—The whole plant. To prepare a powerful mother-tincture, we must commence with a dry trituration of the seeds (*the black dust*), and to this add alcohol gradually until the trituration commences to be fluid; then add an equal weight of alcohol. The whole to be put away for some days in a dry place, to be left at rest, and afterwards filtered. The season for collecting this fungus for medicinal purposes is in the months of August and September.*

MEDICAL USES (HOMŒOPATHIC).—Bovista is especially indicated in irritable, juvenile, or debilitated systems, with great variability of the circulatory and nervous systems, as well as for florid, scrofulous, or nervo-venous individuals, more especially for such as have a tendency easily to take cold, with disturbance of circulation, or swelling of the glands. In such, Bovista is most especially specific in affections of the skin, and in diseases of the heart. Papulous, squamous, and vesiculous eruptions of the skin. Lichen, especially agrius. Prurigo. Psoriasis, even diffused. Pityriasis. Herpes (with dry and humid spots). Erythema. Intertrigo. Impetigo. Acne. Eruptions at the corner of the mouth, and ulceration of the lips. Ulcers on the fingers. Intermittent fevers. Catarrhal and rheumatic

* Care must be taken to gather the true Bovista, and not the Lycoperdon giganteum or proteus, which is much larger and more *tuberculous*.

affections. Hemorrhage of the nose and teeth, especially when occurring in children suffering from skin eruptions. Toothache, when accompanied by swelling of the lips. Menoclasia from cold. Bronchitis acuta Affections of the heart. Palpitation from organic disease. Numbness and paralytic feeling in the hands, as sequelæ of arthritic or rheumatic disease, or from remains of a heart affection (*Noack and Trinks, Arzneimitt.*, p. 288).

ANTIDOTES.—Camphor. In cases of poisoning by this fungus, recourse must be had to the same means as given for the treatment of poisoning by the Agaricus muscarius.

Plate XII.

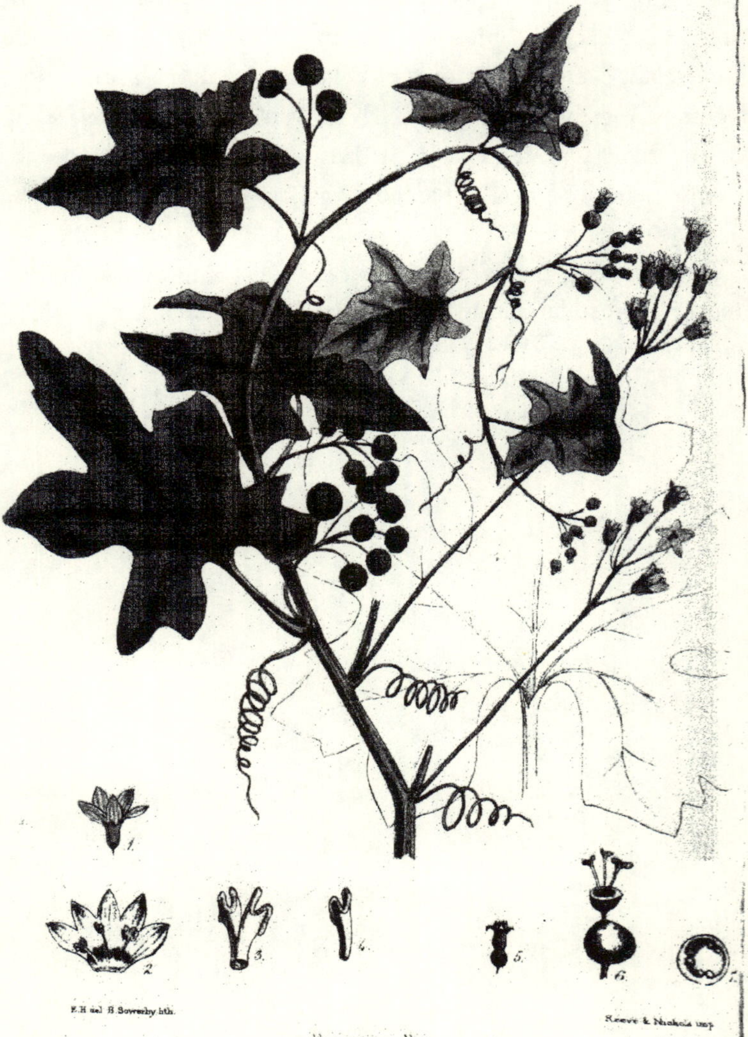

F.H del. B. Sowerby lith.

Reeve & Nichols imp.

Bryonia alba.

XII.

BRYONIA ALBA.

(BLACK-BERRIED WHITE BRYONY.*)

SYNONYMS.—Vitis nigris, *Matthiol.* Bryonia alba vulg., *Linn.* Bryonia dioica, *Jacq.* Bryonia vera. Vitis alba. Uva serpentina, s. anquina colubrina.

FOREIGN NAMES.—*Fr.:* Bryone, Coulevre. *Ital.:* Brionia, Vita bianca. *Span.:* Neuza alba. *Port.:* Norca branca. *Ger.:* Weisse Zaunrube, Stichwurz. *Dut.:* Welde wyngaar, Witte Bryon. *Swed.:* Hundrosva. *Pol.:* Pryestepbiaty.

Nat. Order, CUCURBITACEÆ.—MONŒCIA, MONODELPHIA.

GEN. CHAR.—*Calyx* five-cleft. *Corolla* five-cleft; barren anthers in two pairs, and a single one fertile. *Style* three-cleft. *Berry* three-celled; skin thin; herbaceous climbers, with simple tendrils, and stalked, alternate leaves.

SPEC. CHAR.—*Leaves* cordate, five-lobed, dentate, calloso-scabrous. *Flowers* racemose, corymbose, monœcious. *Calyx,* in fertile flowers, as long as corolla. *Stigma* smooth. *Berry* black.

HISTORY.—The Bryonia was one of the ancient remedies. Dioscorides mentions three kinds: the Αμπελος μελανα, the Bryonia alba of Linnæus; the Αμπελος λευκη, or Vitis alba, the Bryonia dioica; and the Αμπελος αγρια, the Tamus communis, or black Bryony; but this latter he carefully distinguishes from the other two, and considers it mild and edible. He treats of them at considerable length, and recommends the Bryonia alba (Vitis

---

Fig. 1. The calyx and corolla of male flower. 2. Section of ditto, to show the stamen. 3. The anther. 4. Section of ditto. 5. Female flower. 6. The germen, styles, and stigma. 7. Section of the berry, showing the position of the seeds.

* The name is derived from Βρυω, germino, expressive of the vigorous and rapid growth of its annual stems from the perennial root.

nigra), or, as others call it, Bryonia nigram or Chironiam vitam, as "urinas porro cient, menses pellunt;" also in affections of the spleen; in epilepsy (comitialibus), vertigo, and paralysis. The leaves as beneficial, as topical applications in ulcers, etc. The Bryonia alba (dioica) he extols for many virtues, more particularly in gangrenes and wounds, whitlow, apoplexy, cough, induration of the spleen, etc.

Pliny confounds them altogether, and Gerarde gives the following reason for his so doing. "Black Bryonia is called in Greek Αμπελος αγρια; in Latin, Bryonia nigra, Vitis sylvestris, or wild vine; notwithstanding it does not a little differ from Labrusca or Vitis vinifera sylvestris, that is to say, from the wild vine which bringeth forth wine, which is likewise called Αμπελος αγρια. Why both these were called by one name Pliny was the cause, who could not sufficiently expound them in his 23rd Booke, first chapter, but confounded them and made them all one, in which error are also the Arabians."

Joannes Bodæus, in his Commentary on Theophrastus, gives the following definition of the two. "One species" (B. alb. Linn.), he says, "bears black berries; the other" (B. dioica) "red. The root of the one is darkish externally, a pale whitish-yellow internally; the root of the other is white."

Matthiolus makes the Nigra vitis the Αμπελος μελαινα of Dioscorides, the same as the Tamus communis; but the remark of Dioscorides, that the fruit, at first green, when ripe is black, confirms it as the Bryonia alba, the only one of the species that has this peculiarity, the berries of the Tamus being red; he gets over this by saying that, although Dioscorides represents this, yet in his country the berries always remain red. He evidently confounds the two plants, probably never having seen the Bryonia alba, as it is chiefly confined to the north of Europe.

Dodonæus describes the true Bryonia alba under the name of Bryonia nigra; but Bauhin calls it Bryonia alba, and says, "It differs from the common white Bryony only in that the root is of a yellowish box colour of the inside, and the fruit or berries are black when they ripen."

Pereira (*Elem. Mat. Med.*, vol. ii. p. 1153) makes the Αμπελος μελαινα of Dioscorides the Tamus communis; but as we have noted before, the berries of the one are always black, of the other *invariably red.*

Dr. Adams, in his Commentary on Paulus Ægineta, vol. iii., says: "The wild vine is evidently the Tamus communis, the white Bryony the Bryonia dioica, and the black the Bryonia alba of Linnæus."

Mesne recommends the use of Bryonia alba in many diseases, and extols it highly; and Serapion ascribes to it, amongst other virtues, that of producing a great flow of milk. Galen (*De Simplic.*, lib. vi.) says, "the virtues of the Vitis nigra (Bryonia alba, Linn.) are the same as that of alba (B. dioica), but weaker."

Bryonia seems to have been used formerly extensively in many diseases, although at the present time it has fallen into disuse. Dioscorides employed it in epilepsy, vertigo, and melancholia. Galen in gout, especially podagra, hysteria, and hypochondriasis. Cælius Aurelianus in jaundice. Sydenham in disorders of the mind, delirium, mania, insanity, and imbecility. Trautman in arthritic hemicrania. Alexander Trallian in deafness and hypochondria, diarrhœa, dropsy, pleuritis, stitches in the side, sciatica, white swelling and white tumour of the knee. Hartmann in diseases of the womb and tardy delivery. Loniger in asthma, pain in the neck, in hemorrhages and spitting of blood.

To those conversant in homœopathy, the foregoing enumeration is particularly interesting, as the benefit derived from Bryonia, in all these cases, arose from the property it has of producing symptoms similar to these diseases on persons in health; and Paulli (*Quadrip. Botan.*, Argentorati, 1667, p. 35), in allusion to its effects on the uterus, says: "Recensiones practici tanquam, specifico in uteri morbis omnis generis radicibus utuntur, vel ut menses moveant mulierum, vel ut iis fœtum mortuum ejiciant, vel denique ad quem affectum potissimum commendantur, ut ab uteri strangulatur eas vindicent." It was recommended by Harmand Montgarni (*Nouveau Traitement des Maladies dysentériques Verd.*) for inflammatory diarrhœa and dysentery. Horn and Richter, however, advise its discontinuance in these affections, because it is apt to produce such irritating action on the intestinal canal as almost even to excite inflammation.

In Culpepper's Complete Herbal and English Physician at large are the following remarks:—

"Bryonia is one of the furious martial plants, and amongst other virtues, when mixed with honey, doth mightily cleanse the chest of rotten phlegm, and wonderfully help any old and long cough, to those that are troubled with shortness of breath."

Description.—The plant proved by Hahnemann is the Bryonia alba of Linnæus, and not the Bryonia dioica, or white Bryony, so common in the hedges and thickets in many parts of this country. It is a perennial climbing plant, with palmate leaves of bright-green colour, rough to the touch, and the terminal lobe longer then the rest. The flowers are whitish or yellowish-white. The male and female flowers growing upon the same plant, the former on long peduncles. *Stamens* distinct. The *fruit globose* and *black*. Flowers June and July. The chief distinguishing characters between the Bryonia alba of Linnæus and Bryonia dioica are—1st, the leaves of the alba are of a brighter green than the dioica. The berries are *black* in the one, and *red* in the other, and the male and female flowers of the alba grow on the same plant, whilst in the dioica they are on different stems.

Geographical Distribution.—North of Europe, Germany (in many parts more common than the Bryonia dioica), Hanover, some parts of France, Lorraine, Pyrenees, Spain, and north of Italy.

It is not indigenous in this country, although Plukenet described it as not unfrequent about Cambridge. He was evidently mistaken, as it was not observed by Ray, nor has it been found since in that neighbourhood, nor in any other part of Great Britain.

Localities.—Hedges and thickets.

Besides the Bryonia alba, the following are the different species found in various parts of the world, they all probably contain the essential property of the plant, viz., Bryonine.

1. *Bryonia dioica.* Berries red; root yellowish-white within; leaves palmate, callous, scabrous on both sides, alternate, five-lobed; the terminal lobe the largest, and very dissimilar to the others; flowers white, with elegant green ribs and veins; berries globular, scarlet, smooth. The leaves in autumn have the smell of musk. Native of Great Britain and other parts of Europe.

2. *Bryonia palmata.* Leaves palmate; berries yellowish Native of Ceylon.

3. *Bryonia laciniosa.* Leaves palmate; berry globular, green. Native of Malabar.

4. *Bryonia Africana.* Leaves palmate; berry solitary, yellowish.

5. *Bryonia Cretica.* Leaves palmate, rough, with callous points on the upper surface; root large, running deep into the ground; berry red. Native of Candia.

6. *Bryonia Boronensis.* Leaves semi-palmate, resembling those of the common fig; root and stems like those of the common Bryony. Native of Buenos Ayres.

7. *Bryonia variegata.* 8. *Bryonia grandis.* Stem shrubby, smooth, large; leaves roundish, five-angled, not lobed; flowers large, whitish; berry red. Native of India and Cochin China.

9. *Bryonia cordifolia.* Leaves cordate, five-lobed; petioles long, with two teeth at the base of the leaf. Native of Ceylon.

10. *Bryonia maderaspatana.* Native of the East Indies.

11. *Bryonia scabrella.* Native of the East Indies.

12. *Bryonia scabra.* Native of the Cape of Good Hope.

13. *Bryonia nana.* Native of Africa.

14. *Bryonia Abyssinica.* Native of Africa.

15. *Bryonia Americana.* Leaves smooth, deep-green above, rather glaucous beneath, large, cordate; root tender, white, and bitter; stem long, angular, twining, pointed, with a leaf, a tendril, and a flower at each joint; flowers greenish without, white within; berries oval, about the size of an olive, red. Native of the Antilles.

16. *Bryonia Japonica.* Native of Japan.

17. *Bryonia racemosa.* Native of Jamaica.

18. *Bryonia verrucosa.* Leaves cordate, angled; berries globular.

19. *Bryonia latebrosa.* Leaves subtrilobate, hairy, drawn to a point at the base. Native of the Canaries.

20. *Bryonia amplexicaulis.* Stem angular, smooth; berries solitary, the size of a hazel-nut. Native of the East Indies.

21. *Bryonia hastata.* Leaves hastate, edged with little teeth; berry small, red. Native of China, about Canton.

22. *Bryonia triloba.* Native of Cochin China.

PARTS USED IN MEDICINE, AND MODE OF PREPARATION.—The root must be taken before the plant flowers, therefore before the month of June, and the juice is to be expressed from it, and prepared according to the mode previously mentioned of preparing the recent plant. The root has a very nauseating, biting taste and disagreeable smell. It grows sometimes to a great size, and has been sold as the root of the Mandrake by herbalists. The root of the Bryonia alba is somewhat different to that of the Bryonia dioica, being more branched and more covered with tubercles.

POISONOUS EFFECTS.*—Orfila (*Tox. Gén.*, vol. i. p. 679) made the following experiments on the root of the Bryonia upon animals. He applied two ounces four grains of the fine powder of the dry root of Bryonia to the cellular tissue of the external part of the thigh of a good-sized dog. The

* The Cucurbitaceæ are generally harmless. The chief exceptions to this rule are the colocynth, bryonia, and elaterium.

animal died in about sixty hours, without having appeared to experience other symptoms than a very severe pain. On opening the body, there was no lesion of the alimentary canal; the lungs were sound; the membrane operated upon exhibited an inflammation so extensive, that it was terminating in suppuration.

In another experiment, he introduced into the stomach of a small dog half an ounce of the dry root, finely pulverized, and tied the œsophagus. After four hours the animal did not appear to be at all affected, but was found dead the next morning. The blood which filled the ventricle of the heart was coagulated; the lungs, slightly crepitant, were of a reddish colour, and contained a considerable quantity of blood; the stomach, very red at the exterior, contained nearly all the injected powder; the mucous membrane, of a fiery red, presented here and there blackish spots, not ulcerated; the interior of the large intestines was much inflamed; the other parts of the digestive canal were scarcely inflamed. The same experiment was repeated with three ounces of water, in which had been infused for four hours, half an ounce of the root of powdered Bryony. Thirteen hours after, the animal did not seem to experience any other symptoms than a great state of debility; he made but few efforts to move, but had no vertigo; he died in the night. On examination the next day, the heart was distended by a considerable quantity of blood, partly coagulated and partly fluid; the lungs, a little red, contained fluid blood; the mucous membrane of the stomach was of a cherry-red over its whole extent, including the rectum. The other intestines, except the commencement of the duodenum, were nearly in a normal state.

Symptoms on Man.—In a communication in the *Gazette de Santé*, Sept. 1816, there is an account of a woman who had just been confined, and the village doctor had ordered her, for the purpose of stopping the milk, a draught composed of about an ounce of Bryony root, in a pint of water, and a lavement made of a concentrated decoction of the same substance. Four hours after she died. On inspection of the matters which had been passed, it was perceived that the whole of the lining membrane of the rectum had come away. An inspection of the body was not allowed.

Pyl mentions a fatal case of poisoning with it at Cambray in France. The subject was a man, who took two glasses of an infusion of the root to cure ague, and was soon after seized with violent tormina and purging, which nothing could arrest, and which soon terminated fatally (*Neues Magazin*, t. 3, p. 557).

Many observers attest that the administration of Bryony is followed by violent vomitings, accompanied by faintings, severe pains and abundant serous alvine dejections, thirst, etc.

These facts lead us to think—1st, that the Bryony acts on man as upon animals; 2nd, that the effects appear to depend upon the inflammation that it developes, and upon the sympathetic irritation of the nervous system upon its absorption; 3rd, that it is in the soluble portion in the water its deleterious property resides.

Bryonia owes its power to an extractive matter discovered by Brande and Firnhaber, to which the name Bryonine is given. According to the experiments of Collard de Martigny, Bryonine acts on the stomach and on a wound exactly as the root itself, but more energetically; when introduced into the cavity of the pleura, it causes rapid death by true pleurisy, ending in effusion of fibrin (*Nouv. Bibliothèque Médicale*, 1827, p. 221).

MEDICAL USES (HOMŒOPATHIC).—"The resemblance of the effects of Bryonia to those of Rhus cannot be mistaken. Bryonia also totally changes the disposition of the mind. The fever it causes is chiefly manifested by chilliness; its symptoms appear, and are increased in a peculiar manner while the body is in motion, although it is not uncommon to perceive its alternate effects in the relief of the symptoms by repose.

"From this it follows that, in the use of Bryonia, cases may occur in which the medicine, though perfectly homœopathic, and given in a small dose, does not produce the expected results for twenty-four hours, because there has appeared only one series of symptoms, which correspond with its alternate effects. In this case, a second dose, given at the end of twenty-four hours, produces amelioration, and the opposite range of effects, in the same manner that a second dose of any other medicine given directly after the first, terminates its action.

"Very few other substances present this phenomenon, but it is not unusual with Bryonia. When Bryonia is not perfectly homœopathic, the injurious consequences occasioned by it are generally removed by Rhus, or some other appropriate medicine, or at least by Camphor.

"According to the ample list of symptoms excited by Bryonia in healthy persons, we may form various states of artificial disease, corresponding exactly with many of the common maladies, especially with certain fevers, and many kinds of spasms, pertaining to women; upon which may be founded the expectation of homœopathic success. The curative effects of Bryonia are therefore very extensive" (*Hahnemann, Mat. Med. Pura*, art. *Bryonia*).

Clinical Observations.—*Noack and Trinks* (l. c.): Bryonia is especially suitable to nervous, dry, slender, and bilious individuals, with a choleric temperament; to people with brown complexion, brown or black hair, irritable character, and disposition to inflammation of the dermous tissues. In diseases of women and children, Bryonia is especially serviceable, as it corresponds with great irritability, little energy, constancy of reaction, inclination to effusions and accumulations of lymph, nervous diseases, and likewise active congestion. Bryonia excites both the peripheral nerves and capillary vessels, giving rise to symptoms intermediate between inflammation and nervous irritation. It is especially indicated in affections where resorption is necessary; in typhoid infiltrations, serous effusions, and sugillations. It is most serviceable in affections where the catarrhal, pituitous, and rheumatic character prevails, or where synochal symptoms pass into the nervous stage; likewise in affections of a typhoid character. Morbid affections, brought on by catching cold in dry cold weather and sharp wind. Bad consequences of chagrin, anger, excessive bodily exertion, and a sedentary mode of life; conditions which are accompanied by ill humour, and chills and coldness of the body. In diseases of a rheumatic-bilious and catarrhal nature. Arthritic affections. Arthritica nodosa. Acute rheumatism. Dropsical conditions. Hysteric convulsions. Some cutaneous affections. Rheumatic and rheumatic-gastric fevers, with great action of the circulatory system, and increased sensibility. Acute rheumatism, especially when concentrated in wrist, elbow, knee, and ankle joint, with hot and burning swellings. Intermittent fevers, with gastric disturbance, with rheumatic affections, increased by motion, and inclination to constipation. Tertian ague. Fevers, mostly in the cold stage. Gastric, bilious, mucous, and nervous fevers. The synochal fevers verging on typhus. Febris nervosa versatilis. Abdominal typhus (alternating with Rhus). Different kinds of fevers, gastric, bilious, and typhus. Irritative sensibility of the tongue (everything tastes salt). Loss of appetite and taste. Milk fever. Headache, brought on by affections of the mind and from cold. Cephalalgia and tearing headache in females. Megrim and hemicrania. Frontal headache. Encephalitis, meningitis, and arachnitis. Cerebral affections, the sequelæ of cholera. Bleeding of the nose from cold, with gastric affections. Epistaxis of an active kind. Rheumatic inflammatory toothache, Stomacace. Gastric affections. Chronic cardialgia. Sub-acute inflammation of the liver. Jaundice. Chronic abdominal affections. Colic, especially of an inflammatory kind; attacks of colic of pregnant and lying-in women. Hysterical spasms. Peritonitis muscularis. Peritonitis. Puerperal peritonitis (after Aconite). Diarrhœa, brought on from cold, and in spring and autumn. Obstinate constipation. Cholera Asiatica, when the liver is the chief seat of the affection. Spasmodic labour-pains. Metrorrhagia. Galactorrhœa (after Belladonna has been tried without avail). Mastitis, when the mammæ are very hard;

painful knotty breasts, owing to suppression of the secretion of milk in nursing women. Bronchial catarrh. Inflammatory affections of the organs of respiration, especially when accompanied by darting, stitching pains. Acute and chronic bronchitis. Influenza, with cough, and when coughing, much headache. Chronic cough, when excited by the least irritation. Convulsive cough, with stitching pains in the chest during and after the attack. Rheumatic inflammations of the chest, lungs, and pleura, with a low, nervous condition, and gastric complication. Serous or muscular pleurisy. Parenchymatous pneumonia. Pneumonia after the inflammatory symptoms have been subdued by Aconite. Pneumonia biliosa. It must be borne in mind that Bryonia will not be sufficient, without the help of Aconite in these affections, and other medicines in alternation. Asthmatic conditions. Acute rheumatism of the joints. Phlegmonous inflammation of the feet.

ANTIDOTES.—Aconite. Chamomilla. Ignatia. Nux vomica. It antidotes Alumina and Rhus. According to Dulong, Tincture of Gall-nuts is an antidote against the poisonous effects of Bryonia. As in all cases of poisoning by irritants, all emetics, vinegar, etc., must on no account be administered.

XIII.

CALENDULA OFFICINALIS.*

(MARIGOLD.)

SYNONYMS.—Caltha officinalis, *Matth.* Caltha vulgaris, *Bauhin.* Solseginum aureum. Solis sponsa. Flos omnium mensium. Verrucaria.

FOREIGN NAMES.—*Fr.:* Le Souci de Jardin. *Germ.:* Die Gemeine Ringelblume, Todtenblume. *Dut.:* Goudbloem. *Ital.:* Calendula, Fiore d'ogni mese. *Span.:* Calendula. *Russ.:* Nogotki.

Nat. Order, CORYMBIFERÆ, *Juss.*—SYNGENESIA, POLYGAMIA NECESSARIA.

GEN. CHAR.—*Calyx* simple, nearly upright, with numerous linear-lanceolate, nearly equal divisions. *Corolla* radiate; florets of the disk numerous, tubular, semi-quinquefid, the length of the calyx. The *Ray* strap-shaped, very long, three-toothed, hairy at the base, without nerves, with pistils only. *Stamens* of the disk: filaments fine, capillary, very short; anthers the length of the floret, inserted in a hollow cylinder. *Pistil* of the disk: germen oblong, three-cornered; style thread-shaped, scarcely the length of the stamens; stigma obtuse, bifid, straight. *Pistil* of the ray: germen oblong, three-cornered; style thread-shaped; stigmas two, oblong, acuminate, reflexed. *Pericarp:* the permanent calyx converging and depressed. *Seeds* in the centre of the disk, none; in the circumference sometimes, but rarely, solitary, membranous, inversely heart-shaped, compressed; in the *ray* solitary, layers oblong, incurved, triangular, with membranous angle, marked on the outside longitudinally with the figure of a vegetable. *Down* none. *Receptacle* naked and flat.

SPEC. CHAR.—*Receptacle* naked. *Down* none. *Calyx* with many divisions. *Seeds* in the circumference of the disk membranous.

Fig. 1. Floret of the ray. 2. Floret of the disk. 3. Seed-vessel (magnified).

* The word Calendula is derived from Calendæ, the months, because the plant flowers all the year through.

Plate XIII.

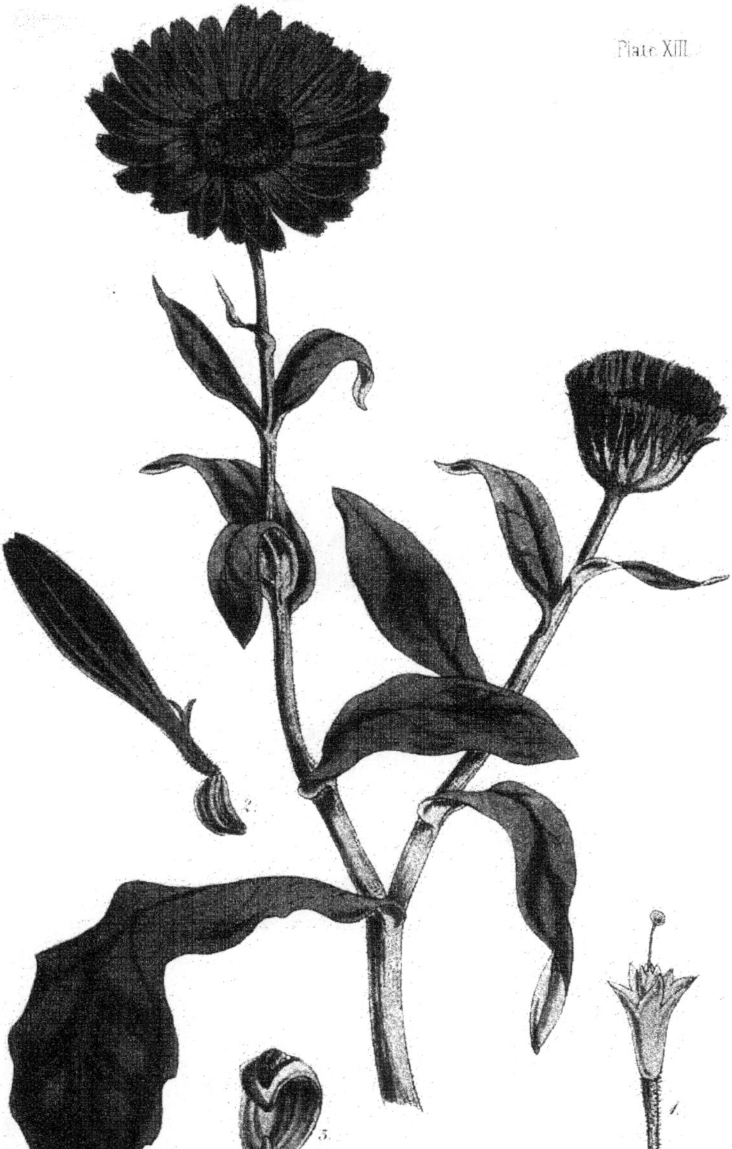

S. Sowerby, del. et lith.

Reeve & Nichols, imp.

Calendula officinalis.

HISTORY.—The ancients considered the Calendula a deobstruent remedy, exerting a great influence on the circulation. Dioscorides recommends it in cancer; and Fuchsius (*Hist. Stirp.*, 1546) prescribed the juice of it against toothache.

Virgil (*Bucol.*, *Eclog.* ii.) mentions it:

> "Tum Cassia atque aliis intexens suavibus herbis
> Mollis Luteola pingit vaccinia Caltha."

Gerarde, also, in describing its virtues remarks, "that the flowers and leaves of Marigold being distilled, and the water dropped into red and watery eyes, ceaseth the inflammation and taketh away the pains."

Calendula was formerly in much request as a medicine, and was used more especially in carcinoma and scirrhus; according to Westring, with great effect in the third stage, particularly in diminishing the pain, and rendering the pus less corroding; but on further experiment by others, the same effects were not produced, and therefore it was thrown aside. It was also used in chlorosis, hysteria, epilepsy, jaundice, and some kinds of dropsy. Schneider found it of great efficacy as a lotion to fresh wounds, inducing union by the first intention. Zorn considered Calendula of great service in throwing out the eruption of measles and small-pox; and as a topical application to stop the bleeding in hæmorrhoides fluentes. It was a favourite remedy with Boerhaave, who employed it in uterine diseases, in diseases of the kidney, and jaundice. Its chief use, however, was for cancer, and it was the principal ingredient in the famous Rust Pill, which consisted of oxide of iron, colewort, and extract of Marigold. W. Carter found the extract of Calendula of great assistance in obstinate vomiting; and De Camp, in a case of cardialgia, where all medicines, etc., were vomited up, owing to a great irritability of the stomach. Muhrbeck used the extract of Marigold, in chronic vomiting, with great success, in a case where violent pains were felt at the same time in the region of the uterus; it was remarked that these pains increased when the dose exceeded thirty-four grains in the twenty-four hours. It is interesting to note that Elgafaki states that violent vomiting ensues after taking four drachms of the juice of Marigold. Dr. Stein extols the efficacy of this plant in cancer of the skin; he prepares the juice from the green plant and its blossoms, and makes an ointment with butter and charcoal, which is applied to the ulcer.

Description.—Calendula officinalis is one of the most common annuals in our gardens; has a short divaricated stem, dividing low into numerous bushy branches, a foot or two in height, pubescent, and pale green, as well as the leaves; these are long, a little sinuated, the lower and middle ones oval and blunt, the upper ones lanceolate. The *flowers* are radiated, and of a golden colour, coming out at the ends of the branches. Flowering the greater part of the summer; the flowers being open from nine in the morning to three in the afternoon.

Geographical Distribution.—Native of France; and found in cultivated grounds over the greater part of Europe.

Parts used in Medicine, and Mode of Preparation.—The Leaves and Flowers. For internal use, the tincture is prepared as is described under Aconite. For external application, Dr. Thorer recommends the following:—One preparation was obtained by filling one-third of a clean bottle with the leaves of the plant, and the other two-thirds with fresh, clean well-water. This mixture was exposed to the rays of the sun for two or three days, taking care to cork the bottle well, the moment of fermentation being carefully watched. In this way a water having a slightly aromatic smell was obtained, which was immediately poured off, and, in bottles hermetically sealed, was at once carried into a cool cellar. Another preparation is obtained by mixing two-thirds of equal parts of alcohol and water with one-third of the flowers of Marigold. This second preparation should be used diluted, lest the alcohol should irritate the wound.

The chief employment of Calendula has been as an external

application on incised wounds, and is considered a specific for sugillations, bloody and serous infiltrations of the cellular tissue in open wounds and ulcers. It also deserves notice in treatment of diseases of the glands; in traumatic inflammation of the eyes; and, according to Dr. Thorer, Marigold is useful in scrofulous and sclerotic tumours. He notices some interesting cases of the healing virtues of Calendula in extensive laceration of the soft parts. One case involving the tendons; others, the skin, cellular tissue, and muscles. He considers the Marigold far superior to Arnica in healing recent wounds and lacerations, with or without loss of substance; and Arnica more specific in contusions, bruises, and sprains. Another important character of Calendula is, that it effects the healing of wounds without leaving any prominent eschar.

The following interesting case, treated by Dr. Thorer, will exemplify the beneficial use of Marigold. A boy, aged sixteen years, was caught in the cogs of a wheel in a mill. The following injuries were received: a compound fracture of the left upper arm, the ends of the bone protruding through the skin; a deep flesh-wound in the bend of the elbow; the forearm was entirely deprived of its muscular coating, so that the ulna and radius were laid bare for about six inches; the hand was nearly torn off, and was adhering to the arm by a small piece of flesh; the skin and anterior muscles of the right leg were torn off, exhibiting a large and deep flesh-wound which penetrated to the bone; there were a number of small flesh-wounds on the face. The arm was amputated at once above the splintered part; and the fleshy parts of the right leg were covered with compresses moistened with Calendula tea. These compresses were continued till the cure was completed. Granulation took place without suppuration; whereas the usual suppurative process set in in the stump of the upper arm, which had been subjected to the usual surgical treatment. On seeing the effects of the Calendula on the leg, Dr. Thorer applied it to the arm, and the cicatrizing process at once commenced and went on as favourably as it did in the leg. Every wound healed admirably, closed by granulation, and was covered with a new skin. The boy entirely recovered in seven weeks.

W. C. had his fingers caught in the wheel of a mill; the anterior joint of the index-finger, and two joints of the ring-finger were entirely torn off, and the fleshy part of the tip of the middle finger was likewise carried away; a small portion of the bare bone of the second joint of the ring-finger had remained, and the patient was very anxious to have it amputated. It was left, however, with the hope that the granulation might be favourable, and cover this little remnant of the joint with fleshy particles. The Calendula was applied on the second day after the occurrence of the accident. The result of the application was very satisfactory. The wounds did not suppurate, and the granulation went on undisturbed to the termination of the cure. The little spiculum of bone on the ring-finger had exfoliated slightly at the tip, but that portion of the bone which was adhering to the joint had become covered with flesh.

Dr. Schulz has used the Calendula with the most satisfactory results, in compound fractures of the limbs, etc. It will suffice to remark, that in all cases where the fleshy parts have been carried away, and the edges of the wound cannot be brought together by plaster, the Aquæ Calendulæ is the best application as a wash. The suppurative process, which is so exhausting in large wounds, is either entirely prevented or very much shortened and diminished by the Calendula wash. Calendula may also be useful in induration of stomach and uterus.

Plate XIV.

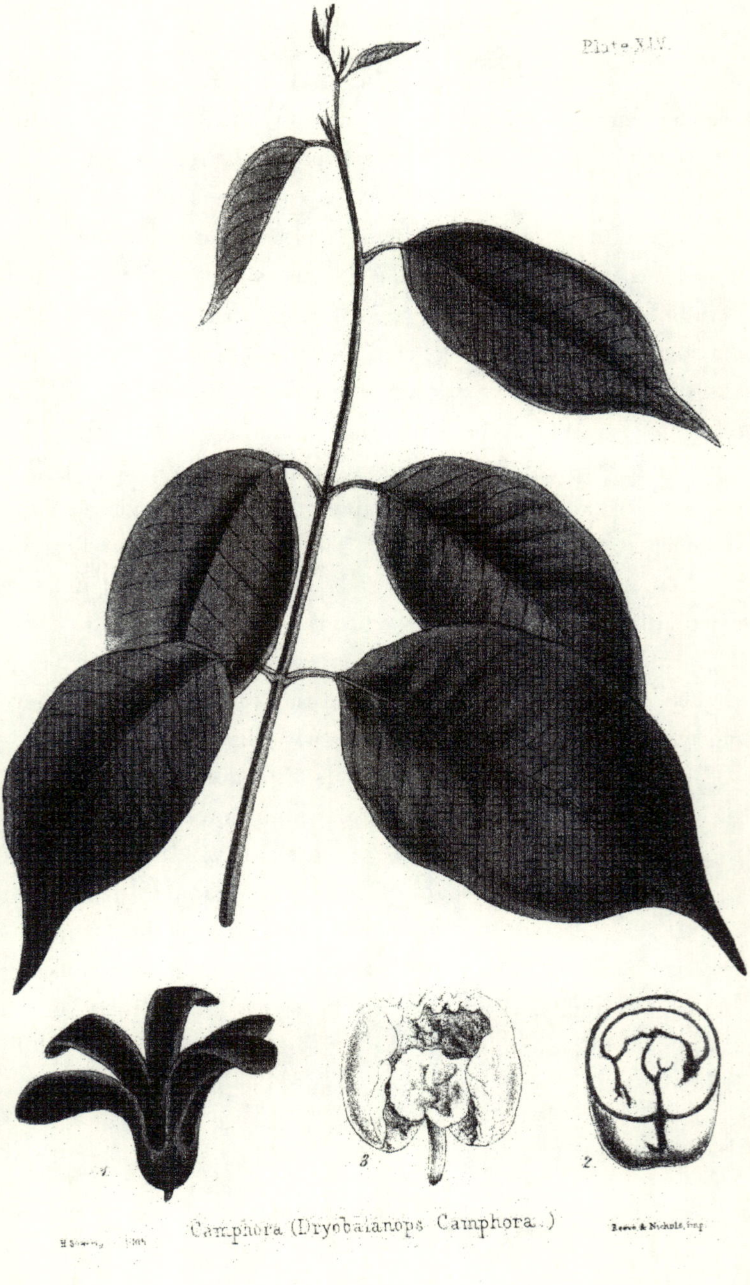

Camphora (Dryobalanops Camphora.)

H. Sowerby lith. Reeve & Nichols, imp.

XIV.

DRYOBALANOPS CAMPHORA.*

(THE CAMPHOR-TREE.)

SYNONYMS.—Dryobalanops Camphora, *Colebr.* Dryobalanops aromatica, *Gärtn.* Shorea, Camphorifera, *Roxb.* Pterygium teres.

FOREIGN NAMES.—*Fr.:* Camphre. *Ital.:* Canfora. *Span.:* Alcanfor. *Germ.:* Kampher. *Dut.:* Kamfer. *Swed.:* Kamfert. *Dan.:* Campher. *Russ.:* Kamphor. *Sanscrit.:* Carpura. *Arab.:* Cafúr. *Hind.:* Capur. *Malay.:* Kapurbarus.

Nat. Order, GUTTIFERÆ.—POLYANDRIA, MONOGYNIA.

GEN. CHAR.—*Calyx* one-leaved, permanent, enlarged into a gibbous cap, with five ligulate, long, scamose wings. *Corolla* five-petalled. *Capsule* three-valved, one-celled. *Seed* solitary. *Embryo* converse, without perisperm.

SPEC. CHAR.—*Leaves* superior, alternate, inferior ones opposite, elliptic, obtusely acuminate, entire. *Petioles* short. *Stipules* in pairs, subulate, caducous.

HISTORY.—Camphor was unknown to the ancients, but the Arabian physicians Avicenna and Serapion speak of it under the name of Kaphor. Sprengel (*Hist. de la Méd.*, t. ii. p. 238) considers that Simeon Seth (*De Aliment. Facult.*) gives the earliest record of it. No medicine has been so much used in various diseases as Camphor: it has been generally an ingredient in almost every prescription, and advised for affections

---

Fig. 1. The perianth and capsule. 2. The capsule, transverse section. 3. The embryo.

* Camphor is found in many plants, but only in two in any great quantities, viz., Dryobalanops Camphora and the Laurus Camphora, or Camphor Laurel, which was supposed formerly to be the only plant which yielded the Camphor of commerce.

the most opposite in their character: in fevers, in inflammatory diseases, in the exanthemata; in mania, melancholia, and other forms of mental disorders; in spasmodic affections; irritation of the urinary and sexual organs; poisoning; chronic rheumatism and gout; cholera; and as an external remedy for a variety of diseases.

The following remarks, translated from Noack and Trinks' introduction to art. Camphor in *Hom. Arzneimittellehre,* are extremely interesting. According to Sundelin (*Handbuch Spec. Heilmittel.,* 2nd edit., p. 146) and others, Camphor excites flow of blood from the nose, ears, kidneys, and uterus; but Richter (*Com. Pharmacol.,* vol. iii. p. 370) recommends it against hemorrhages; and Ettmuller cured a dangerous metrorrhagia with it. Neümann (*Spec. Pathol. et Therap.,* 2nd edit., vol. i. pp. 106, 797) says: "It has been demonstrated that Camphor excites perspiration; nevertheless, we see among persons with acute rheumatism, who deliquesce without alleviation, that this perspiration ceases as soon as they take Camphor;" and again: "The operation is certain; the violent sweat and fever moderate themselves almost immediately; the greatest diaphoretic remedy lessens diaphoresis." Greiner also, besides many others, recommends it against colliquative sweatings. Siemerling observed very profuse sweatings after the use of Camphor.

Schmucker praises Camphor as a prophylactic of hydrophobia (*Schneider's Warnh. aus d. Wünd. Arz.,* vol. ii. p. 114). Selle makes it an ingredient of his potio antilyssa. G. A. Richter (l. c., p. 375) remarks that it appears likely to be of great service in symptomatic hydrophobia; and Alix asserts having cured a declared hydrophobia with Camphor (*Obs. Chir.,* Fasc. iii. p. 177; *E. Krügelstein, Die Gesch. d. Hundwuth, etc.,* p. 555). Brumwell relates of a dog evincing signs of hydrophobia after having Camphor given him (*Med. Observ. and Inquir.,* vol. vi. p. 229; *Murray,* l. c., p. 476). The animals on which Carminati and Menghini experimented with Camphor were taken first with giddiness, then with rage, stupor, dread, rattling in the throat, sighing, screaming, foaming at the mouth, sobbing, trembling, convulsions, and even epilepsy (Comp. *Murray*, l. c., pp. 475, 480, 487, 504, 517, 519, etc). Pereira (*Materia Medica*, vol. ii. p. 792) mentions that Camphor dissolved in oil and administered to dogs, has produced tetanic convulsions. Purkinje and Alexander fell into convulsions on swallowing Camphor. Simmons saw in a maniac, to whom he gave Camphor in gradually augmented doses, an epileptic fit come on, after passing through which the patient recovered his senses (*Richter's Chir. Bibl.*, vol. vii. p. 771). Nevertheless, Camphor has acquired a great name in spasmodic diseases, in tetanus, epilepsy, and St. Vitus's dance. Murray says of Camphor: "Spasmos solvit," and "Epilepticis bene multis opem fert" (l. c., pp. 485, 496); he even cites a case (*Lockeri Obs. Pract.*, p. 42), where an epilepsy of three years' standing had been cured by Camphor. That Camphor produces inflammations of the organs is as well known as that it disperses them. Barthez recommends it as an antiphlogistic in spreading inflammations: "In inflammationibus internis summo cum fructu propinari, quotidie videmus" (*Spielmanni Instit. Mat. Med.*, Argentor. 1774, p. 311). Dörffurt observes: "In general, Camphor is said to have been employed with great success in all inflammatory diseases where there is a quick and lively pulse, and the blood circulating with difficulty" (*Dissert. on Camphor*, Wittenb. and Zerbst, 1793, p. 211). On the other hand, Geoffroy mentions that Camphor disposes the blood to inflammation (vol. ii. p. 781). Murray (l. c., p. 370) relates that Carminati and Menghini found, on dissecting the animals destroyed by Camphor, that the membranes of the brain, the lungs, heart, vessels, and intestines were inflamed; while he himself adds, at p. 477: "Protractiori autem actione inflammat tam partes, in quarum immediato contactu est, quam alias remotiores;" but at p. 494, he says again: "Levat et eximie internas inflammationes." Pouteau calls Camphor a specific in all erysipelatous inflammations, and many other practitioners down to the present time agree with him (*Mélanges de Chir.*, p. 180). Vogt, however, presupposes that it is universally known how injurious Camphor cushions are on actively inflamed, erysipelatous parts; also in erysipelas accompanying wounds and ulcers. Horn, again, says that in some inflammations Camphor has, it is true, acted beneficially, but he says it must be borne in mind that most inflammations, whether with or without fever, depend upon a diminution of the vital activity (*Handb. d. Pract. Pharm.*, Berlin, 1805, p. 222). Supposing that to be really the case, why should bleedings then be ordered in the greater number of inflammations, which accords least of all with diminished vital activity? Stahl (*Materia Medica*, Dresden, 1744, vol. i. p. 78) has demonstrated that Camphor is a suppurative. The dissecting reports of Carminati, Menghini, and Orfila prove that it produces corrosions and gangrenous ulcers. P. T. Schneider, Paulus, and others expressly mention that it excites inflammation, mortification, and gangrene; yet what medicine has been more extolled for gangrenous tumours than Camphor? Camphor has been found to be an important remedy in inflammatory as well as nervous and typhoid fevers. In this respect, Murray says (l. c., p. 485): "Quamvis calidæ indolis sit, in quibusdam febribus tamen eminet," and (p. 492), "De inflammatoriis febribus præcipue sub ea pulsus velocitate vigoreque et stasi sanguinis, quæ tum obtinet, dubitari posset, si ratiociniis unice inhærere fas esset. Ast metum jam minuit explorata Camphoræ in inflammationibus externis discutiendis virtus." According to Fr. Home (*Clin. Vers. Trans.*, Leipsic, 1781, p. 40), one can expect no advantage from the use of Camphor (which renders very good services in diseases of an inflammatory kind) in nervous fevers, as being diseases of an opposite, so to say, anti-inflammatory nature; he therefore concludes Camphor would be injurious even in nervous fever. Of a contrary opinion are Stoll, Vogel, Reil, and many others. Friedländer calls, therefore, Camphor a Heros in malignant, putrid, and typhoid fevers. Jörg expresses himself thus, in his *Materein. Künf. Heilmitt.*, p. 271: "In consequence of the quality of irritating the brain, and causing accumulation of blood in it, Camphor has certainly often done great injury in typhus, when this has put on more the character of inflammation of the brain." It is true, Camphor excites apoplectic, soporous states, but it is also known to have been employed for removing the same. Hunnius cites a case of sopor at its highest pitch, cured by injections of Camphor into the median veins (*Hufeland's Journal*, vol. xxii. st. 4, p. 44). But G. A. Richter observes (l. c., p. 380): "Camphor must, generally speaking, be employed with some caution in apoplexy, as it operates almost narcotically in large doses." Here we have it distinctly stated that in large doses it produces, as it were, apoplexy; but when employed with caution, that is, in small doses, it brings about cure! Camphor is an acknowledged chief remedy in mania and melancholy; yet it has avowedly in many instances excited or aggravated both those forms of disease. Simmons effected the cure of a maniac with Camphor, after an aggravation of the state had been first induced by it. Cullen (*Mat. Med., trans. by Hahnemann*, Leipsic, 1790, vol. ii. p. 338) relates a case of madness (not of an asthenic kind) in which the cure was brought about by Camphor; and Hahnemann remarks thereupon that he had witnessed two similar cases, but that, in melancholic madness combined with general debility and sluggishness of the whole body, he had in several cases obtained no help from Camphor. "Adversus maniam fere specifici titulum obtinuit Camphora"—"affirmat tamen *Kinnear* quod saltem frigidis corporibus conveniat, calidis contra et plethoricis noceat et morbum omnino augeat" (*R. A. Vogel, Hist. Mat. Med.*, edit. nova, Francof. et Lips., 1764, p. 312). We read in Stahl (l. c., p. 79): "Among those who suffer from phrenitis, and rave, Camphor has been given with benefit." But Quarin says: "Sunt qui magnas doses non ferunt sine acceleratione nimia pulsus, congestionibus ad caput, convulsionibus et phrenitide lethali" (*Method. Medend., Febr.*, p. 57). According to Pinel, Esquirol, and others, Camphor is serviceable in certain kinds of mental disorder, and in others injurious. In Murray (l. c., p. 504) there is the following passage: " Non miror aliquos Camphora sumta in majorem furorem raptos, vel quietos ante jam repente delirasse vel convulsivos fuisse, prout ille æger, cujus Carminati meminuit, ex scabie retrogressa maniacus." Burserius von Kamtfeld advises Camphor to be applied where the sensibilitas nervea is diminished, and not where the irritabilitas is augmented; Friedländer observes thereupon: " But who does not know that in maniacis the sensibility of the whole body is diminished, being augmented in its principal seat, the brain. Were one to administer Camphor in this state, madmen would be driven into raving madness." T. Lenhard says: " It is hardly to be believed that medical men should be capable of such imbecility as to prescribe Camphor for patients in madness; by the use of Camphor these patients are only rendered more frantic, deranged, and melancholy" (*Dörffurt,* l. c., p. 232). According to Neümann (l. c., vol. iv. p. 451), it is perhaps in no variety of mania possible to suppress the malady so easily in its first commencement, as in the mania puerperalis that occasionally breaks out in child-bed, and that by means of Camphor. According to Kraus (*Philos. Pract. Pharmacol.*, Goett., 1831, p. 478), the recommendations of Camphor for cramps in child-bearing, for mania, particularly mania libidinosa, and for diseases of seminal irritation in general, as also for narcotism, particularly when proceeding from opium, are products of servile implicit faith. Siemerling observed after Camphor "intoxication of the second degree;" the phenomena that Camphor produces in the organism have an extraordinary analogy with those produced by spirituous liquors. Barkhausen (*Observations on Drunken Madness*, Bremen, 1828, p. 112) has nevertheless seen Camphor often used, and has himself used it, with benefit in delirium tremens. Quarin (l. c., p. 57) warns against too large doses of Camphor, as it, among other things, produces also "oculos torvos inflammatos." Murray (l. c., pp. 495, 523) praises the latter in inflammations of the eyes and eyelids; wherein many agree with him, and among others, Most (*Encyclop. Pocket Vocab. of Pract. Pharm.*, Rostock and Schwerin, 1841, p. 209), who advises the use of Camphor for "recent and old ophthalmia catarrhalis and rheumatica." According to Moreau, Camphor acts in ophthalmia militaris, alternately stimulating and calming, by exciting in the part it comes into contact with, warmth, redness, and such burning pain that the eye instantly swims in tears, and whereas the burning and tears are only transitory, the redness and irritation disperse, and the bulbus returns to its normal condition (*Annales d'Oculiste et Gynécologie*, vol. i. livr. 20, in *Schmidt's Annuary*, vol. xxviii. No. 1). "In otalgias," says Kraus (l. c., p. 479), "one can only expect aggravation from the customary putting of Camphor into the ears, which also generally proves to be the case." That Camphor induces salivation has been evidenced by the experiments of Vincenzo Menghini (*Comment. de Bononiens, Scient. et Art. Instit.*, p. 199); but that it removes salivation, particularly the mercurial, is also well known. Friedländer calls the specific virtue of Camphor against mercurial salivation, and strangury after cantharides, fictitious; and adds: "By the idea of *specific* there can be nothing else understood than the action of a substance on a formation of the body; now this action is at all times, by the organic laws of animal life, stimulation; consequently Camphor ought rather to augment than restrain the agencies of both the above substances; meanwhile, if such is the case, the phenomenon must then proceed from another healing principle of Camphor." The fact contested by Friedländer is established, and (as is partly evidenced by the above) the principle of homœopathy explains the incident. Camphor produces inflammatory irritation in the urinary organs. According to Scudery, Camphor causes strangury (*Annali Univers. di Med.*, 1829, Giug.); as also, according to Emmerich and Heberden, who observed in two cases, strangury after the use of Camphor. Yet Camphor has gained a great name for strangury, especially that which is produced by cantharides. Mason Good (*Study of Medicine*, 4th edit., Lond., 1834, vol. iv. p. 350) calls Camphor a diuretic and sedative, and that hence it has often been employed with great benefit in strangury, especially in that produced by cantharides. Rob. Willis (*Diseases of the Urinary System*) considers Camphor indispensable in inflammations from cantharides, and a principal remedy in rheumatic inflammations of the kidney. Home (*Clinical Exper., etc.*, p. 33) says of the antidotary virtue of Camphor against cantharidal strangury: "I should wish we could always guide ourselves by such sure experience in the art of pharmacy." On the other hand, Jörg (l. c., p. 269) opines, grounding on his experience: "Just as little is Camphor able to afford benefit in the inflammatory irritation of the uropoetic organs, which are produced by cantharides, whether used inwardly or outwardly." In Geoffroy (l. c., p. 779) we read the following: "It is the truth, and not to be denied, that there have been some people in whom the natural faculty has been weakened and stifled by too long a use of Camphor; and on the other hand, there are many who have had recourse to this resin for suppressing lustful desires, and have complained of having been, in consequence, much more tormented with those desires." According to Hoppe (*System of Pharm.*, Leipsic, 1837, vol. ii. p. 213), Camphor causes sensual pollutions, and strengthens considerably the urinary and generative organs, but when there is weakness and laxness, it removes the sensibility and irritability. Neümann (l. c., p. 156) observes: "Camphor is considered to act specifically on the diminution of the sexual power; nevertheless we read in the accounts of observers that they have tried it on themselves, and have found it to increase that power." (Compare this with *Murray*, l. c., p. 518.) Jörg (*Handb. d. Krankh. d. Weibes*, 2nd edit., Leipsic, 1821, p. 242) places Camphor almost on an equality with the chief stimulants, and says: "And further we know also now for certain that Camphor possesses no peculiar property of lowering the sexual desire, as several have believed, and as the vulgar still imagine; and therefore the utility of this medicine in the above-mentioned malady (nymphomania) is refuted. The case may, however, occur where Camphor does good service in nymphomania too; but this can only be when it bears the character of debility, and when the generative system is no longer so highly irritated." But if there still exists some irritation, and Camphor being at the same time so great a stimulant, will not then the existing irritation be yet heightened by the Camphor? and if it then nevertheless renders good services, does not that come to pass on the principle of homœopathy? Vogt (*Pharmacodyn.*, l. c., p. 509) recommends Camphor in diseases of the urinary and generative organs with the phenomenon of increased irritation of those parts. Hufeland (*Enchirid. Med.*, Berl., 1836, p. 282) commends the use of Camphor in nymphomania, satyriasis, and onanism: "it is," he says, "truly a specificum antaphrodisiacum, and I have seen even atrophy of the testicles arise from the continual internal and external exhibition of it." According to Selle also (*Medic. Clin.*, 5th edit., Berl., 1789, p. 606), Camphor, used frequently, weakens the generative faculty; hence it was formerly looked upon in monasteries as a so-called *means* of chastity. Joh. Chr. Stark (*Handb. z. Kennt. u. Heil. in N. Krankh.*, Jena, 1800, vol. ii. p. 129) assures that in lewdness much may be effected by Camphor remedies, among others. According to Friedländer, Camphor, "as is known," has no specific virtue against nymphomania. The notion that Camphor is capable of lowering the vitality of the sexual organs, and that it can hence directly benefit in diseases of those parts with increased sensibility, dates probably, according to Jörg (*Ma-*

terial., etc., p. 268), from the fabulous times of medicine, "out of which, it is true, we have at the present day not yet completely issued;" in which latter point, at least, he is without doubt perfectly right. The dissolvent virtue of Camphor has been in many quarters praised and proved; and yet Löseke says, in his *Materia Medica* (6th edit., 1790, p. 162): "It often causes indurations of the glands, particularly confirmed erysipelas; it expels the acrid matter which causes gout and pains in the limbs, from the parts that could stand the virulence thereof, into the vitals, and thereby often cuts short life with the greatest rapidity." And yet has not Camphor been, on the contrary, set forth as an excellent remedy in rheumatismus vagus? To all these controversies it remains to be added, that Camphor was combined with other remedies known to be prejudicial to its workings, and to stand in an antidotary relation to it, namely, with opium, mercury, cantharides, and saltpetre. As regards the latter, Scudery expressly observes that it diminishes the effect of Camphor (*Arch. Génér. de Méd.*, 1829, vol. xxvi. No. 9, p. 143). If this combination was made designedly, then let us hear what Schoene (*Pract. Pharm.*, Berl., 1815, vol. i. p. 117) says to it: "The union with weakening medicines, as saltpetre, etc., recommended in former times, must be considered a folly. Who is there capable of acting so absurdly, and thinking to combine two opposite remedies, when the action of the one nullifies the effect of the other? If the Camphor is thought to act too violently, it is better not to give it at all; but should it be considered necessary to administer it, one should then begin with the smallest dose, and one will be sure never to err. For children, one may divide the grain into several parts, being still assured of obtaining the genuine effect of one's remedy." This is the very thing Hahnemann taught, and had such a course been pursued long ago, the pharmacology of the 2000 years old science of medicine would now have been in a better state than is actually the case; genuine experience would have been gained, all hollow hypotheses banished, and the enormous injury would have been avoided which has been done in consequence of the ignorance of medicaments and the wholesale waste of them. Had Camphor always been administered in suitably small doses, there would have been no reason for complaining so manifoldly of aggravations of diseases, especially since it was had recourse to so surprisingly often in such phases of disease as had been seen to be produced by itself. Horn mentions (l. c., p. 224) that there is no medicament having so many and so frequent idiosyncratic obstacles throwing themselves in its way as Camphor, and he signifies thereby nothing other than homœopathic aggravations, which could only have been avoided by suitable small doses.

The foregoing comparison leads to the following conclusions:

1. The 2000 years-old science of medicine has no ground for being proud of its foundation in pharmacology, when it exhibits such a Babylonish confusion, such absolute contradictions, such partial, perverse notions and abstractions as have been evidenced, where the best observers are accused by others of deception and distortions of facts.

2. Camphor is a medicine which does all honour to homœopathy, since it has acquired the most reputation in those very diseases which it is of itself capable of producing in the greatest similarity, as the poisonings, dissecting reports, experiments on healthy and diseased organisms, and the cures and aggravations observed therein entirely prove.

3. It is the homœopathic physician alone who can possess the sufficient indication for the employment of medicaments, when the experiences made at the sick-bed and the positive symptoms coincide in so surprising a degree (as in Camphor), "where it is Nature that speaks, and not prejudices or the vagaries of hypotheses."

Description.—The Dryobalanops Camphora is a stately forest tree, growing to an immense height. The Camphor is found in masses in cavities of the wood of the trunk and large branches, but is so highly prized by the Chinese that, according to Christison, it seldom reaches this country, that which is found here being the product of the Laurus Camphora.* A single tree will yield from eleven to twenty-two pounds avoirdupois. The younger trees do not yield Camphor, but exude an oily substance when cut.

The precise age when this tree begins to yield Camphor is not known; but the young trees yield an oil which has many of the properties of Camphor. The natives have a peculiar mode of tapping the trees to discover if Camphor exists in the interior.

The trees are cut to the heart, about eighteen feet from the ground, until the Camphor is seen, and hundreds of trees may be mutilated before one is found containing sufficient quantity of Camphor to make it worth the labour of destroying so enormous a tree. It has been asserted, on excellent authority, that some of these trees in the island of Labuan have been estimated at 250 feet in height. When attained, it is felled and cut into pieces about six feet in length, which are again split, and the Camphor is found in the heart, occupying a space of the circumference of a man's arm. The mode of procuring the Camphor from the Laurus Camphora is as follows.

In Japan, the roots and wood of the tree (Laurus Camphora) are chopped up and boiled with water in an iron vessel, to which an earthen head containing straw is adapted, the Camphor sublimes and condenses on the straw.

In China, the chopped branches are steeped in water, and afterwards boiled until the Camphor begins to adhere to the stick used in stirring; the liquid is then strained, and, by standing, the Camphor concretes. Alternate layers of dry earth, finely powdered, and of this Camphor, are then placed in a copper basin, to which another inverted one is luted, and sublimation effected.

* This is not now the case; great quantities of Bornean Camphor now come to this country, and as it is the purest, is given here instead of the Laurus Camphora.

There are two kinds of Camphor (Camphora crudus) known in commerce—1, Dutch, or Japan Camphor, supposed to come from Batavia; and 2, ordinary Crude Camphor, imported from Singapore and Bombay, and is chiefly produced from the Island of Formosa.

Refined Camphor is met with in the form of large hemispherical or convex-concave cakes, perforated in the middle. It is translucent; has a crystalline, granular nature; a strong, peculiar, not disagreeable, aromatic odour; and an aromatic, bitter, afterwards cooling taste. It is solid at ordinary temperatures, soft, and somewhat tough, but may be easily powdered by the addition of a few drops of rectified spirit. It evaporates in the air at ordinary temperatures; but in closed vessels, exposed to light, sublimes and crystallizes on the sides of the bottle. It is combustible in the air, burning with a very sooty flame. It is lighter than water, its specific gravity being 0.9857. Water dissolves but a very small portion of it. Alcohol readily dissolves it, but if water is added to the solution, the Camphor is precipitated. Camphor is readily known by its odour, and it does not blacken in burning.

Geographical Distribution.—The Eastern Archipelago. In the forests of Borneo, Labuan, and Sumatra.

Physiological Effects.—*On Vegetables.*—Solutions of Camphor act in the same deleterious manner on plants as the volatile oils; they destroy the mobility of the contractile parts, without exciting them, and the vapour only is sufficient to destroy fleshy plants and ferns.

On Animals.—The vapour of Camphor proves injurious to *insects* (the tineæ which destroy wool excepted). To amphibials (frogs) the vapour proves hurtful, causing strange movements, hurried respirations, trembling, and stupor. To birds and mammals it is extremely injurious if given in too large doses. It produces tetanic spasms in dogs, with violent convulsions like epilepsy, followed by insensibility and death (*Orfila, Tox. Gén.*, vol. i.) Scudery, of Messina (*Annal. Univers. di Med.*, vol. xxxvi.

p. 102), confirms this, and remarks that the convulsions were attended with a singular kind of delirium, which made the animals run up and down, without apparent cause, as if they were maniacal. He also found that the urinary organs were affected generally, and for the most part with strangury.

On Man.—The symptoms it produces in over-doses on man have not been often observed; its effects are singularly uncertain, at one time producing most injurious consequences, at another, perfectly harmless. It is a narcotico-acrid poison; its narcotic effects were shown in the case of Mr. Alexander (*Experimental Essays*, p. 128, 1763), who, in the course of his experiments on his own person, was nearly killed by this poison. After having proved, by previous experiments, that a scruple did not affect, or cause any particular symptom, he swallowed two scruples, mixed with syrup of roses; in twenty minutes he became languid and listless; in an hour, giddy, confused, and forgetful; all objects quivered before his eyes, and a tumult of undigested ideas floated through his mind; at length he lost all consciousness, during which he was attacked by strong convulsive fits, and maniacal frenzy. These alarming symptoms were dispelled on Dr. Monro discovering the subject of his patient's experimental researches, by an emetic, but a variety of singularly mental affections continued for some time after. The emetic brought away all or nearly all the Camphor, which had been swallowed three hours before.

Dr. Erckhorn, of New Orleans, swallowed three drachms, in small doses, within three hours, the only result was, great heat, palpitation, hurried pulse, and a pleasant sense of intoxication; afterwards, moisture of the skin, followed by profound sleep for some hours, attended with excessive sweating; and lastly, great debility (*American Journal of Medical Science*).

It appears that its local action is that of an acrid. A piece of Camphor held in the mouth for half an hour caused the mucous lining to become red, hot, swollen, and painful; and it is probable that had the experiment been continued much longer, ulceration would have ensued.

Camphor in large doses causes disorder of the mental faculties, the external senses, and volition; the symptoms being lassitude, giddiness, confusion of ideas, disordered vision, noise in the ears, drowsiness, delirium or stupor, and convulsions. In its power of causing stupor, Camphor resembles opium, but differs from the latter in more frequently causing delirium and convulsions. Epilepsy also has been ascribed to the use of Camphor.

Camphor has peculiar antaphrodisiacal properties, the smell of it often producing this effect. "Camphora per nares castrat odore mares." When taken largely in coarse powder, it commonly occasions pain in the stomach, sickness, and vomiting, acting as an irritant; but when in a state of fine division, and dissolved, it excites narcotic symptoms, such as giddiness, staggering, obscurity of vision, confusion of ideas, and delirium.

Medical Uses (Homœopathic).—*Hahnemann's observations:* "Until the present time, physicians had used Camphor in ignorance of its real effects, more especially as they have usually prescribed it either mixed with other medicines, or to be taken at the same time with them; and, what is worse, during the perturbation of morbid symptoms. For what Alexander has observed of its *pure* effects amounts to nothing, and has been expressed only in general terms.

"The action of Camphor is perplexing and difficult to study, even in a healthy subject, because the primitive effects often alternate rapidly with vital reaction, so that in many cases it is hard to distinguish between the primary and consecutive effects.

"Camphor is not less puzzling and surprising as regards the results of its action, for it destroys the violent effects of a great many different vegetable remedies, as well as those of cantharides, and a variety of mineral and metallic substances. It must, therefore, exert a kind of general pathological action, to which we will not give a precise denomination, that we may not lose ourselves in the clouds, where our observations are no longer based upon experience, and we are liable to errors of imagination.

"As I have said, from experience, Camphor removes the too powerful effects of a large number of medicines, whether they have been given unsuitably or in too large doses, but this it commonly does only in virtue of its primitive action, and simply as a palliative. Therefore, when it is employed for this purpose, it must be repeated frequently, in small doses, every five or fifteen minutes; or if the necessity be urgent, every two or three minutes should be given a drop of the saturated alcoholic solution, the eighth part of a grain mixed with two drachms of pure water; or it may be as well to inhale the solution every few minutes. A grain of Camphor dissolved in eight drops of alcohol will unite with 400 grains of tepid water, and by shaking, a complete solution is obtained, notwithstanding the opinion of the authors of the *Materia Medica,* who assert that Camphor is insoluble in water.

"The rapidity with which the action of Camphor passes off, and its symptoms succeed each other, make it unfit for the cure of chronic complaints.

"As the inflammation of the skin called erysipelas (which spreads in rays of a clear, red tint, and disappears for the moment under the pressure of the finger) is only one symptom of disease, proceeding from internal causes, and as Camphor applied to the skin has somewhat of a similar effect, the local application of it may be useful in disorders that come on rapidly, accompanied by erysipelas, provided there is analogy between its symptoms and those of the complaint.

"In the Siberian influenza, Camphor given as soon as feverish heat takes place, acts only as a palliative, but is valuable, because it is a complaint of short duration. It is then given in frequent doses, gradually increased. It does not diminish the length of the disease, but greatly lessens its violence, and brings it to a close without danger. (A single weak dose of Nux vomica will often cure this complaint homœopathically, in a few hours.) When a large dose of Camphor causes danger, opium is the proper antidote, as Camphor is a powerful acid in cases of poisoning by opium; thus each of these two substances destroys the other. Is it not strange, after this, that we should so often find them together in the same prescription?"

Clinical Observations.—*Noack and Trinks:* Vertigo. Loss of consciousness and coldness of the body appear to be the primary symptoms of a dose of Camphor, and point to a diminished afflux of the blood to those parts which are distant from the heart; whereas the rush of blood to the head, heat of the head, etc., are symptoms denoting a reaction of the vital powers, just as forcibly as the former symptoms denoted their diminished action. Slight and recent inflammations which have come on suddenly may therefore be removed by the palliating, cooling effects of Camphor; old inflammations never. The continued use of Camphor will frequently induce obstinate ophthalmia, corresponding to the permanency inherent in the reaction of the organism. "I (Hahnemann) am not prepared to deny the homœopathicity of external applications of Camphor to inflamed eyes in acute cases; but I cannot advocate it, for the reason that I never use external applications in the treatment of ophthalmia."

According to Noack and Trinks, Camphor is, next to bromine, the most volatile remedial agent, and is remarkable for the rapidity with which its effects pass off, and its primary symptoms succeeded by the secondary. It is especially suitable when the sensibility of the nervous system is diminished or suspended; when the muscular fibre is affected with paralytic weakness; when the irritability of the organism, and especially that of the capillaries, are lessened. It is especially suitable to lax, bloated, and particularly rheumatic, catarrhal constitutions, and to the phlegmatic and melancholic temperament; to individuals with cold extremities, slow respiration, and languid pulse; to those affected by changes of weather, and who are advanced in age; and to those who have suffered by protracted illness. Camphor restores the susceptibility of the organism to medicinal substances, and ought to be replaced by other suitable remedies as soon as the vital energies have been restored. Camphor is the principal antidote to a number of vegetable medicinal agents. It has been advantageously employed in many diseases. Amongst others: Catarrhal affections. Epilepsy. Dropsical diseases. General and local asthenic inflammations, both acute and chronic. Passive inflammations, especially when of a rheumatic and erysipelatous character. It may be used as a preventive of a number of severe diseases, especially catarrhal, in the precursory stage, when a general uncomfortableness and chilliness announce the approach of a feverish condition. Typhus in the second stage. Asiatic cholera in the cold stage, with viscid sweat. According to Lobethal, Camphor is specific in the Asiatic cholera, as long as the body has a natural colour, even if the temperature of the body should be ever so low. In the stage of asphyxia, Hahnemann recommends Carbo veget. and Secale cornut., with the frequent use of ice-pills. Purpura senilis, with indications of gangrene in the toes. Delirium tremens. Headache, brought on by the feet getting wet, by catching cold, or by sudden change of temperature, with catarrhal affections of the organs of respiration. Mercurial ptyalism. Diarrhœa, with colicky pains (especially when cholera is epidemic), with symptoms of frequent chilliness, or a sensation as if cold air passed through the unnerved parts. Inflammatory irritation of the urinary organs. Influenza. Violent spasms of the chest, brought on by excessive emotions, etc.

Antidotes.—Spirit. nitr. dulc., coffee, and alcohol increase the effects of Camphor. Camphor increases the action of Nitre. According to Hahnemann's experience, Camphor is no antidote against the violent effects of Ignatia. Opium is an antidote to Camphor; and Camphor is a great preserver of life in cases of poisoning by Opium. Camphor is an antidote to a number of vegetable drugs, especially such as have a drastic effect, and cause vomiting and diarrhœa, paleness of the countenance, coldness of the extremities, and loss of consciousness. Camphor as an antidote, should be administered in frequently-repeated doses.

XV.

CANNABIS SATIVA.

Hemp.

SYNONYMS.—Cannabis sativa, *Linn.* Cannabis indica, *Lam.*

FOREIGN NAMES.—*Fr.:* Le Chanvre. *Germ.:* Die Hanf. *Dut.:* Bloemrut. *Ital.:* Canna. *Span.:* Caña. *Braz.:* Racua-canga. *Malab.:* Kalu-bab. *Arab.:* Kinnub.

Nat. Order, CANNABINACEÆ, *Lindl.;* URTICEÆ, *Juss.*—DIŒCIA, PENTANDRIA.

GEN. CHAR.—*Male—Calyx:* perianth five-cleft; segment oblong, acuminately obtuse, concave. *Corolla* none. *Stamens:* filaments five, capillary, very short; anthers oblong, four-cornered. *Female—Calyx:* perianth one-leafed, oblong, acuminate, opening longitudinally on one side, permanent. *Corolla* none. *Pistils:* germen very small; style two, very long; stigmas acute. *Pericarp:* the permanent calyx closely covering the seed. *Seed:* nut globular, depressed, two-valved.

SPEC. CHAR.—*Male: Calyx* five-cleft, *Corolla* none. *Female: Calyx* one-leafed, entire, opening on one side. *Corolla* none. *Style* two. *Nut* two-valved, within the closed calyx.

HISTORY.—Cannabis was well known to the ancients, but they did not seem to be aware of its narcotic properties. Herodotus designates it under Καννaβις ημερος, and states that the Thracians made a kind of cloth from it. The seeds were also thrown upon red-hot stones, and the perfumed vapour obtained in this manner used for a bath, which excited cries of exultation. Dr. Royle considers it to be the same as the Nepenthes of Homer, "the assuager of grief," given by Helen to Telemachus in

---

Fig. 1. The male plant. 2. The female. 3. Calyx and stamens of male plant. 4. A separate anther. 5. Female flower. 6. The seed.

Plate XV.

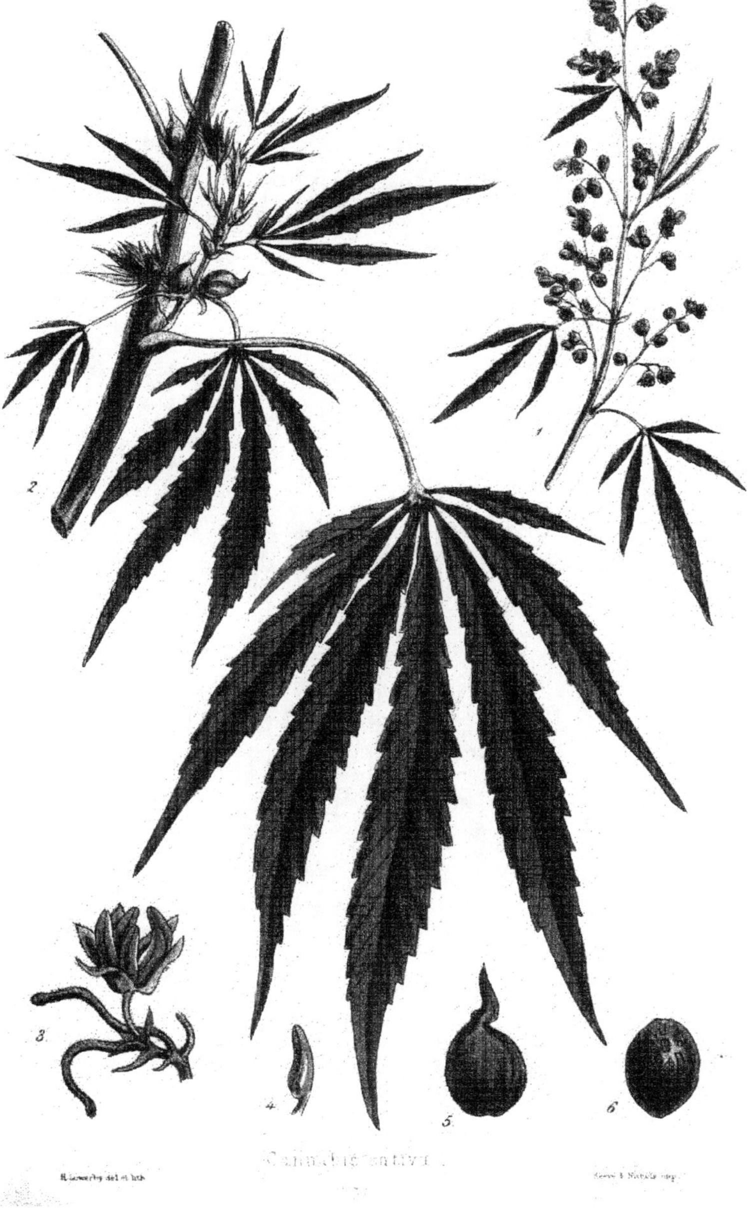

Cannabis sativa.

H. Sowerby del et lith

Reeve & Nichols imp.

honour of Menelaus. Helen is said to have received the plant from a woman of Egyptian Thebes. Galen (*De Simpl.*, lib. vii.) made use of it as a remedy for toothache. Dioscorides recommends it in the form of cataplasms to soothe inflammations and discuss tumours. Pliny mentions it under the name of Cannabis. Paulus Ægineta says the fruit is carminative and desiccative, and the juice of it when green useful for pain and obstructions in the ears. The Arabian physicians Avicenna and Serapion describe it with great accuracy. It is known in India under a variety of vulgar names, such as, "grass of faqueers," "leaf of delusion," "increaser of pleasure," "exciter of desire," "cementer of friendship," "laughter-mover." It was used as an intoxicating substance in very early times both in Asia and Egypt.

Cannabis* has been employed in allopathic practice chiefly in the following cases: Rheumatism. Jaundice. Worms. Catarrhs. Tetanus traumaticus (Cann. ind.) Hydrophobia (Cann. ind.) Weariness of pedestrians. Podagra. Burns (the oil out of the seed, hemp-seed oil?) Measles and smallpox. Erysipelas. Cephalalgia. Rheumatic affections of the eyes. Pains in the ears. Cholera (Cann. ind.) Diarrhœa. Bloody evacuations. Dysentery. Inflammation and suppuration of the bowels. Diseases and painful complaints of the urinary organs. Cystodynia. Urodialysis senilis. Strangury from inflammation of the urinary ducts, for instance, in gonorrhœa or from stones in the bladder and kidneys. (Willis recommends Cannabis and belladonna for obviating the attacks during the passage of the calculi through the ureter.) Gonorrhœa; for the suppressing of it, and for restoring it when suppressed. Want of sexual inclination. Sterility. Excessive sexual irritation. Nymphomania. Suppressed lochial discharge. Leucorrhœa. Catarrhal hoarseness. Hooping-cough (Huland). Dry, irritating cough. Swelling of the breasts.

* Noack and Trinks' *Handbuch für Hom. Arzneimittellehre.*

Medical men and authors of the old school entertain varied views of the action of Hemp. It is described as an astringent and palliative by some; then stimulant and narcotic by others; now an aphrodisiac, then an antaphrodisiac, and so on. It was thought to escape out of this dilemma by dividing those properties between the herb and the seed; but this distinction could not hold good, and observers soon began to doubt. Hence Dierbach, while placing Hemp-seed among the medicamina sedantia seu mulcentia, adds, that the latter does indeed possess something of the volatile, narcotic principle of the herb, as may be inferred from its effect (*Synops. Mat. Med.*, 1842, 2nd part, p. 825). Hope places Hemp in the list of the nervina excitantia and narcotica pura. Arnemann calls the infusion of the leaves a mild, narcotic stimulant (*Pract. Arzneimitt.*, 6th edit., Goett., 1819, p. 333). According to Kraus, linaria is a violently excitatory narcotic, inspiring blood-thirstiness, the Haschisch of the Orientals (*Philos. Pract. Heilmittel.*, Goett., 1831, p. 513). Linnæus designates the Vis cannabis sativa as a narcotica, phantastica, dementans, anodyna, repellens. Sachs says of Hemp: "It decidedly has no especial medicamental efficacy;" that it may be dispensed with, and is only a weak substitute, or rather no substitute at all (!) of opium. (*Handb. d. Pract. Heilmittel.*, Koenigsberg, 1830, vol. i. p. 708). Most puts a mark of interrogation to this conjecture, but affirms that Hemp has not the injurious effects of opium, and is also a harmless aphrodisiac (*Encyclop. Handb. d. Wort. Pract. Heilmittel.*, Rostock and Schwerin, 1841, p. 214). When such contradictions are to be met with in the "practical" pharmacologies, when the caprice existing in the management of the material is exposed to light so unconstrainedly, might one not fancy that the designation of "practical" is a pendant to the Lucus a non lucendo? Kosteletzky says, with good reason, that Hemp belongs to those remedies which deserve all regard, but which have still not been sufficiently investigated in the special mode of action (*Algem. Med. Pharm. Flora*, Prague,

1833, vol. ii. p. 404). For certain cases of disease Hemp has been recommended as a specific: if it be really such, it is so homœopathically. Lonitzer says: "Hemp-water is good for headache proceeding from heat;" and a little further on he says: "the Hemp herb increases headache in those who deal in it" (*Herbarium*, Ulm, 1705). "Si quis in Cannabino agello diu sederit," observes Lindenstolp; "aut dormiverit, non solum inde luscus evadit, sed etiam vertiginosa et ebrius, quod mihi ipsi puero sæpius contigit" (*Liber Venenis*, edit. Stentzel, Francof. et Lips., 1739, p. 541). Junker confirms the same with the words: "Intus summum ventriculum et caput gravat" (*Compend. Mat. Med.*, Hal., 1760, p. 94). Zorn states that Hemp cumbers the head; and in another page that it alleviates headache vi narcotica, and .conduces to sleep (*Botanologia Medica*, Berl., 1714, pp. 160, 161). Schroeder opines: "Some bind the emulsion, prepared from the seed, round the head; but they do wrong, for it causes silliness" (*Arzneischatz.*, Nuremberg, 1693, p. 909). According to Chardin (*Voyage en Perse*, Amsterd., 1711, tom. iv. p. 208), pedestrian travellers in Persia, when exhausted, invigorate themselves with a beverage prepared from Hemp; but how great the paralytic debility and exhaustion is which Hemp itself causes, appears clearly from Hahnemann's *Register of Experiments*, as also from Wibmer's *Report*. Herrmann observes of Hemp: "Orgasmum genituræ maxime compescit et propterea tanquam antaphrodisiacum laudatur" (*Cynos. Mat. Med.*, Argentor., 1710, p. 178). Valentini says that Hemp-seeds are especially given against excessive concupiscence, and that the emulsion may be prescribed for females having furor uterinus (*Herbarium*, Francfort, 1719, p. 567). Olearius, again, affirms exactly the reverse in the words: "Persæ existimant veneris desideria inde cieri et simul sterilitatem produci" (*Travels in the East*, p. 529, in *Murray*). Hence occurs the following passage in Schroeder: "The seed hinders the birth-seed, if often used; whereas the

Persians take this seed, as also the leaves, under the name of Bengi, to arouse the venerem thereby." Zorn also combines both controversies, and confirms the former assertion by several citations, and the latter by the energetic rendering into German of the unbecoming name of Bengi and Kidibengi, by which term also those were designated who made use of Hemp for the purpose of arousing sexual desire. In the same way, Zorn mentions that Hemp possesses the property of fattening, and that it therefore makes the hens who eat of it prolific, so that they lay the more eggs. Geoffroy, however, expresses himself on the same matter thus: "Matthiolus writes, he has found out that Hemp-seeds render hens prolific in eggs. But, then, as Lobel observes, it afterwards makes them unfruitful by reason of the frequent nourishment it affords them" (*Dissert. Mat. Med.*, trans. from the Latin, Leipsic, 1761, vol. iii. p. 389). Hemp is everywhere considered a specific against gonorrhœa; but it is also certain that Hemp produces gonorrhœa, as is proved by the results of experiments put together by Hahnemann.

Here and there one finds the assurance given, that the Hemp-seed emulsion deserves the preference in the irritated state of the urinary organs, only because it does not constipate so easily as other emulsions. If it really has this effect, it would then appear that there are specific relations lying at the foundation of this, which may be reduced to the fundamental law of homœopathy. For was not Hemp formerly employed in diarrhœas, and up to the present day in India for the cholera, precisely on account of its constipating properties. And Wibmer observed on himself so obstinate a constipation and total atony of the intestinal canal, after taking the alcoholic tincture of this herb, that even strong purgatives in large doses were ineffectual for clearing out the existing impurities and flatulencies. In Zorn we read: "Quidam ex hoc semine emulsiones parant et in febribus commendant, vimque alexipharmacum ei tribuunt." Wibmer, again, was thrown into such a fever with congestions towards the head, through the tincture of Hemp, that he had to lose twelve ounces of blood, and to apply leeches and cold fomentations round the head. Morgagni observed tonical spasms, which he attributes to the agency of Hemp, and even a sort of catalepsy has been seen to arise from it. Matthiolus (*in Diosc.*, lib. iii. c. 188), again, says of the Italian women: "Decoctum in morbo comitiali pueris exhibent." And Shaughnessy found, in a case of tetanus, appearing after a moxa, that the tincture of the resinous extract of Hemp produced unexpected results, and that in all cases of tetanus the immediate effect was relaxation of the muscles (*Lancet*, Oct. 1840). According to Neuhold, Hemp causes cataract (*Act. Nat. Cur.*, vol. iii. p. 150). And in Schmidt's *Jahr B. d. Ges. in und Aust. Med.*, vol. xxviii. p. 209, there is mention made of the medicamental virtues of Hemp in cataracta lenticularis.

Its general effects on man are, alleviation of any pain, remarkable increase of appetite, unequivocal aphrodisia, and great mental cheerfulness. Its more violent effects are, delirium of a peculiar kind, and cataleptic condition. Mr. Donovan found it had great power in reducing the most intense neuralgic pains. Mr. Miller considers its virtues consist in the power of controlling inordinate muscular spasms. Dale says (*Pharmacologia*, 3rd edit., 1737), "Semen genitale imminuit usu, continuato, tussi sputulatam, ictero substernuit et caput vaporibus reflet." Murray (*Mat. Med.*, p. 613): "In gonorrhœa recente, infusam seminum horum Theæ potum plurimum virtutis habet ad inflammationem et ardorem urethræ qui istius indicum prœbet, superandum quum oleosa et mucilaginosa seminum, existaverum et leniter anodyna, natura stimulum optime retundet et irritum reddat et aquæ tepidæ. Connubium eundem cum lobo eluat. Valet hoc, non de gonnorrhœa, venerea, sed et arthritica, ut ipse casu, singulari expertus sum."

DESCRIPTION.—Cannabis Sativa is an annual. *Stem* from six to eight feet high or more. *Leaves* petioled, stipulate, digitate, opposite. *Leaflets* five to seven, lanceolate, acuminate, serrated; outer one the smallest. *Male flowers* in small, loose racemes or spikes, at the ends of the stem or branches. *Female flowers,* axillary, solitary, very small; both kinds sometimes occur on the same plant, but always one of them very few in proportion to the other. All the old authors ignorantly call the male flowers female, and *vice versâ*. The leaves in India are chiefly employed for making Bhang and Jubzees, of which the intoxicating powers are well known; but a peculiar substance is collected by the natives pressing the upper part of the young plant between their hands, and then scraping off the secretion which adheres; this is known under the name of Chenus, and is so esteemed by Asiatics that they prefer it to wine or opium. According to Dr. Royle, the Cannabis Sativa and Indica are the same plant, only differing in the effects of its preparation from the difference of climate.

GEOGRAPHICAL DISTRIBUTION.—Herodotus mentions the Cannabis as a Scythian plant. Beerberstein met with it in the Caucasus. Dr. Royle describes it as a plant of Persian origin, and subjected to the severest cold in winter, and the greatest heat in summer. It is well known in Bokhara, Persia, and the Himalayas. Father Hamelin found it in the Illinois in North America. Cultivated in Russia and the north of Europe extensively, for commercial purposes; also in France and the south of Italy. It is observed that a difference exists between plants grown in the plains and those on the mountains, and also when grown thickly together. The peculiar principle of the plant is found wanting or very much weakened in those plants which are grown in a very moist climate and thickly together.

Cannabis Indica, according to Dr. Royle, only a variety of the C. Sativa. Leaves alternate. Stem nearly cylindrical, smaller, more branched, and harder than the preceding species. Leaves all constantly alternate. Leaflets linear, lanceolate, very sharp-pointed; in the male plants five to seven, in the females commonly but three, on a petiole, near the top, entirely simple.

A native of the East Indies. Its hard stem and thin bark render it incapable of being wrought into filaments, and spun like common hemp; it has a strong smell, like that of tobacco. The Indians make of its bark and the expressed juice of its leaves and seeds a liquor, which has an intoxicating quality; and if they wish to produce a stronger effect, they either chew or smoke its dried leaves, mingled with tobacco. A little nutmeg, cloves, camphor, and opium, mixed with its juice, form the composition which the Indians call *Majek*, and which, according to Clusius, is the same as the Malack of the Turks.

PARTS USED IN MEDICINE, AND MODE OF PREPARATION.—The Flowers. To make the homœopathic preparation, the flowering tops of both male and female plants are gathered, and the juice expressed from them, and which is mixed with equal parts of alcohol. Some recommend the female flowers only, because these exhale, during their flowering, a strong and intoxicating odour, whilst the male plants are completely inodorous.

MEDICAL USES (HOMŒOPATHIC).—*Hahnemann's observations:* "Up to the present time, the seeds of the Cannabis have been employed generally only in the form of emulsions and decoctions. Formerly some physicians, viz., Dodoens, Sylvius, and Herliz, found it useful in some kinds of jaundice. The beneficial effects of Cannabis in inflammations of the urinary organs is entirely owing to its homœopathic action, from its having the power to produce an analogous morbid condition in those organs of healthy persons, an effect which has never been doubted by any who have experimented with this medicine. As to the herb itself, it is only employed as a popular remedy. It has been also used by the Persians and others to soothe the fatigue arising from over-walking, as Chardin informs us; this effect is equally homœopathic. We can also employ the Cannabis with great success, in more attenuated doses, in different diseases of the chest, and organs of sense, etc. I usually employ the juice of this plant, mixed with equal parts of alcohol, and not more attenuated, the dose a small part of a drop; but the thirtieth attenuation developes the medicinal virtues of this plant in a much greater degree."

CLINICAL OBSERVATIONS.—*Noack and Trinks*: Cannabis may be employed in the following affections. Hysterical conditions. Convulsions. Tetanus. Acne. Gutta rosacea. Dullness of the mental faculties. Mania. Melancholia. Gonorrhœa. Scrofulous ophthalmia, with excrescences of the lamellæ of the cornea. Specks on the cornea remaining after scrofulous ophthalmia. Old specks and ulcers of the cornea. Incipient leucoma. Pannus. Traumatic cataract. Chronic vomiting. Gastralgia. Induration of the liver. Colic. Ascites. Constipation, with retention of urine. Phymosis. Acute and chronic affections of the urinary organs. Nephritis. Cystitis. Gravel (in alternation with Rosa canina). Dysuria. Hæmaturia. Impotence. Abortus. Sterility. Leucorrhœa. Periodical asthma. Pneumonia, brought on by violent exertion. Short, oppressed breathing, owing rather to aching than stitching pains. Cough, with tough, green expectoration. Palpitation of the heart, with anguish; sympathetic affection of the large vessels. Cramp in the calves of the legs.

ANTIDOTES.—To large doses, a few glasses of very sour Lemonade: to small doses, Camphor.

Plate XVI.

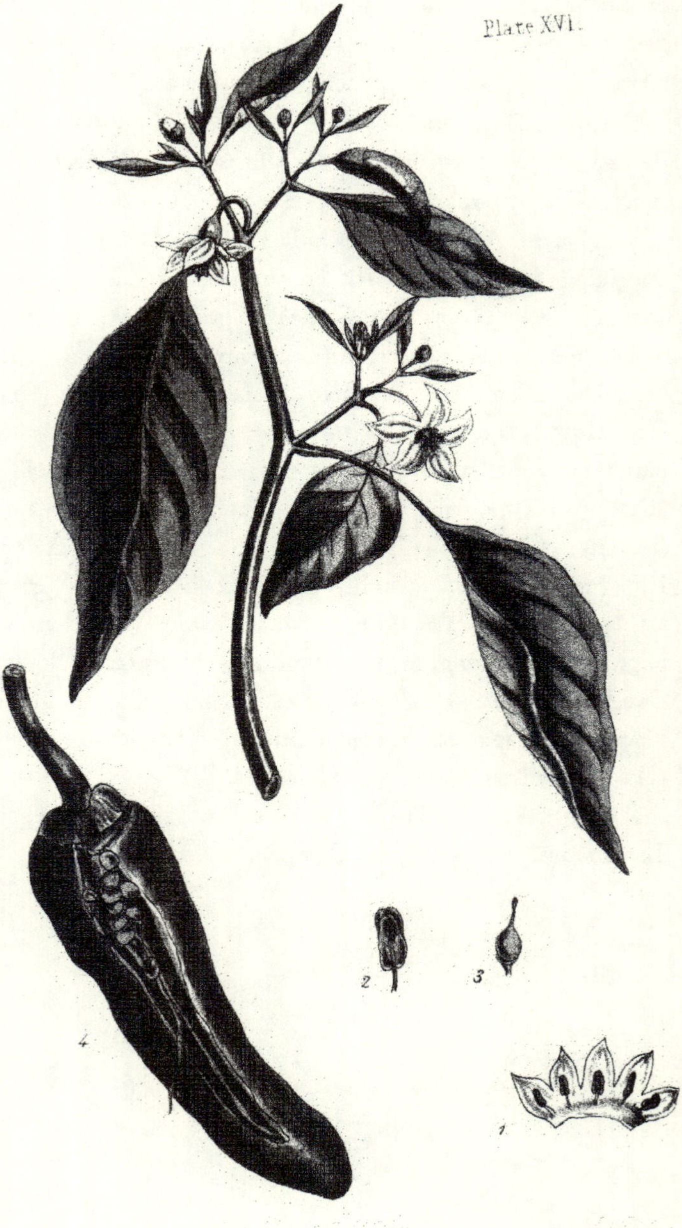

Capsicum annuum.

Reeve & Nichols imp.

L.W. del. H. Sowerby, lith.

XVI.

CAPSICUM ANNUUM.

*Capsicum or Chilly.**

SYNONYMS.—Piper Indicum vulgatissimum, *Bauh. Πιν.*, 162. Vallia. Capo. Molago, *Rheed. Mal.*, ii. tab. 35.

FOREIGN NAMES.—*Fr.:* Poivre d'Inde, Poivre d'Espagne. *Germ.:* Spanischer Pfeffer. *Ital.:* Pepe di Guinea, Peperone. *Span.:* Pimentero annua, Pimiento da Indias. *Port.:* Pimentaa da India. *Dut.:* Spaansche Peper. *Swed.* and *Dan.:* Spansh Pepper. *Russ.:* Perets strulschkovoi. *Arab.:* Fetfel-achmar. *Pers.:* Fulfili-surkh. *Tam.:* Mollagai.

Nat. Order, SOLANEÆ, *Juss.;* LURIDÆ, *Linn.*—PENTANDRIA, MONOYGNIA.

GEN. CHAR.—*Calyx* five-toothed, persistent. *Corolla* rotate, five-cleft. *Anthers* converging, two cells, dehiscing by fissures. *Berry* juiceless. papery, hollow, two to four-celled, many-seeded, naked. *Seeds* naked.
SPEC. CHAR.—*Peduncles* solitary. *Fruit* oblong, pendulous. *Petioles* smooth. *Stem* herbaceous.

HISTORY.—Sprengel (*Hist. Rei Herb.*, vol. i. p. 201) makes the Piperitis or Siliquastrum of Pliny the Capsicum annuum of Linnæus, but Roxburgh doubts this plant being a native of Asia, and considers it exclusively a native of South America, in which case it must have been unknown to the ancients. It has been generally used only as a condiment. As a medi-

---

Fig. 1. The flower cut open, to show the stamens. 2. A separate stamen. 3. The germens and pistil. 4. The seed-vessel.

* Capsicum is derived either from κάπτω, to bite, on account of the biting heat of the seed and pericarp, or from capsa, a chest, from the form and structure of the pericarp.

cine under the allopathic school, it has been chiefly valuable as a local stimulant to the mouth and throat in cynanche maligna and scarlatina anginosa; also in the dyspepsia of drunkards, as a gastric stimulant. It has also been used in cholera, low fevers, intermittents, and dropsies. Dr. Wright (*Med. Facts and Observ.*) extols it as a remedy against the black vomit in fevers of tropical climates.

Description.—Capsicum annuum is an herbaceous annual, from one to three feet high. *Peduncles* solitary. *Fruit* oblong. *Stem* nearly simple, round, a little striated, smooth. *Leaves* egg-shaped, acuminate, entire, petioled, placed in no regular order. *Petioles* long, flexible, generally smooth, but sometimes, as well as the stem, a little pubescent. *Flowers* white, lateral. *Peduncles* long. *Fruit* smooth and shining; very variable in its form and colour—in some instances long, straight, acute; in others, short, thick, and obtuse; in some, red in colour; in others, yellow, and sometimes both colours on the same plant. The dried fruit sold by druggists is flat, more or less shrivelled, blunt, or pointed at one end, while the calyx and stalk are usually attached at the other end. The length of the berry is two to three inches; the breadth one-half to three quarters of an inch; the colour yellowish or reddish-brown; the taste hot and pungent; the epidermis is tough and leathery; the seeds are flattened and whitish.

Geographical Distribution.—According to most authorities, a native of the East and West Indies; according to Roxburgh, a doubtful native of these countries, and originally from South America. It has, however, been used as a condiment in all Eastern countries from time immemorial.

Parts used in Medicine, and Mode of Preparation.—The Capsules and Grains, at maturity, which are powdered, and then infused in twenty parts of alcohol, or the three first attenuations are made by trituration.

Physiological Effects.—Capsicum belongs to the acrid aromatics. Applied to the skin it is a rubefacient and vesicant.

Swallowed in small doses, it creates a sensation of warmth in the stomach; in larger doses, it produces a glow over the body, excites thirst, quickens the pulse, and exerts a stimulating influence over the urino-genital organs; in excessive doses, it will produce vomiting, purging, abdominal pains, and gastric inflammation, according to Vogt (*Pharmakodyn*, Bd. ii. s. 581); and a paralysed and altered condition of the nervous influence, an affection of the head, drunkenness, and giddiness, according to Richter (*Ausf. Arzneim.*, Bd. ii. s. 173). A strong preparation of Cayenne pepper has been known to occasion death (*Lond. Med. Gazette*, vol. xxiii.)

HOMŒOPATHIC USES.—The following are Hahnemann's observations on this plant. "In the two Indies, where the Capsicum (Piper Indicum seu Hispanicum) is indigenous, it is employed only as a condiment. This custom has been imitated in England, France, Italy, and Germany, where they often substitute the Cayenne pepper (Capsicum baccatum), which is still more powerful. The object is to stimulate the palate, and to increase the appetite beyond the bounds prescribed by Nature, and thus undermine and destroy the health. This powerful substance has been but little employed as a medicine. However, Bergius informs us that he has cured several chronic intermittent fevers with three doses of Capsicum, each dose of two grains, but he did not administer it alone; for the old hereditary sin of the ancient *régime* of medicine (of mixing drugs) suggested to him to unite with it laurel-leaves, in the proportion of twenty to three. He does not describe either the intermittent fevers that he has cured, according to the totality of the symptoms, but is satisfied in giving the name, as is the general custom amongst the practitioners of the old school, so that it is impossible to come to any conclusion from the cases he relates. The homœopathic physician proceeds in a manner more certain in the cures he undertakes with the Capsicum. After having studied the pure symptoms that this substance produces on persons in health, he only applies it to those natural diseases in which the symptoms have the greatest possible analogy.

"Those persons in whom the fibre is rigid, are less susceptible to the action of Capsicum annuum."

CLINICAL OBSERVATIONS.—*Noack and Trinks:* Capsicum has been found useful in intermittent fevers. Nostalgia, with redness of the cheeks and sleeplessness. Hysteric cephalalgia and megrim, Prosopalgia. Stomacace. Angina aphthosa. Heartburn in pregnant females. Spasm of the stomach. Tympanitis and flatulence. Colica flatulenta. Diarrhœa and dysentery. Burning and blind hæmorrhoids. Tenesmus of the bladder. Gonorrhœa. Asthma flatulenta. Influenza, etc. etc.

CHARACTERISTIC PECULIARITIES.—Most of the symptoms occur in the evening, and at night. Aggravation of the symptoms by contact, open air, and cold temperature.

ANTIDOTES.—Camphor. Capsicum antidotes Caladium and China.

Plate XVII.

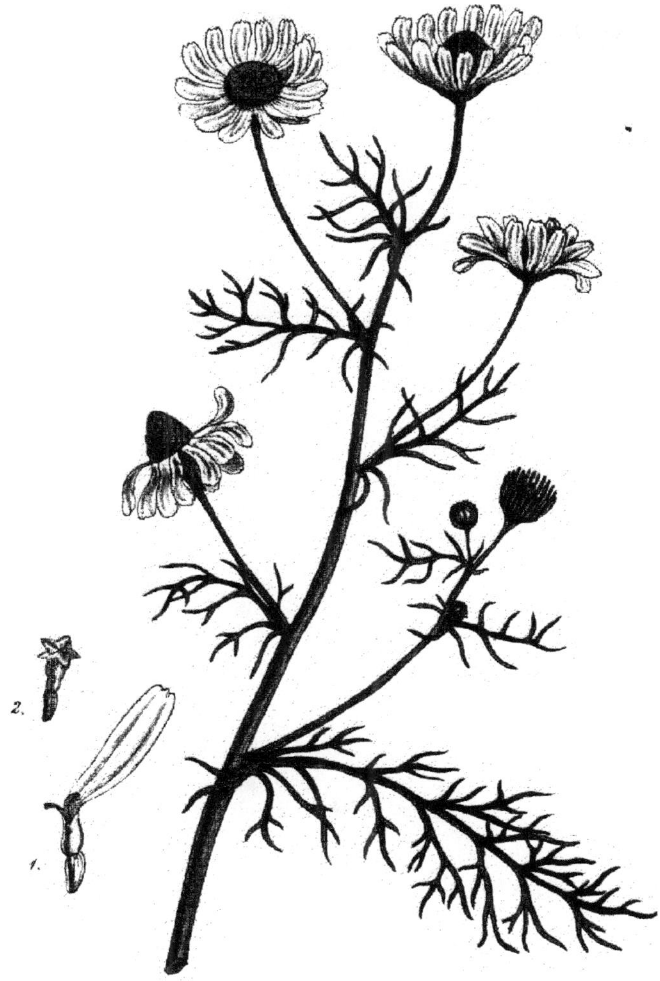

Chamomilla (Matricaria Chamomilla.)

Reeve & Nichols imp

XVII.

MATRICARIA CHAMOMILLA.*

Wild Chamomile, Bitter Chamomile, Corn Fever-few.

SYNONYMS.—Chamæmelum vulgare. Chamomilla nostras. Lucanthemum.

FOREIGN NAMES.—*Fr.:* Camomille commun. *Germ.:* Feld-kamille, Halmercherz, Matricaire, Mutter-kraut. *Dut.:* Maartel. *Ital.:* Matricaria. *Span.:* Matricaria. *Dan.:* Modcrut. *Pol.:* Maruna-ziele.

GEN. CHAR.—*Involucrum* slightly convex, closely imbricated, with several oblong, nearly equal, membranous-edged scales. *Corolla* compound, radiant. *Florets* of the conical disk numerous, perfect, tubular, with five equal, spreading segments. *Florets* of the ray numerous, strap-shaped, spreading, or reflexed, blunt, with three terminal teeth. *Filaments* in the tubular florets only hair-like, very short. *Anthers* in a cylindrical tube. *Germen* in all the florets inversely egg-shaped, angular. *Style* thread-shaped, not prominent. *Stigmas* spreading, blunt. *Seed-vessel* none, but the unchanged, expanding calyx. *Seed* in all the florets inversely egg-shaped, angular, without any border or crown. *Receptacle* naked, almost perfectly cylindrical, hollow.

SPEC. CHAR.—*Leaves* smooth, twice-pinnatifid; the segments very narrow, strap-shaped. *Involucrum* nearly flat; its scales bluntish.

HISTORY.—The Matricaria Chamomilla has been generally passed over as a medicinal plant, the Matricaria Parthenium and Anthemis nobilis being preferred. It is, however, mentioned by Dioscorides under the name of Lucanthemum. Hippocrates extols the virtues of Παρθενιον, which is, according to Sprengel, Matricaria; but Sibthorp considers it to be the Matri-

---

Fig. 1. Floret of the ray. 2. Floret of the disk.

* The name is derived from matrix, from its supposed specific virtues on that organ.

caria Parthenium. It is not mentioned by the Arabian physicians. The Finlanders use an infusion of it in consumptive cases. Gerarde says that "it is neither good for meat or medicine, but is commended against the infirmities of the mother, seeing all stinking things are good against those diseases. It also causeth blisters on the hands of weeders and reapers." Culpeper, in his *Complete English Physician*, gives the following curious account: "Venus commands this herb, and has commended it to succour her sisters, and to be a general strengthener of wombs, and remedy such infirmities as a careless midwife has there caused." It is also, according to the same author, a special remedy against opium when taken too liberally.

DESCRIPTION.—This common annual flowers from May to August. The *root* is rather large, woody, and fibrous. *Stem* upright, from twelve to thirteen inches high, much branched, solid; somewhat angular, striated, smooth, leafy. *Leaves* alternate, sessile, clasping the stem, smooth, deep green; the upper ones simply, the rest doubly pinnatifid (wing-cleft); the segments strap-shaped, very narrow, and minutely pointed. *Flowers* numerous, terminal, solitary, on striated, naked peduncles. *Scales of the involucrum* somewhat dilated outwards, rounded, and bluntish. *Florets of the ray* white, reflexed at night, elliptic, oblong, with three teeth. *Disk* conical, very prominent, of numerous yellow florets. *Receptacle* oblong, nearly cylindrical, naked, dotted. *Seeds* angular, oblique, of a pale brown colour, quite destitute of any crown or border. According to the observations of Linnæus, cows, goats, and sheep eat it; horses and swine refuse it. A blue essential oil is distilled from the flowers.

There are three species of this plant: the Matricaria Chamomilla, the M. Parthenium, and the M. suaveolens; all of which have the same or nearly the same properties. This genus differs from the *Pyrethrum*, in having no crown or pappus attached to the seed.

GEOGRAPHICAL DISTRIBUTION.—Most parts of Europe.

LOCALITIES.—Cornfields, waste grounds, and by the roadside.

PARTS USED IN MEDICINE, AND MODE OF PREPARATION.—The Whole Plant, gathered when in flower. The mother tincture is obtained by expressing the juice of the whole plant, gathered fresh, and mixing it with twenty parts of alcohol. The attenuations are prepared in the same manner as given under Aconite.

MEDICAL USES (HOMŒOPATHIC).—*Hahnemann's observations :* " This has been extensively used as a family medicine in complaints of all kinds, chiefly those that develope themselves rapidly. But physicians have held it too much in contempt, not considering it as a medicine, but only a popular remedy, and allowing their patients to use it, in conjunction with their prescriptions, in large handfuls, for infusions, tea, etc., as external applications ; while, at the same time, they were giving internal medicines, as if it were always a safe and salutary thing, never injurious, or at least quite unimportant. Also they have occasionally substituted for it Anthemis nobilis, the Roman Chamomilla, not considering that it is quite a different species, possessing different properties.

" Thus we may see how far physicians have been blinded with regard to a plant belonging to a class of powerful medicines, when it was their duty to acquaint themselves thoroughly with its properties ; not only that they might themselves make a wise and proper use of it, but put a stop to the general abuse, pointing out when good effects might be expected from it, and, on the other hand, when it should be avoided.

" But physicians have hitherto not fulfilled this duty ; they have rather rivalled the public in prescribing or permitting the use of this powerful remedy, in all cases, without distinction, and in doses of all degrees.

" Yet it requires but a little ray of sense to perceive that no medicine in the world can be proper for all diseases; that each one has its circle of benefit strictly defined, beyond which every powerful medicine, like Chamomilla, must of course exercise injurious action, in proportion to its energy; and, therefore, to avoid quackery, the physician ought to know previously when Chamomilla may be useful and when prejudicial, as also how to proportion the doses, that they may be neither too powerful nor too weak.

"If we did not know, by a thousand other proofs, how inconceivably blind the science of medicine called practical has been for centuries, and how it has emulated the public in being unreasonable, it would be sufficient to examine impartially how it has acted with reference to so powerful an agent as Chamomilla.

"In fact, no medicine, however polychrest it may be, can be useful and salutary in a tenth part of the existing diseases; neither can this prerogative belong to Chamomilla. But, admitting what is impossible, let us suppose that it can cure a tenth part of the diseases of which mankind is susceptible, is it not clear that, if it is employed universally, it must be injurious to the other nine-tenths? Is it right to purchase success in one case, to the injury of the other nine? What do you mean by injurious effects? says the common practitioner; I see none that depend upon Chamomilla. Certainly, I reply; so long as you are ignorant of the effects so powerful a medicine is capable of producing in a healthy person, you cannot perceive it to be the source of the mischiefs that are caused by the manner in which you employ it. These evils you consider to belong to the complaint itself, and attribute them to the malignity of that complaint; and thus you deceive yourself, while you are doing harm to your poor patients. But cast your eyes upon the glass I hold up to you; read the catalogue of symptoms belonging to Chamomilla; and then, if you fall back into your daily sin, if you put no limit to your habitual use of this plant, see how many among the apparent symptoms will be attributable to those belonging to Chamomilla, and judge of the distress and pain that will be caused to the sick in the abuse of this substance in those cases in which it is not suitable, and when given in large doses."

Clinical Observations.—*Noack and Trinks:* Chamomilla is suitable to venous bilious constitutions and to the choleric temperament. It is suitable to an irritable condition of the nervous system and excessive sensitiveness to pain. All evil effects of moral emotions. The consequences of anger, jealousy, and vexation; especially when producing violent spasms of the chest and throat. Different affections of infants. The screaming of infants when lasting for hours, etc. Fainting and weaknesses of hysteric females. Catarrhal affections with or without fever. Inflammatory swelling and induration of the glands. Catarrhal fever. Fever brought on by teething. Diarrhœa of infants. Angina tonsillaris. Gastric and bilious affections. Cramps in the calves of the legs, etc., etc.

According to Hahnemann, a very small dose of Chamomilla seems very much to lessen the excessive sensitiveness to pain, and the effects it produces on the mind. For this reason, it relieves many of the morbid symptoms produced by excessive use of coffee and narcotic substances; and is, on the other hand, less beneficial to those who remain patient and composed under their sufferings.

Antidotes.—Coffea. Ignatia. Pulsatilla. Aconite, when Chamomilla produces dragging and drawing pain, relieved by movement. Coffea removes many of the unpleasant symptoms produced by Chamomilla, when the patient has not been in the habit of taking it. Chamomilla equally destroys the symptoms of Coffea; but if the latter has been taken habitually, it is of no use, and also when the symptoms correspond to Nux Vomica.

XVIII.

CINCHONA OFFICINALIS.

Peruvian Bark.

SYNONYMS.—Cinchona corona. Cinchona cinerea. Cinchona flava. Cinchona cordifolla. Cinchona lancifolia. Cinchona rubra. Cinchona oblongifolia.

FOREIGN NAMES.—*Fr.:* Quinquina. *Ital.:* China-china. *Span.* and *Port.:* Guina. *Germ.:* China. *Dut.:* China wast. *Swed.:* Kina bark, Kinkina bark. *Dan.:* Kina, Kina bark. *Russ.:* Chinaia korka.

Nat. Order, RUBIACEÆ.—PENTANDRIA, MONOGYNIA.

GEN. CHAR.—*Calyx* five-toothed. *Corolla* hypocrateriform, with a five-parted limb, valvate in æstivation. *Anthers* linear, inserted within the tube, and not projecting, except in a very slight degree. *Capsule* splitting through the dissepiments into two cocci, open at the commissure, and crowned by the calyx. *Seeds* girted by a membranous lacerated wing (*Lindley*).

HISTORY.—The history of the discovery of Cinchona is not accurately known. It was first introduced into Europe as a medicine about the middle of the seventeenth century by the Jesuits at Rome, who received it from their brethren in Peru; hence it was called Jesuits' bark, Pulvis patrum, Pulvis Cardinalis de Lugo. Its medicinal effects were certainly unknown to the natives of South America, although many fabulous stories have been handed down to us as to the first mode by which its virtues as a febrifuge were discovered. For example, Condamini relates that the lions of South America, suffering from ague, were cured by eating the bark of a certain tree. Geoffroy gives an account of Indians affected with this malady being cured by drinking at a

Plate XVIII.

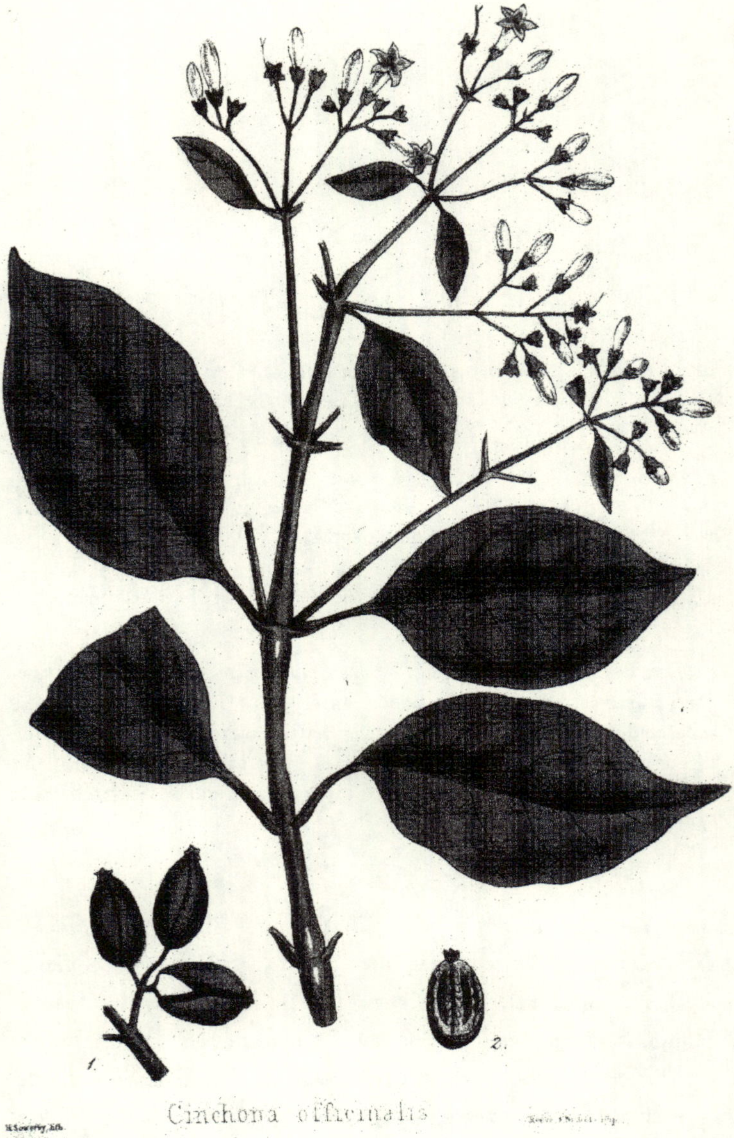

H.Sowerby, lith.

Cinchona officinalis

fountain in which some of the bark of this tree had fallen. He also relates that it was first made known to the Spaniards by a native Indian, grateful for saving his life. Humboldt and Bonpland, and other travellers, however, found the natives of the neighbourhood of Loxa, where the tree grows in great profusion, totally ignorant of its medicinal virtues; and Humboldt tells us of an old tradition, that the Jesuits, having accidentally discovered the bitterness of the bark, used it as an infusion in tertian ague, and in this manner became acquainted with its valuable properties: this he thinks a much less improbable tradition than that which ascribes its discovery to either lions or Indians. It was introduced into Europe in 1632, although the first authentic cure seems to have been that of the Countess of Chinchon, wife of the Viceroy of Peru, in 1640; it hence acquired the name of Cinchona bark and Pulvis Cometiæ. It seems that the Jesuits kept the secret of their wonderful febrifuge for many years, until it was discovered by an English physician, Sir Robert Talbot, who practised in Paris in 1679; he cured Colbert, the Prince of Condé, and the Dauphin of ague, and then sold his secret to Louis XIV., for £1,600 and an annuity of £80 per annum. It was of such value in his time, that it was sold for £5 per ounce. It is one of the specifics of the old school of medicine, and it is a curious fact, that its first introduction was most vehemently opposed by the medical profession. Its specific action in intermittent fevers is well known. It has also been used by the allopathic school, under certain circumstances, in continued inflammatory fevers. In rheumatism and in scrofulous inflammation of the eye. In diseases characterised by atony and debility. In chronic affections of the alimentary canal. In passive hemorrhages and profuse mucous discharges. In cachectic diseases, and as a topical astringent.

Independent of its medicinal virtues, to the homœopathist this medicine has an additional interest, as it is to the peculiar effects it produced on Hahnemann, whilst translating Cullen's

Materia Medica, we are indebted for the discovery of the homœopathic law.

DESCRIPTION.—The whole species are either tall shrubs or considerable forest trees, commonly evergreen and of great beauty, both in foliage and in flower. In consequence of the excessive demand for their bark, they seldom attain full growth. Lindley enumerates twenty-six species, of which twenty-one are well known.

GEOGRAPHICAL DISTRIBUTION. — South America: in the vicinity of Loxa, on the Peruvian frontier of Colombia; Santa Fé de Bogota; from the forests of Huanuco, in Peru, ten degrees south of the line; from the neighbourhood of Apolobamba and La Paz, in Bolivia, or Upper Peru, between five and eight degrees still farther south; in the elevated valleys of the Andes, from 1,200 to 10,000 feet above the level of the sea.

The best bark is produced from trees growing on a dry rocky soil. The bark is collected from May till November, by natives, who are called from this occupation, Cascarilleros. The trees are sometimes cut down for the purpose, but often the bark is stripped from the trees as they stand. The first process is the best, because if the trees are cut down, new shoots speedily spring up, and become in their turn fit for peeling in six or seven years. On stripping the trees, the whole bark, comprising the epidermis, rete-mucosum, cortex, and liber, is removed. The drying is commonly conducted, not in the woods where it is collected, but at the nearest inhabited spot, and great care is observed in the process, as the commercial value of the bark depends upon the brightness of its colour internally, and likewise on the epidermis being uninjured and covered with the lichens which are naturally attached to it. So indiscriminate and reckless was the destruction of this valuable tree, that the Bolivian government found it necessary in 1838 to issue an edict, prohibiting its collection for five years (*Christison.*)

PARTS USED IN MEDICINE, AND MODE OF PREPARATION.—

The Bark of the Crown, or Loxa Cinchona, or of the Cinchona flava, or Regia. The three first preparations are made by trituration, or by infusing the powder with twenty parts of alcohol. This latter is not to be recommended. The best Cinchona bark is known by the following properties.

1. The Crown bark consists entirely of quills, simple or double, straight or nearly so, from six to fifteen inches long, varying in diameter from the size of a crow-quill to that of the thumb, or somewhat larger, and in thickness from the thirtieth to the sixth of an inch. The epidermis is always entire; the external surface is crowded with fine longitudinal furrows, and crossed with transverse fissures; except in the finest quills, it presents various tints of grey, inclining sometimes to liver-brown, and it is generally covered irregularly with minute white lichens, which give it here and there the appearance of silver filagree.

2. The Yellow bark (Cinchona flava) is composed partly of quills, partly of flat pieces. The quills, called in Peru, Calisaya acolada, are generally from nine to fifteen inches long, from one to two inches in diameter, and from an eighth to a third of an inch in thickness; a few, however, are considerably smaller and thinner, but fine quills are never seen like those which form a considerable proportion of crown bark and grey bark; they are generally single and clothed with epidermis. They are much traversed externally by longitudinal wrinkles and transverse fissures, commencing very rough, and in colour greyish-brown, mottled with large greyish-white patches, from adhering lichens. The inner surface is smooth, longitudinally fibrous, clean, and of a yellower cinnamon-brown than the crown bark. The transverse fracture is close, but fibrous and splintery, and the fibres break under trituration into minute sharp spiculæ, which irritate the skin; the taste and odour are as in crown bark, but stronger. The flat pieces, or Calisaya plancha of the Peruvians, sometimes retain their epidermis, but are more commonly striped. Both present all the qualities of the quilled variety, except that

the striped pieces have externally the cinnamon-brown colour of their inner surface, and are free of cracks and wrinkles. They are from eight to eighteen inches long, between a line and half an inch in thickness, and from one to four inches in breadth (*Christison, Disp.*, p. 323).

PHYSIOLOGICAL EFFECTS.—*On Animals.* Dr. Freind (*Comment.*, c. xiv.) states that an ounce and a half of a strong decoction of bark, injected into the jugular vein of a dog, caused violent palpitation of the heart and frequent spasms; half an ounce more produced tetanus and death.

On Man.—The topical effects are astringent or slightly irritant; the constitutional effects are principally manifested by the disordered condition of the vascular and cerebro-spinal systems. In some conditions of the system, Cinchona operates as an irritant or stimulant. Pereira (*Elements of Materia Medica, art. Cinchona*, p. 1091) has the following observations: "If a man in a state of perfect health take a small dose of bark, no obvious effects are produced, or perhaps a little thirst, with some slight disorder of the stomach, or a temporary excitement of the stomach, may be brought on. If the dose be increased, the alimentary canal becomes disordered (indicated by the nausea, vomiting, loss of appetite, thirst, and constipation, or even purging); a febrile state of the system is set up, manifested by the excitement of the vascular system and dry tongue, and the cerebro-spinal system becomes disordered, as is shown by the throbbing headache and giddiness."

MEDICAL USES (HOMŒOPATHIC).—*Hahnemann's observations:* "Next to Opium, China is, of all medicines, that which has been most abused, to the great injury of mankind. It was not only held to be incapable of doing harm, but esteemed the most safe and efficacious of remedies in almost all diseases, especially where there was debility, and it was often given for weeks and months together, in strong doses, repeated several times a day.

"This is evidently proceeding on a false principle, and justifies the reproach I have so frequently cast upon medical practitioners, of seeking in previously-formed opinions, in hypotheses founded on fancy, in theoretical propositions, and in casual effects, that, which in an experimental science should be sought in unbiassed trials, and observations made with extreme care.

"I propose these last means, in order to avoid conjecture and traditional opinions that have not passed through the ordeal of experience; and, with regard to China, I have proved that although it is a certain remedy in many cases, it nevertheless causes in persons in health morbid symptoms, frequently very violent, and of long duration.

"This is sufficient to refute the received opinion that China is never injurious, and perfectly innocent, and that it acts only as a remedy.

"It is not less certain, agreeably to its morbid effects on persons in good health, that its frequent failure, when used by common practitioners, and the aggravation caused by repeated strong doses in many diseases, which are at length rendered incurable by it, are owing entirely to the mischievous mistake of giving it in cases to which it is not applicable, and in large doses; and this is always gratuitously ascribed to aggravation of the natural disease taking place of itself, and not the fault of the physician.

"1. Quinine is one of the most powerful vegetable medicines, when it is employed against a disease to which it is really applicable, and when the subject is severely attacked by that disease. I find that a single drop of the tincture, so much diluted as to contain only the quadrillionth part of the essence of Quinine, is often too strong, but always powerful enough to perform all that this medicine can effect in such a case, and it is very seldom that the patient requires a second dose. Long experience, based on the closest observation, has led me to reduce the dose to this extent, and it has clearly proved to me that even the highest dilutions exercise a more powerful action than is required.

"Thus I have proceeded, diminishing by degrees, till I should reach the point of attenuation sufficient to produce a complete cure, without acting so strongly as to retard it.

"2. A very small dose of China acts but for a very short time, scarcely more than two hours; but the powerful doses commonly given, act for whole weeks, unless vomiting or diarrhœa relieve the system. By this we may judge how far the ordinary practice is justifiable of prescribing immense doses of Quinine, often repeated several times in the day.

"3. If the homœopathic law be true, and its truth cannot be denied, since it is founded in Nature itself,—if medicines can only cure such diseases as are composed of symptoms analogous to those they excite in a healthy person,—we shall find, by studying the symptoms produced by Quinine, that it really pertains to but few cases, and also, that its exceedingly powerful action often enables a single small dose to effect an almost miraculous cure.

"By cure, I understand re-establishment of health, not impaired by any consecutive complaints. Do medical men attach to this word any other sense unknown to me? · For instance, do they say that an intermittent fever is cured, when it has been suppressed by Quinine, in a case not analogous to it?

"I know that all maladies of a regular type, and almost all intermittents, even those to which China is not analogous, are suppressed and silenced by the over-mastering influence of this medicine, in immense and often-repeated doses. But are the unfortunate patients by this means really restored to health? Has not the remedy, by not sympathising with the existing disease, merely transformed it into another (though it does not return by distinct and regular fits), more continued and less apparent? True, the patient can no longer complain that his paroxysms recur at fixed intervals; but observe the long train of sufferings, bodily and mental, caused by the remedy, to which death itself, in some instances, were a blessing.

"Is this health? I confess it is not an intermittent fever, but no one can affirm that it is really health. It is another disease, excited by Quinine, which was more potent than the intermittent, and without which it could not have been beaten down and suspended. If, in some instances, the constitution throws off this new disease after many weeks, the intermittent fever, which was only suspended, reappears in a more severe form, because the organism has been so much injured by the treatment it has undergone.

"If the China is long continued, to prevent the return of the intermittent according to received opinions, then a chronic Quinine disease is established.

"This is the nature of the greater part of the alleged cures effected by Quinine; because our practitioners do not know in what cases this medicine is really appropriate. In the suppression or suspension of the primitive disorder, by exciting a more powerful Quinine disease, they behold only the obstinacy of the former, the development of its symptoms, and its inherent malignity, because they are ignorant of its true source, and do not consider it a fictitious disease, such as it really is.

"The study of the symptoms of Quinine in healthy persons can alone open the perception of those who are not deaf to the voice of conscience, and who seek to benefit their fellow-creatures. But what is least excusable, is the abuse of Quinine, in all cases of debility, as is practised and esteemed rational by the prevalent school.

"As all diseases are followed by weakness, and may by allopathic treatment be brought to the point of total exhaustion, there are scarcely any in which attempts have not been made to fortify the strength by large doses of Quinine, either as infusions, decoctions, extract, electuary, or in powder. It is lavishly used for weeks and months as the chief blessing of the invalid.

"If the tables of mortality could speak, they would terrify us by the recital of the mischiefs caused by this abuse. Nor should we be less shocked, if we could see the list of those condemned for the remainder of their lives to the torments of asthma, leuco-phlegmasia, and jaundice, to spasmodic affections, organic lesions, diseases of the bowels, and wasting fevers.

"I appeal to the good sense of practitioners. How can they thus indiscriminately prescribe Quinine in all cases accompanied by debility? How can they expect to give strength to any one whose disease is unsubdued? Have they ever known a man recover quickly by proper means, without seeing his strength return of itself, as his complaint disappeared? But if weakness can only cease by the cure of the complaint, how absurd to attempt to remove it, without removing its cause! that is to say, by giving wine and bark to an invalid under the influence of disease. To be able to cure all weakness, Quinine must be the universal medicine; but sad experience proves that it is not such, for the symptoms it excites also prove that it possesses the character of a remedy, or really curative properties, in but a few cases.

"It is true that, upon first taking Quinine, it revives for a short time the powers of an invalid, under the most formidable illness. He raises himself in his bed, as if by enchantment; he wishes to get up and dress himself; his voice is stronger; his manner firm; he tries to walk, and is eager for food. But a close observer will perceive in this an unnatural excitement. After a few hours the disease gains power anew, and frequently death approaches with redoubled speed.

"The suspicious strength that the patient feels for a short time is always followed by bad effects, unless in cases where Quinine is the true remedy. Then we shall perceive the disease and the weakness cease together; but this is not a common case, because there are but few diseases that Quinine is capable of curing promptly, durably, and absolutely. In all other cases it is pernicious, in proportion to its great medicinal power. In fact, it is *a rule without exception, that all medicines that fail to cure, because they are not properly adapted to the complaint in question, do harm, according to their potency and the largeness of the doses.*

"It is therefore necessary for medical men to study effects upon healthy persons, and see the changes produced upon them, before they attempt to cure disease and debility by an agent so exceedingly powerful. They should acquaint themselves with the various forms of Quinine disease, before they can determine in what cases it is the fitting remedy; for it is only such as resemble its own entire symptoms, that can be cured by it. In not following this rule, we stray from the right road, and do more harm than good.

"But when we make a conscientious investigation, and do not allow ourselves to be guided by theories, by deceptive names of diseases, and uncertain authorities, when we find this substance to be the true remedy, that which is really and perfectly adapted to the case in question, then Quinine imparts true strength. It fortifies, because it cures; for it is only a frame freed from disease that can regain its powers; they cannot be infused into it by decoctions of wine and bark.

"Under some circumstances, debility is the disease itself, then Quinine gives real strength, because it heals. This happens when the affection depends upon causes of exhaustion. Then almost all the other symptoms coincide with China; in another case, if no other disease exists increasing that loss of the humours, etc., this debility, becoming a disease, yields to one or two weak doses, provided one is careful at the same time to enforce upon the patient a suitable way of living, nourishing regimen, pure air, amusement, etc. Then small doses are as beneficial as large ones, repeatedly taken, are prejudicial.

"The well-known value of Quinine in cases of weakness caused by the abundant loss of various humours, has tended to put medical practitioners upon a system most universally adopted.

"This method consists in *creating* weakness, by the abstraction of humours, under the idea of causing the offending matter to be more easily expelled. When such treatment, especially that based upon aperients, has continued some time, not only the irritation of the intestinal canal has created a disease that suspends the former one until, if acute, it has reached its termination, but a state of weakness has been produced in which Quinine is really efficacious. But no one is aware at what a fatal price this cure is obtained.

"Thus, among other things, spring tertian fevers, which, if left to themselves, would last some weeks, require upon this system treatment for months; at the end of which the patient rejoices that his life has been spared, while a few days would have sufficed for the cure of his first disease. Hence the rule so often inculcated, not to give Quinine, in intermittent fever, until the body has been thoroughly cleared from all morbific matters, or, what is the same thing, until the intestinal disease produced by art has exceeded the natural term of duration of the fever; so that weakness alone remains to contend with, against which Quinine is naturally successful, after the patient has endured long sufferings.

"This was and is still called, in many instances, acting in a methodical and rational way. It is as much so as would be robbing the widow and the orphan to enrich the poor-box.

"Quinine, having for its first consequence an aperient effect, will be found for that reason very useful in certain cases of diarrhœa, provided the patient has no other symptoms in opposition to it.

"In studying cases of moist external gangrene, one may perceive, in the general habit of the patient, morbid symptoms resembling those of Quinine, which explains why Peruvian bark is so valuable in such circumstances.

"I have sometimes seen pains, which a mere touch or the least movement increased to intensity, and which, as described by the sufferer, greatly resembled those caused by Quinine, yield at once and finally to a little dose of diluted tincture, although the attacks had often recurred; the evil was cured homœopathically, and health restored as by enchantment. No other medicine in the world could have produced such an effect, because no other is capable of causing this symptom.

"Quinine is seldom effectual, unless it disturbs the rest of the patient at night, as it does that of persons in health who make trial of it.

"There are some cases of suppuration in the lungs, but few in number, principally such as are accompanied by shooting pains in the breast, excited or increased by external pressure, that have been cured by Quinine, under the condition of resemblance in other symptoms. Then one or two weak doses, separated by a long interval, have produced the cure.

"There are also some few cases of jaundice resembling the symptoms of Quinine. These yield as by magic to one, or at most two doses of the tincture, and health is completely restored.

"An intermittent fever must bear a very close resemblance to the Quinine symptoms, for this medicine to be the true remedy; in which case the disease is conquered by a single dose. But it is best to give it immediately after an attack, before nature has had time to prepare the next. Whenever physicians aim, by large doses, to cut short a fever to which it is not appropriate, they give it just before the attack—the period when that violence, so much to be dreaded in its after-results, produces the most certainly the effect expected from it.

"Quinine makes a permanent cure of an intermittent marsh fever only if the patient can change the air during the treatment, and until his strength is restored. If he remain in the marshy effluvia, the cause of his illness continues to act upon him, and the remedy, though repeated, produces no more effect. In the same manner, the complaints caused by the abuse of coffee yield readily to the proper remedy, but reappear from time to time, if that beverage be not discontinued.

"But how can we reconcile the extraordinary manner in which Quinine has been employed, with the idea of substituting other drugs for this substance, which differs so decidedly from all other medicines, by the way in which it modifies the health of a person, and the energy with which it acts upon him? How can we expect to find a succedaneum for Quinine, that is, to meet, among substances differing so greatly from it, with one possessing the same virtues? Every species,—animal, vegetable, or mineral,—is it not a distinct being or substance that cannot be confounded with any other, even in external appearance? Was there ever a man so shortsighted as to mistake the Peruvian bark for a willow-tree, or an ash for a horse-chestnut?—trees that have so little resemblance to each other. These distinctions apply to *one* sense alone; how must they be multiplied by using all, and still more, when the various substances are tested by trying their effects on persons in health?

" I acknowledge that substances that have been proposed as substitutes for Quinine, from the lofty ash to the humble lichen, from arsenic to sal ammoniac, have all suppressed intermittent fevers. But observers have stated, in speaking of them, that each has frequently succeeded when Quinine has failed, or done harm. Is it not clear that these fevers did not resemble each other? Had they been homœopathic to Quinine, it would have cured them, and no other medicine could have done so.

It is not only in the bitterness, the astringency, the aroma of Quinine, but in its whole substance that the indivisible and dynamic property of modifying the state of health resides; in regard to which, it differs from every other known medicine.

Each of the medicinal substances that have been boasted of against intermittent fevers, exercise upon mankind, by the laws of nature, a special action peculiar to itself.

The Author of all has appointed that each medicine should differ in proportion from all others, that the diversity of modes of action should suffice to meet all the symptoms of the innumerable diseases to which mankind is subject.

If every febrifuge, while it failed in some cases, has really cured others, as I grant, in instances where it has been used singly, it must have been when the disease was appropriate to it alone, and different from that which another has cured. Consequently, those fevers which are cured by different remedies must be different from each other, as well as the remedies themselves, which cannot therefore be considered equivalent, or capable of taking place of each other.

"Nature is far more various in the properties with which she has endowed medicines, than the compilers of Materia Medica have imagined. Also, she is infinitely more varied in the diversities she causes in the human system, than pathologists are aware of in the few dozen forms of diseases, of which even they cannot make a faithful picture.

"It would signify little that in mixing, as they do, Quinine and Iron together, physicians produce a mixture of disagreeable appearance and taste, which is like ink; but they must be told that the result is a substance, possessing neither the virtues of bark nor of iron. This is because iron sometimes acts as an antidote in cases where Quinine has been injurious; while Quinine has put a stop to effects caused by iron wrongly given.

"Iron, however, can only destroy a part of the hurtful properties of Quinine, such as have analogy to the symptoms caused by the former in a healthy person.

"After long treatment, in which large doses of Quinine have been given, many inconveniences often remain, which require other medicines. Very often, these Quinine diseases are carried to such a degree of exasperation, that it is difficult to free the sufferer from them, and snatch him from death. In such cases, ipecacuanha, more frequently arnica, and sometimes belladonna are given, according to the nature of the symptoms. Veratrum album is suitable, when Quinine has caused chilliness of the body, with cold sweats, provided there is also accordance between the symptoms of the disease and those of the medicine."

Clinical Observations.—*Noack and Trinks:* The general action of China results in a state of asthenia. Exhaustion of the vital powers of the whole organism, or of single parts, organs, and systems, accompanied by excessive sensitiveness and irritability of the nerves, or with relaxation of the solids. Deficiency of animal heat. Disposition to passive hemorrhage, from every orifice of the system, and decomposition of the organic matter. Diseases with periodical type point to China. China is particularly suitable for debility, occasioned by a great loss of animal fluids, particularly after excessive and frequently repeated venesections, and after hemorrhage (in this case, also Aur. ?); after exhausting cathartics and purgatives (it will therefore, frequently be found useful in acute affections which have been treated in old-school fashion). In galactorrhœa after long nursing, which is frequently attended with anæmia, œdema of the feet, emaciation; after excessive loss of the fluids, profuse sweat; ptyalism, suppuration; in diarrhœa, arising from weakness and atony of the digestive apparatus; in lienteria, arising from a similar cause; after long-continued sitting up at night; after heavy, acute diseases; in affections resulting from the continuance of immoderate passions, mental exertions, and want of sleep. In all such cases, some of the following symptoms are generally present: excessive sensitiveness of the whole nervous system; debility, exhaustion, intolerance of noise; extreme anxiety and apprehensiveness; hypochondria; paralysis; singing, ringing, and roaring in the ears, paleness of countenance; swoons; sweat after the slightest exercise, particularly in the nape of the neck, and back, chest, and thighs; restless night's sleep, disturbed by frightful fancies and dreams. Atrophy. Asthenic passive inflammations. Rheumatic affections. Hæmorrhoidal sufferings. Arthritic affections. Hydrargyrosis. Dry and humid gangrene. Fevers. Rheumatic fevers. Asiatic cholera. Slow fevers. Intermittent fevers. Chilliness; short chilliness, without thirst; chilliness, followed by heat; thirst, succeeded by chilliness; chilliness, without thirst; internal heat and external coldness; heat, with burning thirst. Bleeding of the nose. Nervous and rheumatic prosopalgia.

Gastric derangement. Gastric and bilious affections. Gastralgia and cardialgia. Tympanitis. Bilious diarrhœa. Yellowish diarrhœa. Diarrhœa passing off without being aware of it. Amenorrhœa. Long-lasting lochial discharge. Leucorrhœa. Hæmoptysis. Pleuritis. Pneumonia. Palpitation of the heart. Acute articular rheumatism, etc.

ANTIDOTES.—To small doses, Arsenicum. Arnica. Belladonna. Calcarea. Capsicum. Carbo vegetabilis. Cina. Ferrum. Ipecacuanha. Mercurius. Natrum. Nux vomica. Pulsatilla. Sepia. Sulphur, and Veratrum. Selenium aggravates the pains caused by China.

XIX.

CICUTA VIROSA.

Poisonous Cowbane, Water Cowbane, Long-leaved Water Hemlock.

SYNONYMS.—Cicuta aquatica, *Murray, Bergius, Wepfer*. Sium alterum olusatri facie, *Lobel, Ray*. Sium erucæ folio, *Bauh.* Πιν. Sium majus angustifolium, *Park, Hall, Flor. Dan.* Cicuta virosa, *Huds. Flor. Ang., Engl. Bot.*

FOREIGN NAMES.—*Fr.:* Cigue vireuse, Cicutaire vénéneuse, Cigue d'eau. *Germ.:* Der Wütherich. *Dut.:* Water-scheerling. *Ital.:* Cicuta virosa. *Port.:* Cegude. *Dan.:* Vand skarntyde. *Russ.:* Omeg.

Nat. Order, UMBELLIFERÆ.—PENTANDRIA, DIGYNIA.

GEN. CHAR.—*Flowers* uniform, perfect, and nearly regular. *Calyx* five-toothed, somewhat leafy margin. *Corolla* of five inversely heart-shaped petals, with an inflexed point. *Filaments* five, thread-shaped, spreading, about as long as the corolla. *Anthers* roundish. *Germen* inferior, hemispherical, compressed, ribbed. *Styles* two, thread-shaped, short, upright, scarcely tumid at the base; subsequently elongated, spreading, and permanent. *Stigmas* blunt, almost capitate. *Floral receptacle* depressed, withering. *Fruit* roundish, contracted at the sides. Double *carpels*, with five flattish, equal ribs, of which the two lateral ones form a margin. *Channels* (interstices) with single *vittæ*, which fills them even in a dried state, but then less elevated than the ribs. *Commissure* (juncture, or point of union) furnished with two *vittæ*, under a loose membrane. *Carpophore*, (receptacle of the fruit) two-parted, transverse section. *Seed* nearly round. *Universal involucrum* of few leaves, or wanting; *partial*, of many leaves. *Flowers* white.

SPEC. CHAR.—*Trunk* of *root* hollow, divided into cells by transverse dissepiments; fibres disposed in whorled fascicles. *Leaves* twice ternate. *Segments* spear-shaped, serrated. *Umbels* opposite the leaves, and terminal (*Baxter*).

Fig. 1. The flower. 2. Bract. 3. Calyx. 4. Germen, calyx, and pistils, all magnified.

Plate XX

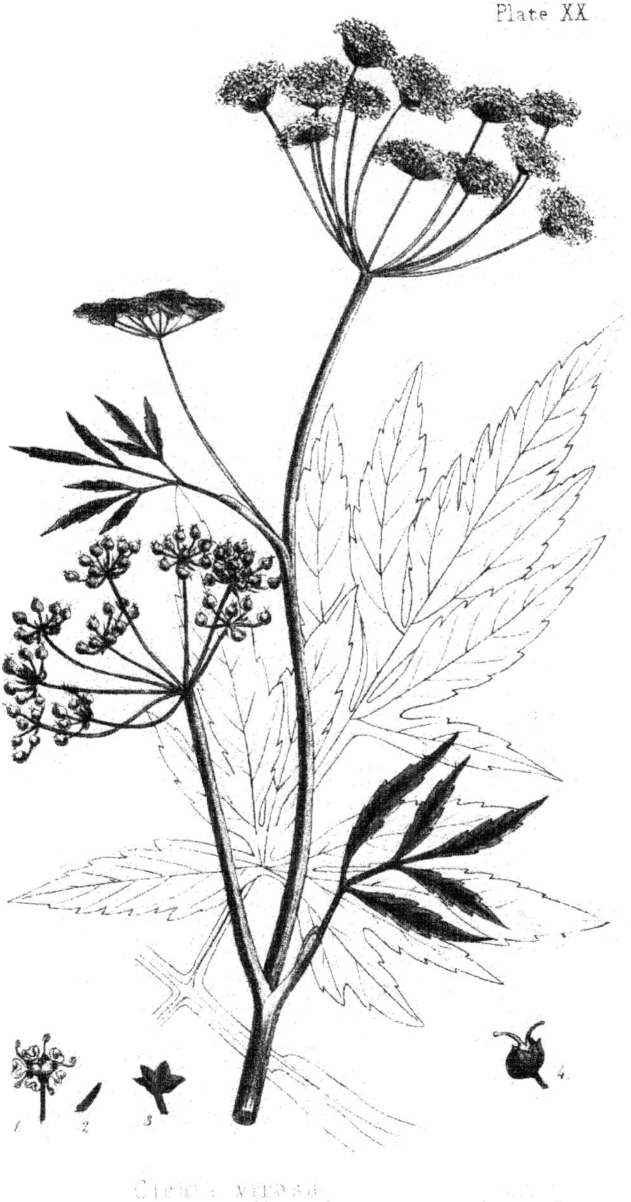

Cicuta virosa

History.—The Cicuta Virosa has been considered by some authors, and amongst them Haller, to be the κωνειον of Dioscorides, and the herb from which the poison used by the Greeks to kill their criminals was extracted; others suppose that a mixture of different substances was employed. However, it is not at all unlikely that this plant, being, from its excessive virulence, a more fit instrument of death, was used in preference to the Conium. Socrates drank *Cicuta,* as also did Phocion; recent commentators, however, consider that the Athenian Cicuta and Conium are identical. Although formerly prescribed, its use now is universally superseded by the Conium maculatum, and it is at present only occasionally employed, under the old school, as a poultice to relieve gouty and rheumatic pains.

Description.—The Cicuta Virosa is a perennial plant. Flowers in July and August. The *root* is tuberous, hollow, divided into cells by transverse partitions; fibres cylindrical, slender, in whorled fascicles. *Stem* from two to four feet high, hollow, leafy, branched, furrowed, smooth, often reddish; its lower part divided by transverse partitions into large cells. *Leaves* on long petioles, twice ternate, bright green. *Leaflets* spear-shaped, pointed, sharply and deeply serrated, from one to two inches long, more or less remarkably decurrent; those of the upper leaves very narrow. *Umbels* upright, large, many-rayed, partly terminal, partly opposite to the leaves. *Umbellules* of very numerous, slender rays. *Partial involucrum* of many small, pointed leaves. *Flowers* white. *Petals* small, equal, much inflexed. *Anthers* and *style* reddish. *Fruit* compressed, roundish, smooth, ribbed, almost black. It is one of the rankest of our vegetable poisons.

Geographical Distribution.—A native throughout all Europe and Siberia; and of North America, between lat. 54° and 64°.

Localities.—In ditches and about the margins of rivers and lakes. Not common in this country; its chief localities being in *Bedfordshire,* Oakley Springs. *Cambridgeshire:* fens between Ely and Prickwillow; in the river about a mile below Prickwillow Bridge. *Cheshire:* Pits near the Little Moor, a mile from Stockport; Pond, two miles from Northwich on the road to Chester, and Brereton Mere; at Pool, near Nantwich. *Cumberland:* Keswick; banks of the Irthing at Walton and Irthington. *Herefordshire:* Hereford, on the river banks, in the Walks. *Kent:* between Canterbury and Ashford. *Lincolnshire:* in the East Fen, chiefly on the edges of the narrow channels called Rows. *Middlesex:* near Hounslow; Denham; and in one of the ponds near the road at Hayes. *Norfolk:* in the river above Norwich; about Yarmouth; Old Walsingham; Hoveton Common. *Northumberland:* Learmouth. *Notts:* in Nottingham Park, etc. *Shropshire:* near Hatton; at Bildwas; Whiston Marsh; Ellesmere Mere; Oxen Pool, near Shrewsbury, etc. *Somerset:* in some boggy grounds near Shepton Mallet and in Burtle Moor; in the canal at Bathhampton. *Staffordshire:* Kingston Pool, near Stafford. *Suffolk:* near Temple Bridge, Cavenham; banks of the Waveney, between Eccles and St. Olave's; about Yarmouth, not uncommon. *Surrey:* about Battersea. *Yorkshire:* near Thirsk and Northallerton. Scotland: in the counties of *Berwick, Dumbarton, Dumfries, Edinburgh, Fife, Forfar, Lanark, Roxburgh,* and *Stirling,* but not common. In Ireland, but rare.

Parts used in Medicine, and Mode of Preparation.—The fresh Root, which is thick, white, fleshy, elongated, transparent, full of hair, and hollow; gathered at the beginning of the flowering, and from which a yellow juice, of a strong and disagreeable odour, and of an acrid, caustic taste, is expressed. This is mixed with equal parts of alcohol, and the various attenuations prepared as before directed.

Physiological Effects.—*On Animals.* Although perfectly innocuous to some animals, as goats, horses, and sheep, to others, viz., horned cattle, dogs, etc., it proves a most virulent and fatal poison. Wepfer (*Cicutæ aquaticæ, Historia et Notæ,* pp. 135-76, 1679) gave an ounce of the root of this plant, cut into small pieces, to a dog; in half an hour the animal foamed at the mouth and vomited; violent convulsive movements ensued; at one time emprosthotonos, at another opisthotonos; inability to remain still, and, on endeavouring to walk, falling on one side: this state lasted two hours. After death, livid spots were found along the whole of the alimentary canal. The same author made various experiments on dogs, wolves, and eagles, both with the root and the juice, and all gave analogous results. On examination after death, the alimentary canal was found inflamed, and sometimes gangrenous; the cavities of the heart were filled with blood, sometimes fluid, at others congealed. The lungs, often infiltrated and gorged with blood, seemed inflamed, as also was the liver. The cavities of the brain contained but little serosity; the vessels of the brain were distended with black blood.

Linnæus gives the following account of the powerful effects of Cicuta on horned cattle:—

"Here I was informed of a disease which had made great ravages amongst the cattle in this neighbourhood, and which was of so pestilential a nature that though the animals were flayed even before they were cold, wherever their blood had come in contact with the human body it had caused gangrenous spots and sores. Some persons had had both their hands swelled, and one his face, in consequence of the blood coming upon it; many people had lost their lives by it, insomuch that nobody would now venture to flay any more of the cattle.

"Everybody at Tornea was continually talking to me of a distemper to which their horned cattle are subject, and which kills many of them in the course of the winter, when they lose from fifty to one hundred head of cattle almost every year. On walking to examine the meadow into which they are first turned out to grass, I found it was a bog or marsh where the Water Hemlock, *Cicuta aquatica* (*Cicuta virosa*, Engl. Bot.), grew in abundance, and had evidently been cropped plentifully by the animals feeding (*Linnæus, Lachesis Lapponica*, vol. ii. pp. 136-40; *trans. by Sir J. E. Smith*).

"This disease made no regular progress, nor was it communicated by infection from one animal to another. The cows are driven altogether in the spring to feed in a meadow near the town. The symptoms differ in different cases; but all the cattle feeding indiscriminately are seized with swelling of the abdomen, attended with convulsions, and die, with horrid bellowing, in a few days. No person dares venture to flay the recent carcases, it having been found by experience that not only the hands but evēn the face, in consequence of the warm steam from the body, became inflamed and gangrenous, and that death finally ensued. * * * *

"I had scarcely landed from the boat in which I was taken to the meadow, than the Cicuta presented itself before me, and explained the cause of all this destruction. The slightest observation teaches us that brute animals distinguish by natural instinct such plants as are wholesome to them, from such as are poisonous. The cattle, therefore, do not eat this hemlock in summer or autumn; but when first turned out in the spring the herbage is short, and insufficient to satisfy them; probably, also, immersed under water, and scarcely perceptibly scented, they are unable to distinguish the wholesome from the pernicious kinds. I remarked that everywhere the radical leaves only were cropped, and no others, which confirmed what I asserted. In a neighbouring meadow I saw this plant cut with the hay for winter food, so that it is no wonder if in that state some even of the more cautious cattle are destroyed by it" (*Linn. Flor. Lapp.*, 2nd edit., p. 76).

On Man.—Many fatal accidents have occurred from eating the root of the Cicuta Virosa in mistake for that of the common parsnip. The whole of the plant, however, is poisonous. The symptoms produced by the roots are vertigo, dimness of sight, headache, and difficult respiration; burning pain at the stomach, and vomiting, accompanied by heat and dryness of the throat;

and in some cases convulsions, preceding death. The mucous membranes were found congested, and dark fluid blood in the sinuses of the brain. Wepfer (l. c.) mentions the case of a man who had eaten largely of the root, being found with his face greatly swollen, and his eyes protruding, breathing with great difficulty, and foaming at the mouth. He was seized with a severe epileptic fit, his limbs assumed a tetanic stiffness; there was spasmodic breathing, with perfect unconsciousness, which state was soon terminated by death. The only marked appearances were fluidity of the blood, and patches of redness on the mucous membrane of the stomach.

Four children, between five and seven years of age, ate the roots of this plant instead of parsnips; within half an hour they were all seized with extreme nausea, burning pain at the epigastrium, and colicky pains in the bowels. They all complained, on reaching home, of sickness, for which warm milk was given them. Efforts to vomit were induced; in one there was full vomiting, but in the other three nothing was ejected from their stomachs. In two of them the pains gradually increased, and in about two hours from the time of their eating the roots they were labouring under complete coma, with tetanic convulsions, the jaws rigidly fixed, profound stertor, and the whole face puffed and bloated, having precisely the appearance of the head of a person who had been some hours under water; pulse intermitting, sometimes imperceptible. Emetics were given without effect, but enemata of castor-oil and oil of turpentine were employed, with great relief. One of the children died in three hours, the others recovered" (*Badgeley, Montreal Med. Gaz.*, June, 1844).

Dr. Schleiser met with the following case:—A girl, aged eight, had eaten this plant; was found quite insensible, her respiration was feeble and rattling, the pulse soft, small, and scarcely perceptible, the pupils dilated and fixed, the face pallid, limbs flaccid, abdomen distended, and there was general coldness of the surface, with an entire loss of the power of swallowing. The patient died in about sixteen hours (*Canstatt's Jahrb.*, 1844, v. 296).

A boy, aged six years, ate some of the root of the Cicuta aquatica, which he mistook for parsnip; in a very short time he suffered from great anxiety at the præcordia, spoke a few words, and fell to the ground. A short time afterwards, horrible convulsive movements came on; he lost the use of his senses, and his mouth was firmly closed; he ground his teeth; the eyes were turned up in an extraordinary manner, and blood was discharged from the ears; he tried to vomit, without being able to open his mouth; his head was constantly thrown back, and there was severe opisthotonos. The convulsions gradually ceased, and he expired about half an hour after the first invasion of the symptoms. The abdomen and face were swollen after death, and there was slight lividity about the eyes (*Wepfer*, l. c., pp. 5-9).

Medical Uses (Homœopathic).—*Hahnemann's observations:* "More profound and complete investigation will show that this remedy is beneficial in uncommon cases, to which no other medicine is homœopathically adapted, and, above all, in chronic cases, for I have seen its action continue for three weeks even in small doses. Until now, it has never been given internally, for whenever Hemlock was prescribed, as it frequently was some years ago, Conium maculatum was always understood.

"The juice of Cicuta virosa was only used externally, as recommended by Linnæus. It enters into the composition of the Hemlock plaster of the Danish Pharmacopœia, which was applied to soothe gouty pains.

"The juice of the fresh root (for when dried it is less powerful) is so active, that in the common practice no one dares to give it internally, as it is usual to give none but large doses. It has therefore been set aside, and its healing qualities disregarded.

"The homœopaths only take advantage of its virtues, making use of the thirtieth dilution."

Clinical Observations.—*Noack and Trinks:* Cicuta may be usefully exhibited in convulsions in women and children, hence eclampsia, also spasms during delivery, and during confinement. Convulsions brought on by the abuse of opium. Hysteric spasms and tetanus. Catalepsy. Opisthotonos. Trismus. Tremor of the limbs. Lichen agrius. Achor. Impetigo sparsa. Porrigo larvalis. Herpes furfuraceus. Herpes labialis. Long-lasting pustulous, confluent, cutaneous eruptions, forming thick, yellow crust, with burning pain. Mentagra. Cholera Asiatica, when violent tonic spasms of the pectoral muscles and distortion of the eyes alternate with vomiting, and the diarrhœa is scanty and rare. Mental affections. Amblyopia amaurotica, with cerebral affections. Spasms of the œsophagus. Swellings of the throat, threatening suffocation. Gastric affections, etc.

Antidotes.—To large doses, Tobacco. Strong emetics given as soon as possible; enemata of Oil of Turpentine, with Castor Oil. To small doses, Arnica. Cicuta antidotes Opium.

XX.

CINA.

(ARTEMISIA CONTRA.)

Tartarian Southernwood, Wormseed.

SYNONYMS.—Artemisia santonica, *Linn.* Semen cynæ, seu Sinæ, seu Contra vermes, seu lumbricorum. Semen sanctum. Semen zedoariæ. Sementina. Semen zinæ. Artemisia austriaca. *Jacq.* Absinth. austriac. tenuifolium, *Clus. Hist.* Ab. ponticum tenuifolium, *Bauh.* Πιν. Ab. tridentinum herbarior, *Lob.* Ab. seriphium, *Dod.*

FOREIGN NAMES.—*Fr.:* Semen contra, Barbotine, Sementine, Graine de Zedoariæ. *Germ.:* Zitttersaame, Wurmsaame. *Ital.:* Seme-sanuto. *Pol.:* Cytwarosoe-nasiene.

Nat. Order, CORYMBIFERÆ, *Juss.;* SYNGENESIA, POLYGAMIA SUPERFLUA.

GEN. CHAR.—*Receptacle* either hairy or naked. *Pappus* none. *Calyx* imbricated, with rounded converging scales. *Florets* of the ray none.
SPEC. CHAR.—*Stem-leaves* pinnate, linear, multifid. *Branches* undivided. *Spikes* one-ranked, reflexed. *Flowers* composed of five florets.

HISTORY.—The Artemisiæ, to which subdivision belongs the drug known as Cina in the homœopathic Materia Medica, held a prominent place among the medicinal substances of the ancient physicians, from Hippocrates to Serapion. They were chiefly recommended as febrifuge, stomachic, and anthelmintic. In modern times, under the allopathic school, Cina has entirely gone out of use. The modern Greek Pharmacopœia contains two species,

---

Fig. 1. The root. 2. Involucrum. 3. Floret of the centre. 4. Floret of the ray. 5. One of the divisions of the involucrum.

Plate XIX.

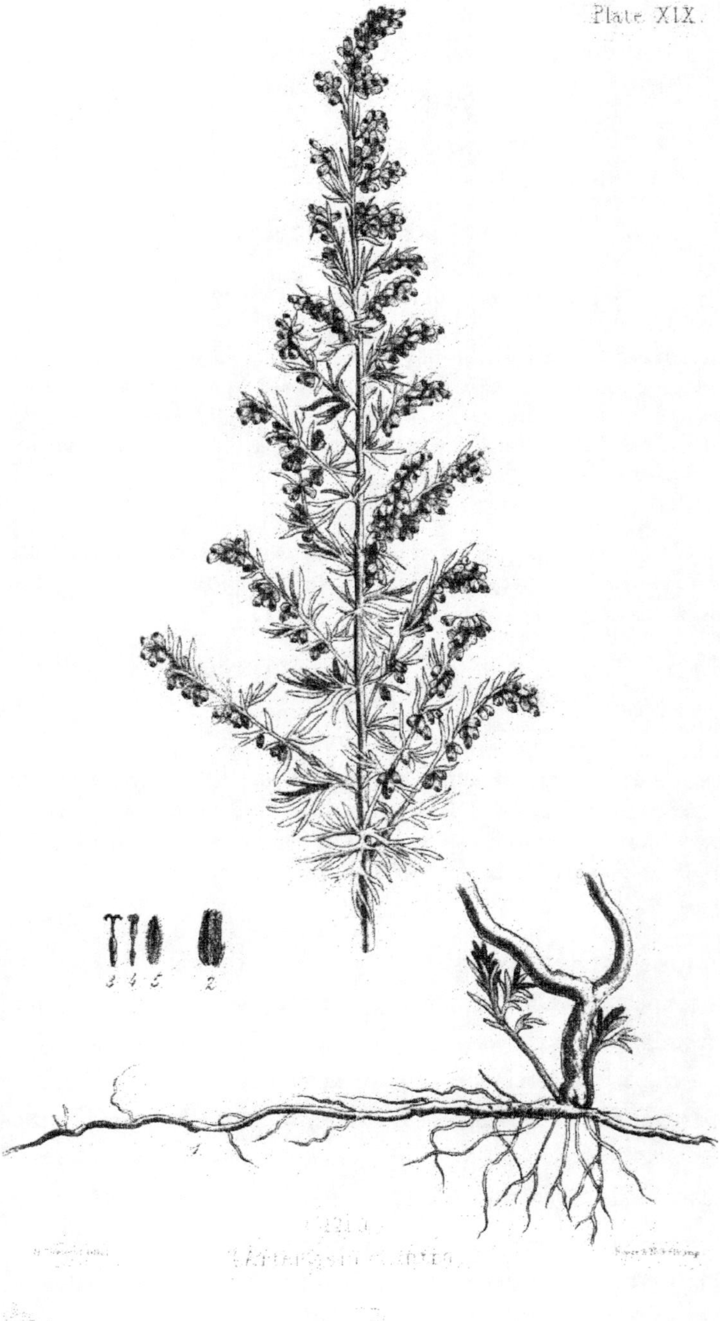

which are described under the names Artemisia absinthium and Artemisia Contra. This latter is the A. santonica or Contra of Linnæus, its name being an abbreviation of Contra vermes. Lindley (*Veget. Kingdom*, p. 705) says that the drug called Semen contra or Semen Cinæ is made up of the flower-heads of many species of Artemisia; those which form the principal part of this substance are A. Sieberi, A. Larcheana, A. Contra, and A. pauciflora: the flower-heads of A. Vahliaria also furnish one of the kinds of Wormseed, called Semen Cinæ Levanticum, or Semen Cinæ in grains. It was formerly supposed that the virtues of the Artemisia Contra as a vermifuge resided in the bitterness of the extract; but, according to the experiments of Baglivi and Redi, lumbrici immersed in the infusion of this substance were killed in five to seven hours; whilst in an infusion of wormwood they continued to live for thirty hours and upwards. So that the vermifuge effects could not wholly depend upon the bitterness of this substance.

Description. — The plant is a hardy shrub, perennial, and flowering in the autumn. The drug is made up of undeveloped flowers, calyces, and fragments of peduncles, mixed with foreign matters. It is imported from Barbary and the Levant; the latter being deemed the best, being less adulterated, and of a greenish hue, and smooth; while that from Barbary is grey and downy. M. Tournefort gives the following account of this drug in the second volume of his Travels: "The Sementine or Worm-powder is not gathered like our seeds. The plant grows in the meadows, and must be let ripen; and the mischief is that, as it grows near to maturity, the wind scatters a good part of it among the grass, where it is lost, and this makes it so dear. As they dare not touch it with the hand, for fear of making it spoil the sooner, when they would gather what was left in the ear, they have recourse to this expedient: they take two hand-baskets, and walking along the meadows sweep the baskets, the one from right to left, the other from left to right, as if they were mowing; by this means the seed is shaken out into the baskets." The adulterations are the seeds of the Tansey (Tanacetum vulgare) and the Mugwort (Artemisia vulgaris). The latter are known, from being of a bright yellow colour, and resembling powdered hay.

Geographical Distribution.—Asia Minor; the Levant; Africa; Barbary; Persia; frontiers of Muscovy. The different species over most parts of Europe.

Parts used in Medicine, and Mode of Preparation.—The whole substance as imported, freed as much as possible from impurities. One part is infused in twenty parts of alcohol, to prepare the tincture, but it is recommended to prepare the three first attenuations by trituration, as more likely to preserve and develope the virtues of this plant.

Medical Uses (Homœopathic).— *Hahnemann's observations:* "However important the properties of Cina may be, it has for ages been used exclusively for children, to expel worms, in doses of ten, twenty, thirty, and sixty grains. I pass over in silence the frequent fatal effects of such doses; nor do I urge that some kinds of worms, in children otherwise healthy, are not to be considered very serious, and that frequently their presence does not lead to any great inconvenience, while psora remains latent. But it is certain that when these creatures exist in great numbers, they indicate a morbid state of body and of developed psora; without the cure of which, they will not fail to reappear, in spite of Cina; so that their expulsion avails nothing, and a treatment so ill-directed often results in the death of the child, after having been long tormented.

"Cina has healing virtues most precious in other circumstances, as we may be convinced by studying its symptoms in persons in health.

"Experience will prove, for instance, that it has a powerful effect in whooping-cough, and in certain intermittent fevers, accompanied with vomiting and canine hunger. I omit other cases in which it is equally advantageous, and which the homœopathic physician will readily discover."

Clinical Observations.—*Noack and Trinks:* Cina may be administered in the following affections. Convulsions. Epilepsy (from worms). Eclampsia. Worm symptoms of children, with febrile symptoms, etc. Quotidian and tertian fevers, recurring after large doses of Quinine: 1. Chilliness, without thirst, followed by heat, with thirst after the heat, sweat. 2. Chilliness, with much thirst. 3. Fevers, where the thirst is present only during the cold stage, and where the patient vomits once or twice. Cina has also cured intermittent fevers, when vomiting without diarrhœa, or diarrhœa without vomiting is present, the remedy being indicated by the dilatation of the pupils and the clean tongue. Chronic vomiting of children, who suffer from worms. Involuntary nocturnal enuresis in children suffering from atrophy. Whooping-cough, particularly in scrofulous children having worms. Whooping-cough in the convulsive stage, particularly when the spasmodic cough ends in vomiting, when the body becomes rigid during the paroxysms of coughing, and particularly when a gurgling noise from the throat down into the abdomen is heard after the paroxysm. Dr. Gray notes that Cina deserves attention in the bronchial catarrhs which remain after measles, especially such as have a kind of hectic fever with them.

Antidotes.—Bryonia. China. Hyoscyamus. Ipecacuanha.

XXI.

CLEMATIS ERECTA.

Upright Virgin's Bower.

SYNONYMS.—Flammula Jovis. Flammula recta, *Bauh.* Πιν., p. 300. Clematis sive, Flammula surrecta alba, *F. Bauh. Hist.*, vol. ii. p. 127; *Tourn. Inst.*, 294. Flammula Jovis surrecta, *Gerarde*, p. 333; *Park. Theat.*, p. 382; *Raii Hist.*, p. 621. Clematis caule erecta, foliis pinnatis ovato lanceolatis, *Flor. Aust.*, tab. 291; *Storck, Libella. de Flam. Jov.* Clematis recta, *Linn.*, Sp., pl. ii.

FOREIGN NAMES.—*Fr.:* Clematite deorte. *Germ.:* Bren waldrebe. *Ital.:* Clematite. *Span.:* Clematide. *Dut.:* Clematis. *Pol.:* Powoy. *Dan. and Swed.:* Clematis.

Nat. Order, RANUNCULACEÆ, *Juss.;* POLYANDRIA, POLYGYNIA, *Linn.*

GEN. CHAR.—*Calyx* (*corolla*) inferior, of four, rarely five, six, or eight, regular oblong sepals; in the bud, either valvular or folded in at the edges. *Corolla* none. *Filaments* numerous, swelling upwards. *Anthers* terminal, of two oblong lobes, bursting laterally. *Germens* superior, sessile, egg-shaped, collected into a round head. *Styles* terminal, longer than the stamens. *Stigmas* simple. *Pericarps* (seeds of Linn.) indehiscent, numerous, egg-shaped, compressed, one-seeded, placed on a capitate receptacle, and terminated by a long, mostly feathering tail.

SPEC. CHAR.—*Leaves* pinnated. *Leaflets* ovato-lanceolate, quite entire. *Stem* erect. *Flowers* tetrapetalous and pentapetalous.

HISTORY.—This plant, although employed as a remedy by the early physicians in some affections of the liver and diseases of

---

Fig. 1. The pericarps, with their feathering tails.

* Clematis, from κλημα, riticula sarmentum, because it climbs trees by means of its pliant twigs.

Plate XXI

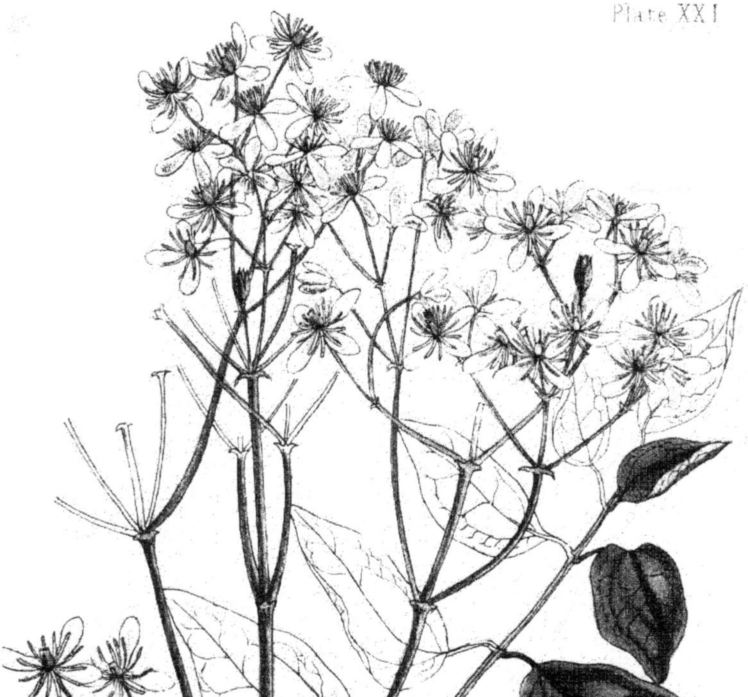

H. Sowerby lith. Clematis erecta. Reeve & Nichols imp.

the skin, fell into disuse until the time of Baron Störck, in 1769,* who first recommended it as a useful internal remedy in many obstinate complaints; chronic diseases of the skin, ulcers cancers, and severe headaches; and in a remarkable case of melancholia (vide *Störck, Lib. de Pulsat.*, p. 57). Notwithstanding its success, it has seldom been employed by other physicians, although it found a place in one of the earlier editions of the *Edinburgh Dispensatory.* The secret of Baron Störck's success consisted in his having unwittingly prescribed this drug according to the homœopathic principle, this medicine producing on persons in health the very symptoms which accompanied the diseases in which he employed it so successfully; and it is worthy of observation, that the same result, from the same cause, occurred more than once to Störck, with drugs which entirely failed in other hands.

At the present time, Clematis does not enter into any of the allopathic prescriptions.

DESCRIPTION.—The *root* is perennial, white, and fibrous. *Stem* three feet high, leafy, striated, herbaceous, greenish, or reddish. *Leaves* large, opposite. *Leaflets* from five to nine, pubescent underneath, petioled. *Flowers* white; in upright, stiff, terminal umbels. *Peduncles* several times ternate. *Petals* oblong, obtuse, somewhat villous, a little longer than the stamens. *Seeds* few, dark brown, smooth, orbicular, much compressed; tails long, yellowish, plumose. Flowers July and August.

Like some of the other species of this genus it is extremely acrid, on which account it was called Flammula by the old botanists. Gerarde gives the derivation of the name *Virgin's Bower*, "by reason of the goodly shadow which they make with their thick bushing and climbing, as also for the beauty of the flowers and the pleasant scent or savour of the same."

* He published several cases of its successful employment, particularly in inveterate syphilitic complaints, which had produced headache, pains in the bones, nodes, ulcers, cutaneous affections, etc. (*Libell. de Flammula Jovis*).

Geographical Distribution.—South of France, Spain, Switzerland, Austria, Gallicia, Hungary, Tartary, and Greece.

Localities.—On uncultivated hills, along hedges, and on woody hills.

Parts used in Medicine, and Mode of Preparation.—The Juice expressed from the leaves and stem of the plant, gathered when commencing to flower, and mixed with equal parts of alcohol; after forty-eight hours have elapsed, the clear liquid is to be separated from the dregs and prepared to the ninth attenuation.

Physiological Effects.—As one of the Ranunculaceæ, we should expect to find irritating properties from the juice of the Clematis, although it cannot be considered as a poison. The recent leaves, on being chewed, excite a burning heat in the tongue and fauces, and if retained long in the mouth, produce blisters and ulceration. The leaves have also been used by mendicant impostors to produce ulcers on the legs, to excite charity.

Medical Uses (Homœopathic).—*Hahnemann's observations* (*Chronic Dis.*, vol. iii.): "The various potencies of its acrid juice, which ought to be extracted from the fresh leaves shortly before the plant begins to blossom, may be used against a number of affections which have their origin in the abuse of mercury, and are complicated with psora; in dangerous eruptions of the head and skin, and various kinds of troublesome inflammation of the eyes. Dr. Stapf found this remedy useful in orchitis and indurated swellings of those organs. At a more remote period, its virtues have been praised by Störck in cases of cancerous ulcers of the lips and mammæ; spongy excrescences; tophi; inveterate eruptions of the skin; peculiar kinds of chronic headache, and melancholia."

According to Noack and Trinks, Clematis is suitable to torpid cachectic individuals, and scrofulous constitutions; swelling and indurations of the glands; rheumatism of the joints; arthritic nodosities; mercurial disease; urticaria; inveterate psoriasis; pains in hollow teeth, especially at night; orchitis, etc.

Antidotes.—Camphor moderates the too violent effects of the drug. Bryonia is said to appease the toothache caused by Clematis.

XXII.

COCCULUS.

(ANAMIRTA COCCULUS.)

The Cocculus Indicus Plant.

SYNONYMS.—Menispermum cocculus, *Linn.* Cocculus suberosus, *Decand.* Anamirta cocculus, *Wight and Arnott.* Anamirta paniculatum, *Colebr.* Menispermum monadelphum, *Roxb. in E.I.C.M., tab.* 130.

FOREIGN NAMES.—*Fr.:* Coque du Levant. *Germ.:* Kokkels körner, Fischkörner. *Swed.:* Kokkelkörn. *Tam.:* Kakacollie verei.

Nat. Order, MENISPERMACEÆ, *Dec.;* MONŒCIA, DODECANDRIA.

GEN. CHAR.—*Flowers* diœcious. *Calyx* of six sepals, in a double series, with two close pressed bracteoles. *Corolla* none. *Male stamens* united into a central column, dilated at the apex. *Anthers* numerous, covering the whole globose apex of the column. *Female flowers* unknown. *Drupes,* one to three, one-celled, one-seeded. *Seed* globose, deeply excavated at the hilum. *Albumen* fleshy. *Cotyledons* very thin, diverging (*Wight and Arnott*).

HISTORY.—The first notice of the Cocculus indicus is in the works of some of the Arabian physicians, but it was chiefly employed as a poison for fish, stupefying them and making them easy of capture. It has been but rarely employed as a medicine, and then chiefly as an external application in scabies, and in ringworm of the scalp. The importation of the drug into this country is considerably less in quantity than formerly, and is seldom used unless it is for the illicit adulteration of beer and

---

Fig. 1. Male flower and stamens. 2. Transverse section of the seeds. 3. The berry. 3. Transverse section of the berry. 5. The embryo.

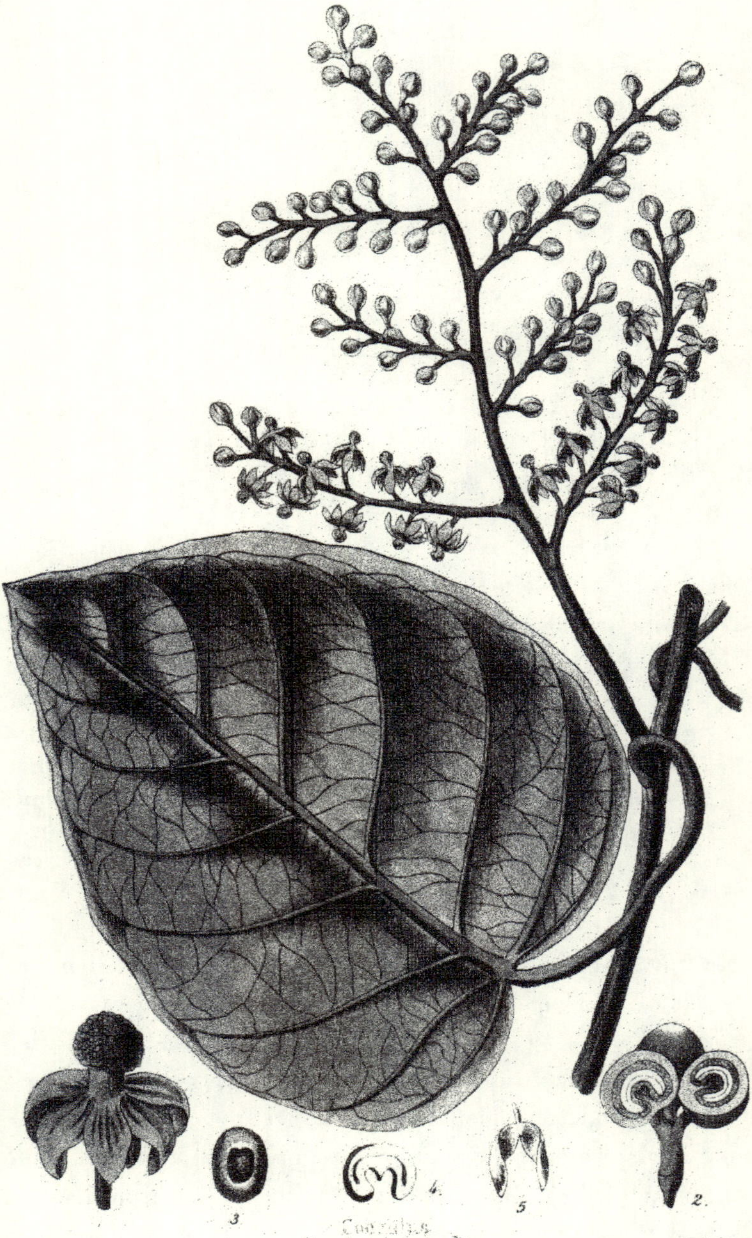

Cocculus
Anamirta Cocculus.

porter in low public-houses; for this purpose it was in great request some years since, notwithstanding the severe prohibitory laws against its use. Morrice (*Treatise on Brewing*) orders "three pounds of Cocculus indicus to be added to ten quarters of malt. It gives an inebriating quality, which passes for strength of liquor; it also prevents the second fermentation of beer, and the bursting of the bottles in warm climates." It is the ingredient used by thieves and other bad characters for the purpose of hocussing their victims.

Description.—The Anamirta Cocculus is a strong climbing plant, with a corky bark. *Leaves* more or less cordate, ovate, leathery, striped, large, from eight to twelve inches long. *Petiole* a little shorter than the leaves. *Fruit* roundish, umbicular, somewhat larger than a large pea, and with the structure of a drupa. The officinal part is the berry which is met with in commerce; it resembles the berry of the bay-tree (bacca lauri). It consists of a dry, roundish, thin, blackish-brown, rugous, acrid, and bitter layer, which involves a thin, bivalved, white, ligneous shell (endocarp). In the middle of this shell rises a central placenta, which is contracted at its base, but enlarged and divided into two cells superiorly; between the placenta and the shell is an oleaginous, yellow, very bitter nucleus (seed), of a semilunar form. This nucleus never wholly fills the cavity of the shell, at least in the Cocculus indicus of commerce, for by keeping, it gradually becomes atrophied, and in old samples it is not uncommon to find the shell almost empty: this change is observed also in other oleaginous seeds. By this character alone, Cocculus indicus may be instantly distinguished from the bay berry (*Pereira, Elem. of Mat. Med.*, p. 1325). The active principle exists in a substance termed Picrotoxine (Picrotoxic acid).

Geographical Distribution.—The coast of Malabar, and the Indian Archipelago.

Parts used in Medicine, and Mode of Preparation.—The Seeds. One part of the seeds, bruised to powder, is mixed with twenty parts of alcohol; apply a slight heat for twenty-four hours, and then dilute to the thirtieth attenuation.

Physiological Effects.—*On Animals.* It is poisonous to most animals. According to Orfila (*Tox. Gén.*, vol. ii. p. 410), it acts as an irritant, and imparts its deleterious effects to the flesh of animals or fish poisoned by it, but this depends on the quantity of poison used: when ten to fifteen grains were used, and the fish afterwards given to animals, the noxious effects were as strongly marked as if they had swallowed the poison (*Ann. d'Hyg.*, 1843, i. 343). All kinds of fish are killed by it, the barbel taking the longest to die. The symptoms on animals are, trembling gait; eyes protruding and haggard; agitation of the muscles, followed by convulsions and contortions of the whole body; falling backwards and forwards; opisthotonos; entire loss of consciousness; foaming at the mouth; tongue and gums livid; respiration quickened and laboured. These spasmodic symptoms remit for a few minutes, and then return with redoubled violence until death relieves. On opening the body after death, in the left ventricle of the heart was found a clot of blood of a brownish-red colour, of a tissue more compact than usual, and of a colour deeper in patches. In other cases, there was vomiting of yellow and liquid matter (*Orfila*, l. c.)

From these symptoms, Orfila (l. c.) considers that the Cocculus exerts its influence like camphor, on the nervous system, and more particularly on the brain; that the active parts of the poison is the picrotoxine; that when it is introduced slightly divided, it limits its effects to the production of nausea and vomiting; and lastly, that the vomiting appears to be the best means to counteract the evil effects whilst the poison remains in the stomach.

On Man.—"From some accounts I have received from an excise-officer, who has been repeatedly subjected to beer adulterated with it, its action appeared to be rather on the voluntary muscles than on the intellectual powers" (*Pereira*, l. c.)

The seeds in powder and decoction give rise to nausea, vomiting, and griping pains, hiccough and anxiety, followed by stupor and intoxication. The shell acts as an emetic; the kernel contains the picrotoxine, in which resides the poisonous qualities.

The following cases of poisoning with this drug have been recorded.

"A boy, aged twelve, swallowed two scruples of the composition used for poisoning fish; it contained Cocculus indicus. In a few minutes he perceived an unpleasant taste, with burning pain in the œsophagus and stomach, not relieved by frequent vomiting, as well as pain extending over the whole of the abdomen. In spite of treatment, a violent attack of gastro-enteritis ensued, with much febrile excitement, followed by delirium and diarrhœa, and he died the nineteenth day after taking the poison. On inspection, the vessels of the pia mater were found filled with dark-coloured liquid blood. In the abdomen there were all the marks of peritonitis in an advanced stage. The stomach was discoloured, and its parietes thinner and softer than natural" (*Canstatt's Jahresbericht*, 1844, v. 293).

"A druggist, of fine sensibility and otherwise healthy, although recently convalescent from an acute disease, some years ago wished to ascertain the taste of the Cocculus seed, and as he considered it a powerful substance, he weighed out a single grain of it, but did not take quite half of this into his mouth, rolled it about with his tongue over his palate, and he had not swallowed it two seconds when he was seized with the most dreadful apprehensiveness. This anxiety increased every moment; he became cold all over; his limbs stiff as if paralysed, with drawing pains in the bones and in the back. The symptoms increased from hour to hour, until, after a lapse of six hours, the anxiety, the stupefaction, the senseless stupidity, and the immobility had risen to the greatest height, with fixed sullen look, ice-cold sweat on the forehead and the hands, and great repugnance to all food and drink; at the slightest increase of temperature of the air (75° Fahr.) he expressed his displeasure; every loud word put him in a passion. All that he could still say was, that his brain felt as if contracted by a ligature, and that he expected speedy dissolution. He gave no indication of inclination to vomit, of thirst, or of any other want in the world. He wished to sleep, as he felt a great inclination to do so; but when he closed his eyes, he immediately started up again, so frightful, he asserted, was the sensation he felt in his brain on going to sleep, like the most hideous dream. The pulse was very small, but the frequency was not altered.

"In these frightful circumstances I was called in. A few drops of Thebaic tincture appeared not to agree with him; this led me to fix upon a strong camphor emulsion, of which I administered to him a tablespoonful about every minute. I soon observed a happy change in his expression, and after he had thus taken fifteen grains of camphor, his consciousness was restored, the anxiety gone, the heat natural. In something less than hour he perspired a little, during the night slept pretty well; but the following day was uncommonly weak, and all the parts which during the direct action of the Cocculus were yesterday painful internally, were to-day uncommonly painful externally to the slightest touch. The bowels remained constipated for several days. It is very probable that all these after-sufferings could have been prevented if, in place of giving fifteen grains of camphor, I had at once given thirty. During the increase of the symptoms from the Cocculus, he attempted to smoke tobacco, with considerable aggravation; they also increased from taking coffee, though not so strikingly as from the other" (*Hahnemann's Lesser Writings*, p. 378, *trans. by R. E. Dudgeon, M.D.*)

MEDICAL USES (HOMŒOPATHIC).—*Hahnemann's observations:* "No one before me has used this medicine as an internal remedy. I have now introduced it into the Materia Medica, after having studied its dynamic effects on persons in health. It possesses many curative virtues, as is proved by the symptoms it produces. A high dilution of the tincture is indispensable in many frequent diseases, in which the symptoms are analogous, particularly in some kinds of low, nervous fevers; in abdominal spasms; and in spasmodic pains in different parts of the body, which produce melancholy, particularly in females; in many cases of paralysis of the limbs, and in moral affections.

CLINICAL OBSERVATIONS.—*Noack and Trinks:* Amongst many other affections, Cocculus has been found chiefly beneficial in spasms of hysteric females from different causes. Suppression of the catamenia, etc. Total and partial spasmodic paralysis. Paralysis of the lower limbs, with insensibility of the parts. Paralysis of the larynx. Fainting fits of hysteric females. Acute arthritis. Fever, with gastric and bilious symptoms. Bilious fever after vexation. Inflammatory typhoid fever, particularly when characterised by predominant nausea, with tendency to produce fainting. Typhus, with giddiness and delirium. Febris lenta, with great nervous weakness, particularly after acute diseases. Typhus abdominalis, first stage, with great and constant nausea, producing a disposition to faint; second stage, characterised by heat. Erethism of the circulation. Debility and asthenia (in alternation with Rhus). Vertigo, with disposition to vomit, and actual vomiting. Megrim and hysteric headache, with nausea and vomiting. Spasm of the stomach. Bilious colic. Spasmodic and flatulent colic. Dysmenorrhœa. Sudden spasms, from retention or suppression of the catamenia. Some cases of hernia. Spasms of the chest, and palpitation of the heart in hysteric females, etc.

ANTIDOTES.—Camphor. Nux Vomica. To poisonous doses: Emetics, emptying the stomach as soon as possible. Acetic acid has been supposed to act as an antidote. The treatment, after the poison has been got rid of, must be the same as for gastro-enteritis.

XXIII.

COFFEA* ARABICA.

The Coffee Tree.

SYNONYMS.—Coffea arabica floribus quinquefidis dispermis, *Linn. Spec. Plant.*, *2nd edit.* Jasminum arabicum lauri folio cujus semen apud nos Coffé dicitur, *Juss. Act. Gall.*, 1713, p. 388. Jasminum arabicum castaneæ folio, flore albo odoratissimo, *Till. Prif.*, *tab.* 32. Evonymo similis ægyptici fructu baccis lauri simili, *Bauh.* Πιν., 498; *Pluk. Phyt.*, 272. Arbor Bon cum fructu suo buna, *Prosp. Alpin.*, *Venet.*, 1591.

FOREIGN NAMES.—*Fr.*: Le Caffayer. *Germ.*: Der Kaffebaum. *Dut.*: Koffy boom. *Ital.*: Il Caffé. *Span.*: El Cafe. *Russ.*: Kofé. *Pol.*: Kawa. *Arab.*: Cauba. *Egypt.*: Caova, Choava.

Nat. Order, RUBIACEÆ, *Juss.*; PENTANDRIA, MONOGYNIA.

GEN. CHAR.—*Calyx* five-toothed, teeth deciduous. *Corolla* salver-shaped. *Stamens* on the tube. *Anthers* arrow-shaped. *Berry* superior, two-seeded. *Seeds* arillate, flat on one side, convex on the other.

SPEC. CHAR.—*Flowers* five-cleft. *Berries* with two seeds.

HISTORY.—Pietro del Valle, the Roman traveller, in his "Viaggi in Turchia, Persia e India, dal 1614 al 1626," maintains that Coffee is the same as the Νηπενθης of Homer. Others, namely, Sir Henry Blunt, Sandys, and Howell, in a letter prefixed to Ramsay's "Organon Salutis" (in which work the liquor is styled "the Turks' Physic of Cophic,") will allow the Coffee no place in antiquity but as the black broth of the

---

Fig. 1. Magnified view of the flower. 2. Corolla, opened, to show the stamens. 3. Germen and pistils. 4. The berry. 5. Transverse section of the seed. The drawing was taken from a natural specimen in the hothouse at Longleat, Wilts.

* According to Bruce, its true name is Caffe, from Caffa, the south province of Narea, in Africa, where it is indigenous in great abundance.

Pl XXIII.

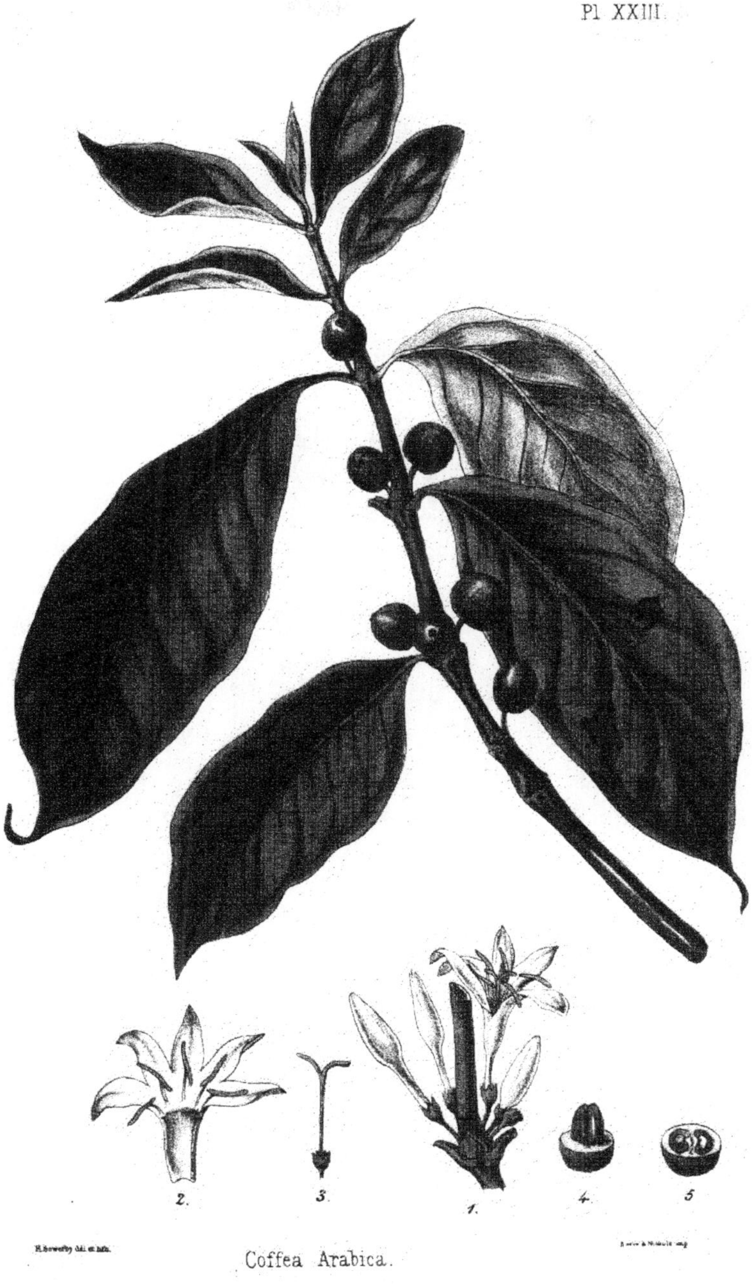

H. Sowerby del. et lith.

Coffea Arabica.

Lacedemonians" Burton (*Anatomy of Melancholy*, folio, 388) has the following notice of Coffee: "The Turks have a drink called Coffa (for they use no wine), so named of a berry as black as soot, and as bitter, like that black drinke which was in use among the Lacedemonians, and perhaps the same which they sip still of, and sip as warm as they can suffer" (vide *Ency. Metrop., art. Coffee*). The first European writer who mentions Coffee is Rauwolf, of Augsburg, who visited the Levant in 1573; he calls it *Chauba*. Then Prospero Alpini, a Venetian physician, mentions it in his work "De Plantis Ægypti," 1592.

The earliest account we have of Coffee is taken from an Arabian MS. in the Bibliothèque Nationale of France, No. 944, and is as follows.

Schehabeddin Ben, an Arabian author of the ninth century of the Hegira, or fifteenth of the Christians, attributes to Gemaleddin, mufti of Aden, a city of Arabia Felix, the first introduction into that country of drinking Coffee. He tells us that Gemaleddin, having occasion to travel into Persia, during his abode there, saw some of his countrymen drinking Coffee. In hopes of receiving some benefit from it, he determined to try it on himself, and after making the experiment, not only recovered his health, but perceived other useful qualities in that liquor, such as relieving the headache, enlivening the spirits, and, without prejudice to the constitution, preventing drowsiness. This last quality he determined to learn to the advantage of his profession; he took it himself and recommended it to the dervishes, or religious Mahometans, to enable them to pass the night in prayer and other exercises of their religion with greater zeal and attention. The example and authority of the mufti gave great reputation to Coffee; some men of letters and persons belonging to the law adopted the use of it. These were followed by tradesmen and artisans that were under the necessity of working at night, and such as were about to travel late after sunset. At length the custom became general in Aden, and it was not only drunk at night by those who were desirous to keep themselves awake, but in the day, for the sake of its other agreeable qualities. Before this time Coffee was scarcely known in Persia, and very little used in Arabia, where the tree grew. But, according to Schehabeddin, it had been drunk in Ethiopia from time immemorial, and where tradition says its power of causing wakefulness was first noticed by a shepherd from the effects on his goats. It not long after reached Mecca, where it was introduced as at Aden by the dervishes, for the same purposes of religion.

It seems, however, that after a time the people of these cities became so fond of this beverage, that it was drank publicly in houses set apart for the purpose, where there was singing, dancing, and music; these were called coffee-houses. The use of it gradually extended to all parts of Arabia, particularly to Medina, and then to Cairo, in Egypt. Coffee-drinking advanced afterwards through Syria, and was adopted at Damascus and Aleppo; and one hundred years after its introduction at Aden, namely, in 1554, it was first drunk at Constantinople, two private individuals having opened coffee-houses for the public sale of this beverage. At length the more rigid Mahometans began to disapprove of its habitual use, as occasioning frequent disorders, and for nearly resembling wine in its effects. The chief mufti declared that roasted Coffee was a kind of coal, and therefore forbidden by the law of Mahomet. Government found it necessary to interfere and restrict the use of it, but this prohibition was soon abandoned.

"M. Galand says it is of greater use in uniting men in society in stricter ties of amity than any other liquor; and he observes, that such protestations of friendship as are made at such times are far more to be depended on than when the mind is intoxicated with inebriating liquors. He computes that as much is spent in private families, in the article of Coffee at Constantinople, as in wine at Paris; and relates, that it is customary there to ask money to drink Coffee, as in Europe for money to drink your health in wine or beer" (*Ellis's Histor. Account of Coffee*, Lond., 1774).

It is supposed that the use of Coffee passed from Constantinople to the western parts of Europe, by Venice, about 1615, as Pietro della Valle, in writing to his friend in Venice, from Constantinople, says, that upon his return he should bring him some Coffee, which was a thing unknown in his country.

We next hear of it at Marseilles, in 1644, where it was brought by some gentlemen who accompanied M. de la Haye to Constantinople, who not only brought the Coffee berry, but the vessels for making and drinking it.*

It was brought to Paris, in 1657, by the celebrated traveller Thèvenot, but was more generally introduced, in 1669, by Soliman Aga, the ambassador from the Sultan Mahomet IV. It was introduced into England, in 1657, by Daniel Edwards, a Turkey merchant; and here, as in the East, it was opposed by the religious prejudice of the day. Many sermons were written both against coffee-drinking and smoking, and the following extract from an old sermon shows the vehemence with which it was attacked. "They cannot wait until the smoke of the infernal regions surrounds them, but encompass themselves with the smoke of their own accord, and drink a poison which God made black that it might bear the devil's colour." Charles the Second placed a duty of fourpence upon every gallon of Coffee made and sold, to be paid by the maker. Ray, in his "History of Plants," published in 1688, says that there were then in London as many coffee-houses as in Grand Cairo itself. He also supposed that the Arabs destroyed the vegetative qualities of the seed, so that it should not be

* La Roque says that "the Arabians, when they take the Coffee off the fire, immediately wrap the vessel in a wet cloth, which fines the liquor instantly and makes it cream at top, and occasions a most fragrant steam, which they take great pleasure in snuffing up, as the Coffee is pouring into their cups. People of the first fashion use nothing but Sultana Coffee, which is prepared chiefly from the outward husks or dried pulp."

grown in other countries. The Dutch were the first to attempt to transplant and grow its seed, as Boerhaave, in his Index to the Leyden Garden, informs us that Nicholas Witsen, burgomaster of Amsterdam, and governor of the East India Company, instructed Van Hoorn, governor of Batavia, to procure from Mocha the Coffee berries and grow them in that colony; this was in 1690. In 1714, the magistrates of Amsterdam sent a plant to Louis XIV., which is supposed by Du Tour to be the parent of all that has been cultivated in France and in the French West India islands. In 1722, the French governor of Cayenne procured a plant (it is said by stealth) from the Dutch colony of Surinam, which in 1725 had produced many thousands. In the year 1732, Coffee was cultivated in Jamaica, and an act passed to encourage its growth in that island.

For medicinal purposes it has not been in much request, except as a dietetic. Lord Bacon says: "It comforteth the brain and head, and helpeth digestion, and condenseth the spirits, and makes them strong and alacre."

Lewis (*Exp. Hist. of Mat. Med.*) says: "It strengthens the stomach, promotes secretions; is said to be serviceable in phlegmatic, corpulent habits; but injurious in thin habits and bilious temperaments, in melancholic and hypochondriacal disorders, and to persons subject to hemorrhages." It has been employed to palliate and dispel fits of periodical asthma; also in rheumatic affections. Atonic gout. Epilepsy. Intermittent fevers. Nervous and typhus fevers. Hysteria. Hysterical spasms and headache. Different kinds of toothache, and in inflammations of the gums. Spasmodic and flatulent colic. Spasms of the stomach. Diarrhœa, combined with rheumatic affections. Constipation. Menstrual colic. Whooping cough in the convulsive stage. Bad breath. And as an antidote to the effects of many vegetable poisons, as Belladonna, Cicuta virosa, Acid. hydrocyanicum, Hyoscyamus, Lolium temulentum, Moschus, Opium, Secale cornutum, Stramonium, etc.

Description.—Coffea arabica is an evergreen shrub, about sixteen feet in height, with a straight stem. The *flowers* are of a pale white; fragrant, but rapidly fading. The *leaves* are evergreen. The *fruit* resembles a cherry, and grows in clusters under the axilla of the leaves, at first of a bright red, and afterwards becoming purple. In Arabia, the fruit, when ripe, is shaken from the tree and dried by the sun on mats. In the West Indies, the fruit is gathered by the hand and dried in the sun on platforms. One hundred bushels of fruit will yield on an average 1,000 pounds of Coffee, each plant yielding from one to two pounds. There are thirty species known.

Geographical Distribution.—Coffea arabica is indigenous in Arabia Felix and Ethiopia., Now cultivated in Equatorial America, and many European countries. It was transported by the Dutch from Mocha to Batavia; from Batavia to Amsterdam; from Amsterdam to Paris; from Paris to Martinique, and then extended itself over the adjacent islands, etc.

Parts used in Medicine, and Mode of Preparation.—The Berry. Dr. Quin, in his *Pharmacopœia Homœopathica*, orders it to be prepared as follows. A drachm of the seeds of the best Arabian Coffee is to be reduced to powder in an iron mortar, which is to be moderately heated, occasionally detaching the mass from the sides of the vessel with a horn spatula. To the powder thus prepared add twelve drachms of alcohol, and put it into a glass vessel; let it remain eight days, and then separate the liquor from the sediment. Let this powder which remains at the bottom of the vessel be pressed free from all moisture, and placed in a glass retort with four ounces of distilled water; boil till one ounce only remains, and mix the clarified liquor with the alcoholic tincture; eighty drops of alcohol is to be added to thirty drops of this mixture, and twice shaken. This constitutes the first attenuation.

This medicine is also prepared by trituration; one grain of the powder is triturated with one hundred grains of sugar of milk, and so on to the thirtieth attenuation, by which the power of the medicine seems to be increased.

Physiological Effects.—"Coffea acts as an astringent and antiseptic. When a person unaccustomed to the use of Coffee drinks a moderate quantity, or one accustomed to its use drinks an immoderate quantity, for the first hours the self-consciousness—the feeling of his existence, of his life—becomes more lively. He gets a circumscribed redness of the cheeks, a redness which does not become gradually lost in the surrounding parts, but which presents the appearance of a well-defined red spot. The forehead and palms of the hands become warm and moist; he feels warmer than before. There occurs a kind of voluptuous palpitation of the heart, somewhat resembling that occurring during great joy; the veins of the hands swell. Presence of mind, attention, sympathy, become more active than in the healthy, natural state; all external objects seem to excite a feeling of pleasure. If the quantity of Coffee taken be immoderately great, and the body very excitable and quite unused to Coffee, there occurs a semilateral headache, from the upper part of the parietal bone to the base of the brain. The cerebral membranes of this side also seem to be painfully sensitive. The hands and feet become cold. On the brow and palms, cold sweat appears. The disposition becomes irritable and intolerant; no one can do anything to please him; he is anxious and trembling; restless; weeps almost without cause, or smiles most involuntarily. After a few hours, sleep comes on, out of which he starts with affright. I have seen this rare state two or three times" (*Hahnemann on Effects of Coffee, trans. by R. E. Dudgeon, M.D.*)

Medical Uses (Homœopathic).—Coffee produces in large doses headaches; it therefore cures in moderate ones headaches that do not proceed from derangement of the stomach, or acidity of the primæ viæ. It favours the peristaltic motion of the bowels in large doses, and therefore cures, in smaller doses, chronic diarrhœas; and in like manner, the other abnormal effects it occasions might be employed against similar affections of the human body, were we not in the habit of misusing it. The effects of opium in stupefying the senses and irritating the tone of the fibres, are removed by this berry, in its character of an antagonistic palliative remedy, and that properly and effectually; for here there is no persistent state of the organism, but only transitory symptoms to be combated. Intermittent fevers, too, where there is want of irritability and inordinate tension of the fibres, precluding the employment of otherwise specific bark, it apparently suppresses in large doses, merely as a palliative remedy; its direct action, however, in such large doses, lasts for two days. I saw a lying-in woman who, after a difficult labour, suffered from intolerable after-pains and a great loss of blood; she cried for Coffee, although when she was well she could scarcely endure it. Who told her hemorrhage resulted from atony of the womb, and this from diminished irritability of the fibres, and that the specific remedy for this was Coffee? A few cups of very strong Coffee were given to her, and the hemorrhage and pains ceased suddenly* (*Hahnemann*, l. c.)

Clinical Observations.—Noack and Trinks have collected the following in their work. Coffea may be employed for the precursory symptoms of small-pox, measles, and scarlatina; such as sleeplessness, bilious vomiting, headache, heat, and sweat. Purpura miliaris. Purple rash, when the pains are excessive, and the patient inclines to whine constantly. Cries and restlessness of children, when the child has been roused from its sleep, and would like to sleep again, but is not able. Sleeplessness from nervous irritation. Intermittent fevers. Violent colic; restlessness and tossing during the paroxysm. Puerperal fever, with excessive nervous irritation, when the pains seem intolerable. Intoxication by wine, mania a

* For more extended observations on the uses and abuses of Coffee, the reader is referred to Hahnemann's Lesser Writings, translated by Dr. Dudgeon, pp. 451 et seq.

potu. Sanguineous and nervous apoplexy (using Coffee as a prophylactic). Headache from excessive congestion of blood. Megrim (Coffee shortens the paroxysms, but does not cure them). Toothache from a purely nervous cause. Toothache of persons who use much Coffee. Throbbing toothache, with great nervousness and violent weeping. In some cases of weakness of digestion and overloading the stomach. Diarrhœa. Spasmodic colic. Violent pains in the abdomen in sensitive females. Excessively violent labour and after-pains. Coffee is an excellent palliative in cases of suspended animation in frozen, drowned, or suffocated individuals, when the vital forces require to be speedily roused.

"Coffee will in some cases prove useful in calming the nervous system after operations. One of my patients was operated on for cataract, after which the following group of symptoms presented itself. Violent inflammation of the eye, with a gnawing pain about the eye and whole side of the head; excessive nausea, as if the patient would die with it; involuntary weeping; qualms of sickness, constantly ascending from the stomach to the brain. Subsultus tendinum. I had some strong Coffee made, and gave the patient a teaspoonful of black Coffee every five minutes; after the second dose the patient fell into a sound sleep, which lasted several hours; when the patient awoke, all these symptoms had disappeared, except the pain about the eye, which was, however, much less, and soon disappeared" (*Hempel, trans. of Jahr's Mat. Med.*)

ANTIDOTES.—Aconitum. Nux Vomica. Chamomilla. Ignatia.

Pl. XXIV.

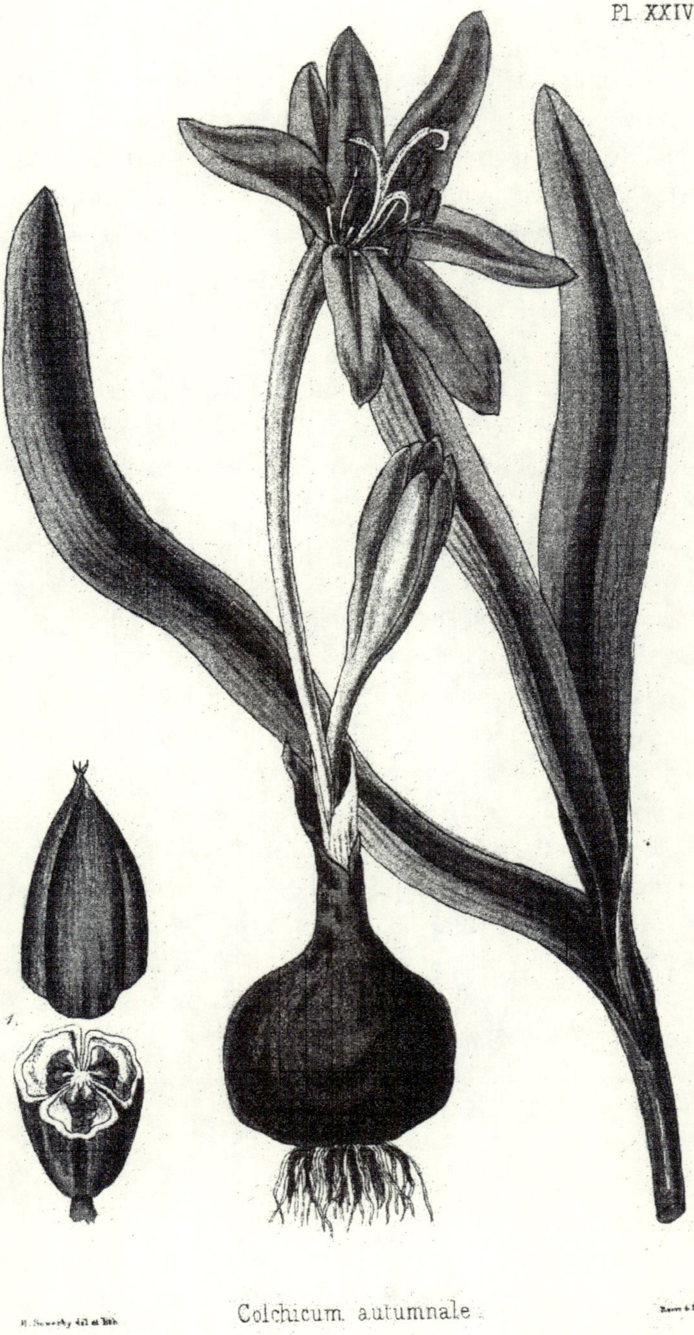

H. Sowerby del et lith

Colchicum autumnale

[illegible]

XXIV.

COLCHICUM* AUTUMNALE.

Common Meadow Saffron, Tuber Root, Naked Lady, Upstart.

SYNONYMS.—Colchicum anglicum purpureum et album, *Johnson's Ger. Em.*, 157. Colchicum commune, *Raii Syn.*, 373. Colchicum vere prodiens, *Camer. Epit.*, 846. Colchicum autumnale, *Linn. Sp. Plant.*, 485; *Willd.*, ii. 273; *Flora Britt.*, *Engl. Bot.*, ii. 133.

FOREIGN NAMES.—*Fr.:* Colchique, Tue-chien, Safran des Près. *Ital.:* Colchico, Giglio Matto, Strozzecane. *Span. and Port.:* Colchico. *Germ.:* Zeitlose, Wiesen-saffran, Lichtblume, Spinnblume. *Dut.:* Tydloosen. *Swed.:* Tidlöse, Nakna Jungfur. *Dan.:* Nogue Jomfrue. *Russ.:* Begvremennik.

Nat. Order, MELANTHACEÆ, *R. Brown;* HEXANDRIA, TRIGYNIA.

GEN. CHAR.—*Calyx* none. *Corolla* of one petal, tubular, very long, with a somewhat bell-shaped, six-parted limb. *Stamens* inserted into the mouth of the tube. *Anthers* oblong, incumbent. *Styles* three, very long. *Capsules* three, inflated, upright, united at the base, many-seeded.

SPEC. CHAR.—*Leaves* flat, broadly spear-shaped, upright.

HISTORY.—The Εφημερον of Theophrastus, the Κολχικὸν of Dioscorides, and the Ερμεδακτυλος of Paulus Ægineta, are supposed by Dr. Adams (*Supplement to Dunbar's Greek Lexicon; Comment. on Paulus Ægineta*), and other commentators, to be identical with our Colchicum autumnale. Pereira (*Elem. Mat. Med.*, p. 628) considers that the Hermodactylus is a species of Colchicum, but not the Colchicum autumnale. Miller (*Gardeners' Dict.*, 1579) considers the broad-leaved Meadow

---

Fig. 1. A tranverse section of the capsules, to show the position of the seeds.

* From Colchis, a province of Asia, where it grows in great abundance.

Saffron, which is indigenous in the Levant, to be the Hermodactylus of the shops. Alexander Trallian, in his work "De Podagra," recommends Hermodactylus as a remedy for gout and other affections, either alone or mixed with scammony, ginger, and other ingredients. He also remarks that the habitual use of this medicine disposes the patients to more frequent attacks of this disease, a peculiar effect likewise of Colchicum, which is corroborated by Sir C. Scudamore (*Treat. on Gout and Rheumatism*, 3rd edit., p. 197).

It appears to have been in great renown in the thirteenth century, and from its supposed virtues in the cure of gout and rheumatism of the joints, it obtained the name of Anima articulorum, "the soul of joints." It was the principal ingredient in all gout specifics; and the famous Eau médicinale is supposed to owe its virtues to a preparation from this plant.*

According to Prosper Alpinus, the Egyptian women ate great quantities of the wasted roots of the Colchicum to fatten themselves, calling them Hermodactyles; but M. Pomet (*Histoire des Drogues*) considers these as the fruit of a large tree; he, however, owns their services in palsies, gout, etc.

This is one of those plants whose violent and singular effects in the bodies of animals engaged the attention of Dr. Störck, in hopes that, by giving it in very small doses, or by due preparation, it might be converted into a medicine, not only safe, but capable of relieving disorders in which the common remedies prove ineffectual. "Sunt multi qui in abstractissimis processibus chemicis quærunt ex metallis medicamenta, et negligunt ea quæ tellus largitur offert, quæ naturæ provida sponte paravit et quæ corpori nostro sunt longe magis analoga" (*Störck, Libell. de Colch. Autum.*)

* Others believe that the chief ingredient in Husson's specific (Eau médicinale) is the Rhododendron crysanthum; the effects of the French medicine are precisely those which are experienced from an infusion of this plant, which the Siberians and Russians regard as an infallible specific in the cure of chronic rheumatism and gout (vide *Paris, Pharmacologia*, 9th edit., p. 122.)

Besides its supposed specific properties in gout, it has been employed by Macleod, Wigan, and others, in rheumatism and rheumatic gout (*Lond. Med. Gazette*, vol. xxi., June 30, 1838). By Störck, in dropsy (l. c.) By Haden, in inflammatory disorders generally (*Pract. Observ. on the Colch. Autumnale*, 1820). By Dr. Hastings, in chronic bronchitis (*Treat. on Inflam. of Mucous Membrane of the Lungs*). By Dr. Lewin, in fevers (*Edin. Med. and Surg. Jour.*, 1837). By Shearman, in syphilis. By Williams, in venereal nodes. By Mr. Raven, in hysteria, hypochondriasis, chorea, and convulsion (*Lond. Med. and Phys. Jour.*, 1817). By Elliotson, in prurigo. By Vogt, in erysipelas. By Müller, in rheumatic headache. By Pereira, in humoral asthma and other chronic bronchial affections (*Elem. of Mat. Med.*, p. 625). In leucorrhœa, by Rulton. In arthritic carditis, by Schönlein, etc.

DESCRIPTION.—Perennial. Flowers in September and October. *Bulb* (*cormus*) solid, resembling that of a tulip, furrowed on one side. *Leaves* strap spear-shaped, blunt, entire, dark green, smooth; a foot or more long, and from one to two inches broad. *Flowers* several, rising from the root, and appearing in succession, pale purple, sometimes white; tube from five or six to eight or ten inches long, white, and surrounded at the base by two or three membranous sheaths. *Limb* cut into six somewhat unequal, oblong, upright, concave segments. *Germen* at the base of the bulb inclosed in one common sheath, and accompanied by the rudiments of the future leaves. *Styles* as long as the stamens, thread-shaped, reaching nearly to the base of the tube. *Stigmas* linear, recurved, channelled, downy. *Fruit* oval, formed of three inflated, many-seeded *capsules*. *Seeds* round, whitish, polished. The flowers appear in September, the leaves and fruit not till the spring following (*Baxter*).*

* "The seeds lie buried all winter within the root, in spring they grow up on a fruit-stalk, and are ripe about the time of hay-harvest. May not the very great length of the shafts account, in some measure, for the delay in ripening of the seeds? As this plant blossoms late in the year, and probably would not have

GEOGRAPHICAL DISTRIBUTION.—Over most parts of Europe, Asia Minor, and North America.

LOCALITIES.—In moist, rich meadows. Sibthorp (*Prod. Flor. Græc.*) found it in Greece, but only on Mounts Parnassus and Thymphrastus, at an elevation of 3,000 to 4,000 feet. In this country, its chief localities are in *Gloucestershire:* in moist meadows. *Hampshire:* in moist meadows. *Oxfordshire:* near Coombe, Heythorp, Stanton Harcourt, Ashford Mills, between Headington and Barton, near Oxford. In meadows near Upper Heyford, Leafield, Wychwood Forest near Filkins, and near Bradwell. *Berkshire:* near Appleton and Cumnor. *Suffolk:* at Little Stonham. *Staffordshire:* Weston Park; by the Trent, near Burton *Suffolk:* near Bungay, both purple and white-flowered varieties. *Warwickshire:* Castle Bromwich. *Worcestershire:* on the banks of the Severn. In moist meadows between Alvechurch and Redditch. *Wiltshire:* near Devizes, a white-flowered variety common. *Yorkshire:* near Rotherham, Richmond, etc. In *Scotland:* near Alloa.

The London market, according to Dr. Pereira, is supplied chiefly from Gloucestershire, Hampshire, and Oxfordshire.

PARTS USED IN MEDICINE, AND MODE OF PREPARATION.—The *Cormus* (or bulb), when gathered at the proper season is about the size of a chestnut, and resembles, externally, the bulb of the common tulip; it is at once distinguished from this and other liliaceous bulbs by being *solid*, the tulip bulb and others being composed of laminæ or scales. It is rounded on one side, somewhat flattened, and grooved on the other; it has two coats, the outer one of a brown colour, the inner of a reddish-yellow. Internally it is white, fleshy, and solid, containing a

time to ripen its seeds before the access of winter, which would destroy them, Providence has executed its structure such, that this important office may be performed at a depth in the earth, out of the reach of the usual effects of frost; and as *seeds* buried at such a depth are known not to vegetate, a no less admirable provision is made to raise them above the surface when they are perfected, and to sow them at a proper season" (*With., Brit. Plants*).

milky juice; it is very feculent, and has an acrid, bitter taste (*Pereira, Elem. Mat. Med.*, 3rd edit., pt. 1, vol. ii.)

Collection of the Cormi (*bulbs*).—The cormus is biennial. It first appears about the end of June or beginning of July; it flowers in the autumn, and produces its leaves in the spring, and its seeds in the June of the following year; it then begins to shrivel, becomes leathery, and finally disappears in the succeeding spring or summer. The activity of the cormus varies at different seasons of the year. It is usually considered to be greatest when the cormus is about a year old; that is, about the month of July, between the withering of the leaves and the sprouting forth of the flowers of the young cormus; at this period the cormus is fully developed, and has not exhausted itself by the production of the young one (*Id.*, l. c.)

Dr. Christison has expressed some doubts as to the propriety of collecting the cormi in July; for though they are plumpest, firmest, and abound most in starch at this period, yet he has found the shrivelled cormi in the succeeding cormi in the following April, to be equally, if not more bitter; and he quotes the analyses of Stoltze to show that while the October cormus yields two per cent., the March cormus yields six per cent. of bitter extract. But there is an error in the quotation, which vitiates the inference intended to be drawn from it. Stoltze found that the October cormus contains 2.17 per cent. of *bitter* extractive, and that the March cormus contained 5.91 per cent. of *sweet* extractive matter, combined with some bitter extractive; and he concludes that the October cormus is much more active, and contains more bitter extractive than the spring cormus (*Id.*, l. c.)

Before drying the cormus, it should be cut transversely into thin slices, the dry coats being previously removed. The slices are to be quickly dried in a dark, airy place, the heat not to exceed 170° Fahr. (*Battley, Lond. Med. Repos.*, xiv. 429). The late Dr. A. T. Thompson recommends the slices to be dried on clean, white paper, without artificial heat; the only objection to this is the time required.

According to Dr. Lindley (*Flora Med.*, p. 589), a quantity of the cormi come to market which have already pushed forth flowers, but which have been broken off, and yet have found a ready sale at the best price.

Quin (*Pharm. Hom.*) and Jahr (*Hom. Pharm. and Posol.*) advise the gathering of the cormi in the spring; but Pereira recommends July as the period of their greatest activity, and objects to Dr. Christison's plan of gathering in October.

The juice is to be expressed from the cormi, and then prepared in the same manner as directed for all fresh plants.

PHYSIOLOGICAL EFFECTS.—*On Animals.* Colchicum acts on many animals as a violent poison. Cattle feeding in meadows where this plant grows are said to be affected in the spring by the seeds which adhere to the coats of the stomach, producing at the several points of their adhesion inflammation, which occasions death; and several pigs having eaten plentifully of the bulbs which had been grubbed up and placed in a yard, died in excruciating agonies, and on dissection the stomach of each was found burst (*Taylor on Poisons, art. Colchicum*).

Sir Everard Home (*Phil. Trans.*, 1816) experimented on some dogs. He injected 160 drops of the vinous infusion into the jugular vein of a dog; all power of motion was instantly lost, and the effect on the pulse was remarkable; at first it could not be felt, in ten minutes it was 84, in twenty minutes 60, in one hour 115, and in two hours 150. The respiration was at one time very slow, at another, on the rise of the pulse, so quick it could hardly be counted. There was much purging and vomiting, and death ensued in five hours. After death the stomach was found universally inflamed.

Orfila (*Toxicol. Gén.*, 3rd edit., vol. ii. p. 257) has constantly given the bulbs of Colchicum, collected in June, to dogs, without perceiving any sensible effect. He therefore considers that climate and season have much to do with its deleterious property. It is said to be harmless to horses; but Mr. Woodward, in "Withering's British Plants" (l. c.), says, that in a pasture in which were several horses, and eaten down pretty bare, the grass was closely cropped even under the leaves, but not a leaf bitten.

On Man.—Störck (*Libellus de Rad. Colch. Aut.*) found that on cutting the fresh juice into slices, the acrid particles emitted from it irritated the nostrils, fauces, and breath, and that the ends of the fingers with which it had been held became quite benumbed; that, applied for two minutes to the tip of the tongue, it rendered the part rigid and almost void of sensation for six hours; that less than a grain wrapped up in a crumb of bread, and taken internally, produced alarming symptoms, a burning heat and pain in the stomach and bowels, strangury, tenesmus, thirst, total loss of appetite, etc., which were greatly relieved by an acidulous mixture of syrup of poppies; that an infusion of three grains of the root in four ounces of wine, slowly swallowed, occasioned a tickling in the larynx and a short, dry cough; soon after, a heat of the urinary passages and a copious discharge of pale urine, without sensibly affecting the other organs of the body; that an ounce of the sliced root being digested in a pound of vinegar for forty-eight hours, and the bottle frequently shaken, the root became insipid, but the vinegar became acrid, irritated the fauces, and produced cough.

According to Dr. Lewins (*Edin. Med. and Surg. Jour.*, vol. xlvii. p. 345), small doses, frequently repeated, produce debility, sensation of malaise, and headache. Dr. Barlow (*Cyclop. of Pract. Med.*, vol. ii. p. 371) has seen twenty evacuations by stool from one dose of Colchicum, without producing corresponding debility. Wood and Bache (*United States Dispensatory*, 3rd edit.) record violent salivation as the result of small doses of Colchicum. Its chief effects, in small and repeated doses, seem to be a tendency to promote the action of the secreting organs, especially of the intestinal mucous membrane, and to produce perspiration. (*Per.*, l. c.)

In large doses, Colchicum acts as a violent poison, and many fatal cases have been recorded. Mr. Fereday (*Lond. Med. Gazette*, vol. x. p. 160) relates a case of poisoning with two ounces of the wine of the seeds of Colchicum taken by mistake for rum. About an hour and a half after swallowing it, acute pain in the bowels came on, followed by copious vomiting of a yellow fluid, tenesmus, small, slow, and feeble pulse. The pain was described as of a knife piercing him; the tongue was natural; the countenance anxious; features sharp; cheeks, lips, and palpebræ purple; sensation of losing his limbs on walking; the vomiting increased; the fluid brought up was like coffee-grounds; and the patient died forty-seven hours after taking the poison. On a *post-mortem* examination, the face, neck, and front of the thorax were found covered with a purple efflorescence. The stomach and bowels were coated with a thick, tenacious, colourless mucus. Blood was effused between the muscular and peritoneal coats; the pleuræ costales were much reddened; the heart was flabby, and its structure easily broken down; two red patches were found, one in the stomach, and the other in the jejunum. Ecchymosed spots were observed on the surface of the lungs, of the heart, and of the diaphragm.

Dr. Ollivier (*Annales d'Hyg.*, 1836, vol. ii. p. 394) records two cases. In the first, continual vomiting, but no purging; pulse thready and slow; intense thirst; severe cramps in the soles of the feet; intellect unaffected; no convulsions or tetanic spasms. The patient died in twenty-two hours. In the second case the symptoms soon set in after taking the poison. There were violent pains in the abdomen; frequent vomiting, but no purging; difficult respiration; pupils not dilated; coldness of the surface; no tetanic spasms, but cramps in the soles of the feet; pulse small; the intellect was not impaired. Death took place in twenty-seven hours. The vessels of the pia mater were much injected; no vascularity of the stomach.

A man swallowed a large quantity of Colchicum seeds; he soon experienced a burning sensation in the throat, with nausea, vomiting, violent colicky pains, and frequent diarrhœa, succeeded by difficulty of breathing, and discharge of bloody urine. After death, patches of mortification were found in the stomach and duodenum (*Pharmac. Times*, Jan. 23, 1847).

A man, aged fifty-six years, of a feeble constitution, and a prey to chronic rheumatism, swallowed, by mistake, one ounce and a half of Vinum Colchici; in about half an hour he was seized with severe pain in the abdomen, and nausea, followed by vomiting and constant alvine dejections, often involuntary; these symptoms continued during the night and the greater part of the following day, then the alvine evacuations ceased, but the nausea continued; the day after taking the poison he was seized with most violent thirst, which continued till his death; the pains in the stomach and intestines were excessively acute; towards evening delirium came on, and he died the following morning. On examination after death, no trace of inflammation could be discovered in the intestines, the stomach only was red (*Edin. Journ.*, April, 1818).

Susan Laing, about thirty years of age, of good health and constitution; she was about two months in pregnancy, and having read in a newspaper that a woman was taken up for causing abortion by taking Meadow Saffron, she determined on getting rid of her burthen by a similar measure. She accordingly bought twopenny-worth and made an infusion of it, which she took on an empty stomach early in the morning of the 10th of March, 1827. I was called to her about four o'clock in the afternoon of the 11th, and on inquiry learned she had miscarried the preceding evening. I found her in a very hopeless state; her extremities were quite cold, and the whole of her body, particularly the hands, feet, and face, livid. The glassy stare of impending death was in her eyes, the respiration was hurried, and the pulse could not be felt at the carotids, and but faintly at the heart. Notwithstanding, the sensorium was undisturbed, and she gave me a clear account of what she had done, her motives for so doing, and the effects the poison had on her.

She said that, in about half an hour after taking it, her stomach became sick, gripes came on, and a violent purging, which continued with great severity. She had had no medical assistance, and had passed a most wretched time from the morning before, and was so tormented with pain and purging, that she had not had a wink of sleep in the course of the night. I administered large draughts of brandy and spices, but to no effect; she died two hours after I came in. The body was opened the next day; all the viscera were found healthy, except that the mucous membrane of the stomach and bowels was dreadfully inflamed throughout its course (*Dillon, in Stephenson and Churchill's Med. Bot.*, vol. ii.)

Garibel, in his "Histoire des Plantes des Environs d'Aix," records that a servant was killed by taking the flowers for an intermittent fever, in which disease they were said to be useful.

H. P. swallowed about an ounce of the tincture of Colchicum, at nine o'clock, p.m., on a full stomach, and at five o'clock the following morning, eight hours after it had been taken, vomiting commenced; as the stomach was emptied the retchings increased in violence, and continued at regular intervals three times an hour for twelve hours; from the sixth hour the violence of the retchings gradually decreased. Acid, pungent taste in the mouth, with more or less bitterness; excessive heat, and great dryness of the mouth and throat; contraction of the chest; breathing quick and difficult; great pain at the pit of the stomach, and in the bowels; frequent purgings, and coldness of the extremities; during the paroxysms, great trembling of the whole frame, and violent pain in the head; afterwards, great prostration of strength (*Communicated to the Author by the patient*).

Medical Uses (Homœopathic).—This drug was not proved by Hahnemann. According to Noack and Trinks (*Handbuch für Hom. Arzneimitt.*), Colchicum is useful in sanguineous constitutions, and in phlegmatic-melancholic temperaments. It is also of especial service in thin, irritable, hysterical, and hypochondriacal individuals, with great disposition to perspiration and acidity, with rheumatism and catarrh. In patients with white, delicate skin, who are liable to perspire on the slightest cause, and with increased irritability. In diseases occurring during a condition of the atmosphere predisposing to rheumatic affections. In rheumatic and gouty conditions, both acute and chronic. Mercurial rheumatism and gout. Dropsy. Anasarca, after the acute exanthemata. Ascites. Dropsy of the joints. Epidemic miliaria. Ptyalism. Rheumatic toothache, with darting, tearing pains, accompanied with a sensation of numbness and cramp in the articulation of the jaw, and is especially painful when the teeth are pressed together, with nightly aggravation of the pains. Singultus. Flatulent colic in hysterical and hypochondriacal individuals. Dysenteric diarrhœa. Chronic dysentery. Epidemic gastric dysentery, prevailing in the autumn. Mucous hemorrhoids. Affections of the bladder and kidneys. Paralytic weakness of the muscles of the urinary organs. Strangury and ischuria. Asthmatic affections. Spasms of the chest (*Ruckert*). Pleurisy, with serous effusion (*Wurm*). Incipient hydrothorax (*Ruckert*). Palpitation of the heart. Rheumatic tearing pain in the shoulder-joints.

ANTIDOTES.—Against large doses, Vinegar and Honey (*Störck*). Caustic Ammonia, six to eight drops, in some eau sucré (*Schönlein*). To homœopathic doses, Cocculus. Nux Vomica. Pulsatilla.

XXV.

CUCUMIS COLOCYNTHIS.

Colocynth, Bitter Cucumber, or Bitter Apple.

SYNONYMS.—Colocynthis, *Gerard. Emar.*, p. 915; *Raii Hist.*, p. 642. Colocynthis fructu rotundo minor, *Bauh. Πιν.*, p. 313. Colocynthis vulgaris, *Park. Theat.*, p. 160.

FOREIGN NAMES.—*Fr.:* Coloquinte. *Ital.:* Coloquintida. *Span.:* Coloquintida. *Port.:* Coloquintidas. *Germ.:* Coloquinte. *Dut.:* Koloquint. *Swed.:* Coloqwint. *Dan.:* Coloqvinder. *Russ.:* Colotsint. *Arab.:* Hunzil. *Pers.:* Hunzil. *Tam.:* Peycoomutikai, Varriecoomutikai.

Nat. Order, CUCURBITACEÆ.—MONŒCIA, SYNGENESIA.

GEN. CHAR.—*Calyx* tubular, campanulate, with subulate segments, scarcely the length of the tube. *Petals* scarcely adherent to each other and the calyx. *Males: Stamina* five, triadelphous. *Females: Stigmas* three, thick, bipartite. *Fruit* (peponida) three to six-celled. *Seeds* ovate, compressed, not marginate. *Flowers* monœcious or hermaphrodite, yellow (*Decandolle*).

SPEC. CHAR.—*Stem* procumbent, somewhat hispid. *Leaves* cordate-ovate, many-lobed, white, with hairs beneath; the lobes obtuse; the petioles as long as the lamina. *Tendrils* short. *Flowers* axillary, solitary, stalked; *females* with the tube of the calyx globose, somewhat hispid; the limb campanulate, with narrow segments. *Petals* small. *Fruit* globose, smooth, yellow when ripe, with a thin, solid rind, and very bitter flesh (*Decandolle*).

HISTORY.—Dr. Adams (*Dunbar, Gr. Lex.*) considers the Κολοκυνθις of the ancient Materia Medica, described by Dioscorides and Galen, to be the Cucumis Colocynthis (Bitter Apple) of the modern Pharmacopœias. But "even in the days of Athenæus, the *literati* complained of the difficulty of dis-

---

Fig. 1. A section of the flower. 2. The anther. 3. A seed. 4. The fruit (pepo).

PL. XXV.

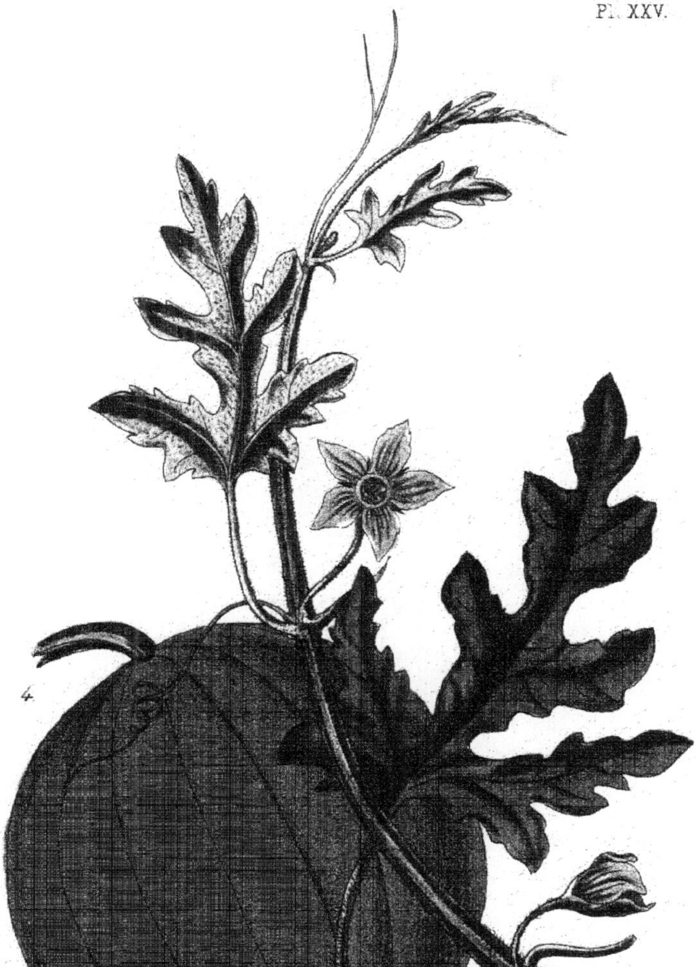

E Sowerby lith. Cucumis Colocynthis. Reeve & Nichols imp.

tinguishing the summer fruits from one another, owing to the confusion of names which had taken place among the authors who had treated of them;" and these remarks may apply to the plant in question, as we find the Colocynth described by Theophrastus put down by Stackhouse as the Cucumis Colocynthis, and by others as the common cucumber. Again, the Κολ. αγρια of Hippocrates has been considered to be the Cucumis Colocynthis by Pereira; the Cucumis sativus by Sprengel and other commentators; and Cucurbita sylvestris, or Wild Gourd, by Gerarde; the latter declares the Colocynth to be the Wild Citrull, and he says: "The Latine translators for Colocynthis do oftentimes set down Cucurbita sylvestris; notwithstanding this differeth from Colocynthis or Coloquintida, for Cucurbita sylvestris is called in Greeke, Κολοκυνθα αγρια."

The Colocynth of modern times is supposed to be the gourd mentioned in the Second Book of Kings, chap. iv., v. 39, when, in the famine in Gilgal, the prophet Elisha showed his divine mission by making the poisonous gourd a wholesome vegetable.

The Arabian physicians called it Alhandal, and were well acquainted with its properties. It is mentioned in the works of Avicenna, Serapion, Mesne, Ebn Baithar, etc.

The Greek physicians employed it chiefly as a drastic purgative in dropsy, lethargy, and in mania, and to produce abortion.

From its violent drastic effects, it has been in general use from the earliest times as an ingredient in most purges, and has been employed chiefly: In alvine obstructions. Habitual constipation. Some diseases of the brain, as apoplexy, mania. In dropsy and in amenorrhœa and chlorosis, as a sympathetic medicine. In chronic gout and rheumatism. Paralysis. Paraplegia and hemiplegia (*Schneider*). Gastric nervous fever (*Hochenberger*). Hæmatemesis. Hemorrhoidal colic (*id.*) Affections of the liver (*id.*) Dysentery (*Araber*). Paralysis of the bladder (*Neumann*). Paralysis of the upper and lower extremities (*Koelpin, Hinze, Vorgtel, Schmur, Neumann*), etc., etc. (vide *Noack and Trinks, Handb. für Hom. Arzneimitt.*)

DESCRIPTION.—This is a trailing plant, with a white, annual, branched root, which strikes deep into the ground. The *stem* is herbaceous, angular branched, covered with rough hairs, and trails along the ground; in its appearance resembling the common cucumber. The *tendril* is filiform, branching opposite each leaf. The *leaves* are triangular, obtuse, sinuated, hairy, of a fine green on the upper surface, rough and whitish underneath. *Flowers* yellow, with greenish veins, and solitary, and appear at the axillæ of the leaves. *Male flowers:* *Calyx* bell-shaped, five-toothed. *Corolla* monopetalous, bell-shaped, divided into five segments. *Stamens* three, short, free; two of which have doubly-bent anthers, or consist of two anthers; in which case, the number of stamens is really five. *Female flowers:* the *calyx* and *corolla* similar to the male flowers. The *ovarium* is round, smooth, inferior. *Style* short, cylindrical. *Stigmas* three; filaments without anthers. *Fruit* (pepo) about the size of an orange, with a thin but solid rind. The flowers appear from May till August (*Woodville and Pereira*).

According to Captain Lyon, the seeds are perfectly innocuous, and highly nutritious, and constitute an important article of food in Northern Africa. But Christison (*Disp.*, p. 357) states that those from the dried fruit brought to this country, however carefully washed, partake slightly of the bitterness of the pulp.

GEOGRAPHICAL DISTRIBUTION.—Japan, the sandy lands of the Coromandel Coast, Cape of Good Hope, Syria, Nubia, Egypt, Turkey, and the Islands of the Grecian Archipelago. Cultivated in Spain. Burckhardt, when travelling in Nubia, found the ground in many parts covered with this plant.

PARTS USED IN MEDICINE, AND MODE OF PREPARATION.—The Fruit (pepo). The following description of the fruit is taken from Pereira's *Elements of Mat. Med.*, p. 1075. "The fruit is gathered in the autumn when ripe and yellow, and in most countries is peeled, and dried either by the sun or by stoves. In commerce it is imported from Spain (Almeria, Gibraltar, Cadiz, Malaga, etc.), Trieste, Malta, Smyrna, Alexandretta, Mogadore, etc. The fruit called Colocynth or Coloquintida (Colocynthis poma Colocynthidis) is imported either *peeled* (generally) or sometimes unpeeled. Its pulp (pulpa Colocynthidis exsiccata) is nearly white, inodorous, light, spongy, porous, tough, intensely and nauseously bitter. The *seeds* (semina Colocynthidis) are smooth, either white or yellowish-white (white Colocynth seeds), or brownish (black Colocynth seeds), bitter, especially the dark-coloured ones, and inodorous. Two kinds of Colocynth, distinguished as *Turkey* and *Mogadore Colocynth*, are known in commerce.

" *Turkey Colocynth: peeled Colocynth.*—This is imported from the Levant, Spain, etc. The usual size of each pepo is about two or three inches in diameter; the shape is more or less globular, according to the evenness with which the rind has been removed, and the degree of contraction in drying; the colour is white or pale yellowish-white. One hundred parts by weight are said to consist of twenty-eight parts pulp and seventy-two parts seeds.

" *Mogadore Colocynth: unpeeled Colocynth.*—The pepo of this kind is larger than the preceding, and is covered with a yellowish, smooth, firm rind. It is imported from Mogadore in small quantities only, and is principally used by druggists for show-bottles."

To prepare it for homœopathic use, the fruit, well dried, is reduced to powder without the assistance of heat, according to the rules given for the preparation of dried plants; set aside for a week, to be shaken twice daily; then attenuated to the thirtieth dilution, and preserved in well-stopped bottles in a dark place. Hahnemann (*Mat. Med. Pur.*) orders the dry fruit to be reduced to powder, twenty grains of which are infused for a week in 400 drops of alcohol, stirring it twice a day. Twenty drops of this tincture contain one grain of the essence.

Physiological Effects.—*On Animals.* Colocynth acts on animals, as on man, as a violent drastic and poison. Orfila (*Tox. Gén.*, 3rd edit., p. 691) made five experiments on dogs: he found that three drachms introduced into the stomach were sufficient to cause death. On examination after death, the mucous membrane of the stomach was found inflamed through its whole extent. The duodenum, jejunum, and ileum, the cæcum, and first portion of the colon were found of a very red colour. According to Viborg (*Pharm. Vet.*, 274), the operation of Colocynth on horses is comparatively slight. Moiroud (*id.*, l. c.) gave four drachms to a small horse, without producing any particular symptoms. He mentions also another curious circumstance, viz., that he found that bryonia (one of the Cucurbitaceæ) had but little, if any, effect on the horse.

On Man.—Colocynth in moderate doses acts as a purge. In full doses, as a violent drastic cathartic and hydragogue. In excessive doses, it has often proved a fatal poison, producing violent vomiting and purging, and other symptoms of gastric intestinal inflammation.

Fordyce (*Fragm. of Surg. and Med.*, p. 66) mentions the case of a woman who was a prey to colic for thirty years, from having taken an infusion of the pulp of Colocynth mixed with some beer.

Tulpius (*Observ. Médicinales*, iv. c. 27, p. 2181) notices the case of a man who was nearly carried off by profuse bloody diarrhœa, in consequence of taking a decoction of three Colocynth apples.

In 1823, a coroner's inquest was held, in London, on the body of a woman who died in twenty-four hours, with incessant vomiting and purging, in consequence of having swallowed by mistake a teaspoonful and a half of Colocynth powder.

Dioscorides (lib. iv. c. 178) had observed that Colocynth introduced into the rectum produced a discharge of blood (dysentery).

A man swallowed three ounces of Colocynth in the hope of getting rid of a gonorrhœa, which he had had for some days. In a short time, violent pains in the epigastrium, with excessive vomiting; in about two hours there were copious alvine dejections; the sight was obscured; he heard with difficulty; slight delirium came on, followed by vertigo. After some slight treatment, the symptoms gradually subsided (*Orfila, Tox. Gén.*, vol. i. p. 695, 3rd edit.)

A locksmith, aged twenty-eight years, subject to bleeding hemorrhoids, complained for some time of pains in the stomach and many other symptoms of dyspepsia. A German workman, his companion, promised to cure him radically by means of a domestic remedy. He took by his advice two glasses of a bitter decoction, which I found afterwards to be Colocynth. The remedy produced frequent evacuations, accompanied by colic; some hours after the patient complained of great heat in his intestines, a sensation of dryness in the throat, and an unquenchable thirst. He came for me at night. The true cause of the disease was hidden from me. I found the patient with a small pulse, very accelerated; the tongue red; the abdomen tender and very painful to touch; the pain was fixed, and very severe near the umbilicus; the stools were suppressed. The next morning the abdomen was more inflated and more painful. The patient was placed in a tepid bath, and six hours after all the pains increased; there was retention of urine, painful retraction of the testicles, and priapism. The third day the retention of urine ceased, but the other symptoms continued; the pulse was small and compressed; hiccough supervened; the extremities became cold; the head and chest were covered with a greasy sweat; in the evening all the pain ceased, and the patient died in the night. On a *post-mortem* examination, the abdominal viscera showed the greatest disorganization; the abdomen was filled with a whitish fluid, full of flocks of the same colour; the intestines were ulcerated, scattered over with black spots, for the most part adhering and covered with false membranes; the internal membrane of the stomach was detached and ulcerated; the peritoneum was almost gangrened; the liver, kidneys, and bladder showed traces of inflammation (*Carron d'Annecy, in Orf. Tox. Gén.*, l. c.)

It is to be remarked that in the experiments with Colocynth and Elaterium, when these poisons have produced death after their introduction into the stomach, this organ and the rectum are found inflamed, whilst the rest of the intestines are found in the natural condition. This applies equally to many other poisonous substances. It appears to depend on the rapidity with which a part of the poison traverses the intestines, and the long time it remains in the stomach and rectum, and not in virtue of a specific action upon this intestine; for it is wanting often when the poison produces death after being injected into the cellular tissue of the thigh (*Orf.*, l. c.)

Medical Uses (Homœopathic).—*Hahnemann's observations* (l. c.): "The ancients brought Colocynth into disrepute by using it in large and dangerous doses as an aperient. Their successors, alarmed at such examples, rejected it altogether, and were thus deprived of its powerful assistance in disease. They ventured upon it only on very rare occasions, after weakening and changing its properties by means of other substances, called correctives, which they considered proper to soften and overcome the venom with which they believed it to be impregnated. They added other aperient ingredients by means of a mucilaginous gum, and diminished its strength both by fermentation and by a continued ebullition with water, wine, etc. But after all these alterations, Colocynth was still dangerous in the large doses they administered.

"How extraordinary it is, that at all times schools of medicine should have shunned reflection, and that, under circumstances like these, the idea should never occur that in cases where medicines of this powerful kind in certain doses are too violent, it may be attributable less to their nature than to the size of the dose, which is capable of being diminished; and this diminution, without taking away the properties of the medicinal agent, will reduce its strength so as effectually to prevent its doing injury, while it allows it to be used successfully. This is, in short, the natural and simple corrective of all medicines endowed with such powerful properties. It is evident that if a pint of alcohol, drank off at once, can kill a man, it is not from any inherent poisonous quality, but from the too great strength of the dose, and that two drops of alcohol would be incapable of hurting the man. It is also clear that if one drop of concentrated sulphuric acid would instantly burn and corrode that part of the tongue on which it fell, it would merely be a mildly acidulated liquor, when mixed with a sufficient quantity of water.

"This is the only way to discover the inestimable value, hitherto unknown, of those powerful (*heroic*) medicines called poisons, in cases which are the most difficult to treat, and to obtain their effects, whether in acute or chronic affections. No schools of medicine have hitherto succeeded in this, because their silly and childish method of softening powerful substances, and rendering them applicable for use failed, and they were obliged to give up the use of the most effective and salutary medicines.

"Guided by the morbid symptoms induced in persons in health, I have succeeded in producing the most happy cures by Colocynth, giving as a dose only a small part of a drop of the octillionth or decillionth dilution of the above tincture.

"To limit myself to a single example, colics of the severest kind are often quickly cured, according to symptoms, when at the same time the other morbid conditions were in some degree analogous to the symptoms of Colocynth."

Clinical Observations.—*Noack and Trinks* (l. c.): According to Professor Martin, Colocynth promotes the secretion of mucus considerably, but not permanently. It acts similarly to spirituous substances. Its primary effects upon the organism are so powerful, that the disturbances which it produces in it are succeeded by secondary symptoms of long duration. Colocynth is especially suitable to sthenic, dry, bilious, atrabilious, sanguineous hemorrhoidal constitutions, and choleric-melancholy temperaments. It is likewise adapted to lax and scrofulous constitutions; to passionate, excitable individuals; women suffering from profuse catamenia, and such as lead a sedentary life. It deserves especial consideration in bilious conditions. Acute sthenic rheumatism. Arthritic conditions. Paralysis. Neuralgia. Arthrocace. Bilious fever, caused by anxiety and grief. Puerperal fever, consequent on vexation. Periodical semilateral headache, returning every day. Megrim, with nausea and vomiting. Violent headaches, accompanied with constriction of the chest. Headache on the left side, with a sensation as if the left half of the head was being torn off (*Gaspary*). Arthritic and other inflammations of the eyes (*Scheller*). Prosopalgia, with violent tearing and burning on one side of the face. Spasmodic, inflammatory, and flatulent colic (*Hartlaub*). Colic from cold, and also from moral emotions, etc. Colic, with diarrhœa after taking food, causing one to bend double. Epidemic dysentery, in the first and second stage (*Scudery*). Dysenteric diarrhœa. Psoitis chronica (*Ruckert*). Coxarthrocace. Ischias nervosa cotunni (with the help of Nux Vomica). Lancinating pains in different parts of the sacrum and hips, obliging one to limp (*Hartlaub*), etc. etc.

Antidotes.—Against large doses, tepid Milk, (?) infusion of Galls, Camphor, Opium. To small doses, Camphor, Causticum, Chamomilla, Coffea, Staphysagria, Tabacum. (?) Colocynth antidotes Causticum and Mercurius.

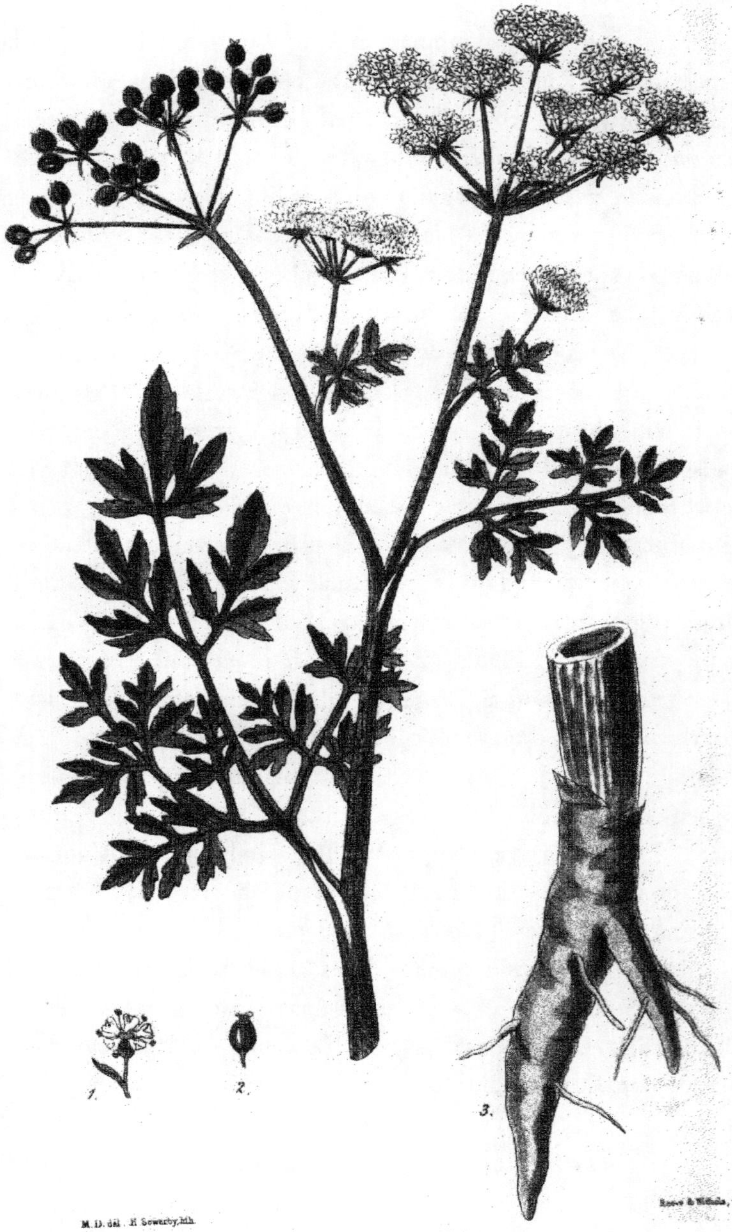

M. D. del. H Sowerby, lith.

Reeve & Nichols, imp.

Conium maculatum.

XXVI.

CONIUM* MACULATUM.

Common or Spotted Hemlock, Homlock, Kex, Herb Bennet.

SYNONYMS.—Cicuta, *Raii Syn.*, 2151; *Ger. Em.*, 1061. Cicuta vulgaris major, *Park. Theat.*, 933. Conium, *Hall Hist.*, vol. i. p. 337. Conium major, *Bauh. Пιν.*, 160. Coriandrum cicuta, *Crantz Austr.*, fasc. iii. p. 100. Coriandrum maculatum, *Roth Germ.*, vol. i. p. 130. Conium maculatum, *Lin.*, *Sp. Pl.*, 349; *Fl. Brit.*, 302.

FOREIGN NAMES.—*Fr.:* Grande Cigue. *Ital.:* Cicuta maggiore, Conio manchado. *Span.:* Cicuta, Ceguda. *Port.:* Cigude. *Germ.:* Geflecte Schierling. *Dut.:* Dollekervel, Scheerling. *Swed.:* Spräklig odort. *Dan.:* Skarntyde. *Russ.:* Botigolor piatnistoi.

Nat. Order, UMBELLIFERÆ.—PENTANDRIA, DIGYNIA.

GEN. CHAR.—*Flowers* all perfect, slightly irregular. *Calyx* obsolete. *Corolla* superior, of five inversely heart-shaped petals, with an acute inflexed point, the outermost rather the largest. *Filaments* five, hair-like, scarcely so long as the corolla. *Anthers* roundish. *Germen* egg-shaped, somewhat compressed, furrowed, wrinkled. *Styles* two, thread-shaped, elongated, spreading, a little swelled at the base, proceeding from the dilated, depressed, wavy, permanent floral receptacle. *Stigmas* blunt. *Fruit* broadly egg-shaped, slightly compressed, with ten prominent, acute ribs, wavy, in an upright state, crowned with the dilated undulated *floral receptacle,* and the shortest, permanent, spreading styles. *Carpel* (seeds of Linnæus) half egg-shaped, tumid, each with five prominent, waved, or crenated *ridges,* becoming finally straight and even. *Interstices* with many striæ, without *vittæ.* *Seed* with a sharp, narrow groove in front. *Universal involucrum* of a few leaves; *partial one* of three leaves on one side. The obsolete *calyx,* the inversely head-

---

Fig. 1. A flower. 2. An unripe fruit. 3. The root.

* From the Greek word *κωνος*, a cone, or a top, whose whirling motion resembles the giddiness produced on a human constitution by the poisonous juice of this plant.

shaped *petals*, the broadly egg-shaped *fruit*, and the *carpels*, with five prominent, waved, or crenated ridges, with the interstices without *vittæ*, will distinguish this from other genera in the same class and order.

SPEC. CHAR.—*Stem* smooth, polished, and spotted, much branched. *Leaves* of involucels spear-shaped, shorter than the umbellules.

HISTORY.—It has been generally asserted that the Conium maculatum of Linnæus is the Κωνειον of the Greeks, and the plant from which the Athenian state poison, which destroyed Socrates and Phocion, was composed; in all probability, they are identical. Dioscorides (lib. iv. cap. 79) describes it pretty minutely, but not clearly enough to distinguish it from other umbelliferæ; nor is Pliny's description sufficient. However, Sibthorp (*Prod. Flor. Græc.*) found it growing in abundance near Athens; and Nicander (*Alexip.*, pp. 34, 35), in describing an account of its effects, enumerates symptoms very nearly analogous to those we are familiar with, as the result of poisoning by Conium maculatum. And the symptoms recorded by Plato, in the following extract from the "Phædo," on the death of Socrates, are very similar to those observed when the poison affects the spinal cord in particular.

"And Crito, hearing this, gave the sign to the boy who stood near; and the boy departing, after some time returned, bringing with him the man who was to administer the poison, who brought it ready bruised in a cup. And Socrates, beholding the man, said, 'Good friend, come hither; you are experienced in these affairs,—what is to be done?' 'Nothing,' replied the man, 'only when you have drank the poison, you are to walk about until a heaviness takes place in your legs; then lie down: this is all you have to do.' At the same time he presented the cup. Socrates received it from him with great calmness, without fear or change of countenance, and regarding the man with his usual stern aspect, he asked, 'What say you of this potion? Is it lawful to sprinkle any portion of it on the earth, as a libation, or not?' 'We only bruise,' said the man, "as much as is barely sufficient for the purpose.' 'I understand you,' said Socrates; 'but it is certainly lawful and proper to pray the gods that my departure from hence may be prosperous and happy, which I indeed beseech them to grant.' So saying, he carried the cup to his mouth, and drank it with great promptness and facility.

"Thus far most of us had been able to refrain from weeping. But when we saw that he was drinking, and actually had drank the poison, we could no longer restrain our tears. And from me they broke forth with such violence, that I covered my face and deplored my wretchedness. I did not weep for his fate so much as for the loss of a friend and benefactor, which I was about to sustain. But Crito, unable to restrain his tears, now broke forth in loud lamentations, which infected all who were present, except Socrates. But he observing us, exclaimed, 'What is it you do, my excellent friends? I have sent away the women that they might not betray such weakness. I have heard that it is our duty to die cheerfully, and with expressions of joy and praise. Be silent, therefore, and let your fortitude be seen.' At this address we blushed, and suppressed our tears. But Socrates, after walking about, now told us that his legs were beginning to grow heavy, and immediately laid down, for so he had been ordered. At the same time the man who had given him the poison, examined his feet and legs, touching them at intervals. At length he pressed violently upon his foot, and asked if he felt it. To which Socrates replied that he did not. The man then pressed his legs and so on, showing us that he was becoming cold and stiff. And Socrates, feeling it himself, assured us, that when the effects had ascended to his heart, he should be gone. And now the middle of his body growing cold, he threw aside his clothes, and spoke for the last time. 'Crito, we owe the sacrifice of a cock to Æsculapius. Discharge this, and neglect it not.' 'It shall be done,' said Crito; 'have you anything else to say?' He made no reply, but a moment after moved, and his eyes became fixed. And Crito, seeing this, closed his eyelids and mouth."

Phocion was poisoned by Κωνειον (*Plutarch's Lives*); but it appears that the Greeks were in the habit of calling poisons by this name, as we find the words πινειν κωνειον, to drink poison (*Lys. c. Eratosth.*); κωνειον πεπωκοτα, having drunk poison (*Plato, Lys.*, 219). Dr. Adams (*Append. Dunb. Gr. Lex.*) says there can be no doubt that it was by a decoction of this plant that Socrates was put to death (see *Macer*, lib. i. c. 8). Haller considers it to be the extract of Cicuta virosa. It is also to be noticed that Plato, in his description of the poison, does not give any particular name, but uses the very general term Φαρμακον, which denotes a strong potion, either poisonous or medicinal. The Latins called the Hemlock Cicuta, a general term used for many umbelliferous poisonous plants; and Lamarck censures Linnæus for having changed the name to Conium, forgetting that Linnæus was only restoring the ancient term; the word Cicuta being entirely of Latin origin, and unknown to the Greeks.

Many Latin authors refer to Cicuta in their writings; and Lucretius (lib. v. ver. 897) exemplifies our old English proverb, "what is one man's meat is another man's poison," in the lines relating to this plant—

"Pinguescere sæpe Cicuta,
Barbigeras pecudes, homini quæ est acre venenum."

It was employed for medicinal purposes in early times. Dioscorides used it as a collyrium mixed with wine, and as a cataplasm in herpes and erysipelas, and as an anaphrodisiac. Pliny (*Nat. Hist.*, b. xxvi. c. 16) says the leaves keep down all tumours, appease pain, and cure watery eyes; and Anaxilaus states that the mammæ, anointed with the juice, never grow afterwards, "et incrementa mammarum et testium cohibere" (*Aretæus de Morb. Acut.*, lib. ii. c. 2.) Avicenna praises it as a remedy for tumours of the breasts. He says (lib. ii. p. 662) it stops bleeding, congeals the blood, and induces lepra. Baron Störck was the first person who introduced it to any extent as a remedial agent; he employed it with great effect in the cures of scirrhus, cancer, ulcers, and many other chronic diseases. The praises he bestowed upon it led to its almost universal adoption, and, of course, to general disappointment; and from the general inefficacy experienced in this country, it was supposed that the Hemlock of Störck was a different plant to ours, but this was proved not to be the case. It has been also used in chronic rheumatism, glandular swellings, and various fixed and periodical pains. Fothergill and Butter (*Med. Observ. and Inquir.*, vol. iii.) recommended its use in hooping-cough, and in painful affections of the face. Rosenstein, in Sweden, President Fisher and Professor Jackson, in America, have found its relaxing effects facilitate the passage of biliary calculi. Bigelow found it useful in jaundice. Bergius extols it in impotency, for its remarkable opposite effects, as an external remedy to those parts. It has been used in nymphomania and satyriasis, from its anaphrodisiac properties. Fothergill, Chaussier, and Dumeril found it successful in tic-douloureux; and it also has been found successful in cases of hemicrania, which are not regularly intermittent; in syphilis by Pearson; and in bronchocele by Gibson, of Pennsylvania. But its chief recommendation, in the allopathic school of medicine, has been in enlargement and induration of the absorbing and secreting glands, and of the viscera; scrofula, obstinate chronic skin diseases, and foul ulcers; also in mammary tumours and profuse secretion of milk (galactorrhœa); for this latter purpose it has been used since the time of Dioscorides. Bayle (*Bib. Thérap.*, vol. iii. p. 618) collected, from various authors, forty-six cases of cancerous diseases cured, and twenty-six ameliorated, by the use of Conium.

Description.—Conium maculatum is a biennial plant, flowering in June and July. The *root* is fleshy, top-shaped, whitish, frequently forked, of a disagreeable smell, and sweetish taste. *Stem* from three to six feet high, upright, round, hollow, smooth, glaucous, shiny, much branched, and copiously spotted or streaked with reddish or brownish purple. *Leaves* large, spreading, repeatedly compound, of a deep, shining green. *Leaflets* egg-shaped, closely and sharply pinnatified. *Petioles* long, furrowed, dilated, and sheathing at the base. *Umbels* terminal, very numerous, upright, compound, occasionally attended by one or two simple axillary ones, all many-rayed and smooth. *General involucrums* of several short, egg spear-shaped leaves, which are membranous at their edges. *Partial* ones (*involucels*) of about three spear-shaped leaves, which are all directed to one side, and much shorter than the umbellules, a character which will distinguish this from the Æthusa cynapium, in which the umbellules are shorter than the involucels (see fig. of Æthusa, pl. 2). *Flowers* numerous, white, all prolific; the outermost slightly irregular. *Fruit* abundant, egg-shaped, slightly compressed, furrowed; the ridges crenated. *Carpels* with five crenated ridges, three on the back, and two on the margins.

The Conium maculatum may be distinguished from other umbelliferous plants by the following characters. The smooth *stem*, spotted with purplish spots; the smooth, dark, and glossy green colour of the lower leaves; the *general involucre* of from three to seven leaflets; the *partial involucre* of three leaflets; the *fruit* with undulated, crenated, primary ridges. The whole herb, when bruised, has a disagreeable smell (compared by some to the odour of mice, by others to that of fresh cantharides). Hemlock has been confounded not unfrequently with the wild celery (Chærophyllum sylvestre); this, however, may be easily distinguished by the stem, which is rough and without spots; the seeds also are not striated. It may also be confounded with the Æthusa cynapium and Anthriscus vulgaris. The Æthusa is smaller; there is no general involucre; there are three long, narrow, unilateral, pendulous leaflets, comprising the partial involucre; and there is entire absence of the peculiar disagreeable smell in the leaves. The Anthriscus vulgaris, or Common Beaked Parsley, is known from Hemlock by the paler colour and slight hairiness of the *leaves*;

by the absence of spots on the *stem;* by the swelling under each joint; by the absence of the *general involucre;* by the roughness of the *fruit;* and by the absence of the strong, unpleasant odour when the leaves are bruised. The Chærophyllum bulbosum has a spotted *stem*, but its swelled joints and rough *seeds* distinguish it from the Hemlock.

Geographical Distribution.—Hemlock is a native throughout the whole of Europe; of the eastern parts of Asia, North America, and Chili, where it has been introduced.

Localities.—In hedges, orchards, waste grounds, and on rubbish and dunghills, especially near towns and villages; frequent.

Parts used in Medicine, and Mode of Preparation.—The Leaves and Flowering Stem, which are gathered in the month of June. The juice is expressed, and treated in the manner ordered for fresh plants.

Physiological Effects.—*On Vegetables.* Marcet (*Ann. de Chim. et Phys.*, xxiv. 219) found that a haricot plant (Phaseolus vulgaris) was almost immediately affected by being placed in a solution of five grains of the extract of Hemlock, and was completely shrivelled up in the course of forty-eight hours.

On Animals.—Although Conium has been found poisonous to swine and other animals, yet sheep, goats, and horses will generally eat it with impunity; and Ray states, that thrushes will eat the seeds, which are more potent than the leaves, even when corn is to be had. Hemlock appears to be more prejudicial to carnivorous than to herbivorous animals.

Rozier (*Tableau*, tom. i. 1773) states that three spoonfuls of the juice given to a cat, killed it in a quarter of an hour. Orfila (*Tox. Gén.*, vol. ii. p. 309) found that the powder and extract were generally harmless when given to animals, but that the juice or leaves of the *fresh* plant produced the most violent symptoms and death. Moiroud (*Pharm. Vét.*, 359) has given three pounds and a half of the plant to a young horse without inconvenience; but in another case, the decoction of four ounces of the dried plant proved fatal. It caused dejection, stupor, dilatation of the pupils, trembling, salivation, nausea, spasmodic contraction of the muscles of the extremities, rolling of the eye, grinding of the teeth, and copious cold sweats.

On Man.—In large and poisonous doses, the symptoms produced by the leaves and seeds are those indicating disorders of the cerebro-spinal system. Dr. J. H. Bennett met with a case which illustrates its effects on the spinal marrow. A man ate a large quantity of Hemlock plant by mistake for parsley, soon afterwards there was loss of power in the lower extremities, but he apparently suffered no pain. In walking, he staggered as if he was drunk; at length his limbs refused to support him, and he fell. On being raised, his legs dragged after him, or when his arms were lifted they fell like inert masses, and remained immovable; there was perfect paralysis of the upper and lower extremities within two hours after he had taken the poison. There was a loss of power of deglutition, and a partial paralysis of sensation, but no convulsions, only slight occasional motions of the left leg; the pupils were fixed. Three hours after eating the Hemlock, the respiratory movements had ceased. Death took place in three hours and a quarter. It was evidently caused by gradual asphyxia from paralysis of the muscles of respiration, but the intellect was perfectly clear until shortly before death.* On inspection, there was slight serous effusion beneath the arachnoid membrane. The substance of the brain was soft on section; there were numerous bloody points, but the organ was otherwise healthy. The lungs were gorged with dark-red fluid blood; the heart was soft and flabby. The stomach contained a green pultaceous mass resembling parsley; the mucous coat was much congested, especially at the cardiac extremity; here there were numerous extravasations of dark blood below the epithelium, over a space about the size of the hand. The intestines were healthy, and these presented

* Compare the symptoms described by Plato in his account of the death of Socrates, pp. 220, 221.

patches of congestion on the mucous coat. The blood throughout the body was fluid, and of a dark colour. A portion of the green vegetable mass was identified by Dr. Christison as part of the Conium maculatum. Some of the leaves bruised in a mortar, with a solution of potash, also gave out the peculiar odour of the volatile principle, Conia (*Edin. Med. and Surg. Journal*, July, 1845, p. 169).

Delirium and convulsions are not common effects of poisoning by this plant (*Taylor*, l. c.)

Two priests ate Hemlock root by mistake; they became raving mad, and mistaking themselves for geese, plunged into the water; for three years they suffered from partial palsy and violent pain (*Wibmer*, *Wirk*, etc., ii. 172).

An old woman suffered for three months with abdominal pain and convulsive movements of the limbs, in consequence of eating Hemlock root* (*Wibmer*, l. c.)

M. Haaf, a French army surgeon, has described a fatal case of poisoning with Hemlock. The subject of it, a soldier, had partaken, along with several comrades, of a soup containing Hemlock leaves, and appeared to them to drop asleep not long after, while they were conversing. In the course of an hour they became alarmed on being all taken ill with giddiness and headache, and the surgeon of the regiment was sent for. He found the soldier, who had fallen asleep, in a state of insensibility, from which, however, he could be roused for a few

* Respecting Hemlock root, we have many different statements; some say that it is highly deleterious; others, that it is perfectly innocuous, but this depends probably on the time of gathering. Ray relates that Mr. Petiver ate half an ounce of the root of Hemlock, and Mr. Healy four ounces, without producing any effect (*Phil. Trans.*, vol. xix. p. 634). Curtis (*Flor. Londinensis*) relates that Mr. Alchorne and Mr. Timothy Lane ate its root with impunity; and Mr. Lane had some boiled, and found them as agreeable as carrots. Mr. Steven, a Russian botanist, states that the Russian peasants eat it with impunity, and it is probable that the colder the climate the less poisonous is the root. Pliny also (*Nat. Hist.*, b. 26, c. xiii.) says, "as for the stems and stalks, many there be who do eat it both green and also boiled, or stewed between two platters."

moments. His countenance was bloated, the pulse only thirty, and the extremities cold. The insensibility became rapidly deeper and deeper till he died, three hours after taking the soup. His companions recovered (*Corvisart, Journ. de Méd.*, vol. xxix. p. 107).

Mr. W. Watson gives an account of two Dutch soldiers, who were quartered at Waltham Abbey, in Essex. "They collected on Sunday, May 6, 1744, in the fields adjoining, a quantity of herbs, sufficient for themselves and two others for dinner, when boiled with bacon; these herbs were therefore dressed, and the poor men first ate of the broth with bread, and afterwards the herbs with bacon. In a short time after they were all seized with violent vertigo; they soon afterwards were comatose, and two of them grew convulsed and died in about three hours. A physician ordered the other two, at that time almost dead, large quantities of oil, by which means they threw up most of what they had eaten, and afterwards grew better. In all of them the effects were the same as those from a large dose of opium. Another soldier ate of the broth made from the Hemlock, with bread, and felt scarce any inconvenience therefrom" (*Phil. Trans.*, vol. xliii. No. 473, pp. 18—20).

MEDICAL USES (HOMŒOPATHIC).—*Hahnemann's observations:* "Press out the juice of the whole plant just before it flowers; mix it with equal parts of alcohol.

"Conium maculatum is one of those medicines in which it is least easy to distinguish between primary and consecutive effects. Among its symptoms are many opposed to each other in certain respects, which must be considered as alternate effects, or perhaps temporary consecutive ones, suspended for a while by some new aggravation of the remedy.

"As to the fatal consequences that follow the continued use of Conium in large doses, with which we have been made acquainted by the unfortunate treatment of Störck, Lange, Andrée, Ehrhardt, Greding, etc. etc., they are true consecutive effects, produced by efforts of nature, fearfully attacked by such large and oft-repeated doses. A relaxation of all the fibres may be observed, accompanied by *asthenic* inflammation, and painful sensitiveness. It seems that the contrary takes place during the primitive effect of Conium, which appears to be a stiffening, setting, and constriction of the fibres, with swelling of the glands, and dullness of the senses, as shown by some cases of glandular enlargement in the neck and lips, occasioned by contusions, and by cataract caused by a blow, which were treated and cured homœopathically. These primary effects, joined to some others, intimate a powerful remedy for that distressing kind of hypochondriasis sometimes seen in men of a retired and strict life, unless it depends upon some primitive miasmatic affection.

Experience teaches us what we ought really to think of the action of Conium in the case (presbytie) of persons advanced in life, and it may possibly be proved that it has the property of destroying this affection (*Hahnemann, Mat. Med. Pur.*)

Clinical Observations.—*Noack and Trinks* (l. c.): The chief tendency of Conium is the liquefaction and dissolving of animal matter, as well normal as abnormal. It is more suitable for the female constitution than the male; to venous, lymphatic, scrofulous, torpid constitutions; to phlegmatic-melancholic temperaments; and also for individuals with rigid light fibres, with an easily excited nervous system. In hypochondriacal and hysterical women, especially to pregnant women. In scrofulosis, tuberculosis, carcinomatous habits, and paralysis, Conium is especially serviceable. Falling off of the hair. Humming and singing in the ears. Weakness of old men (Lobethal considers Conium a panacea of old men). Weak conditions, accompanied by excessive irritability of the body (*Hahnemann*). Old contusions, strains, and contusions of membranous and tendinous formations, consequent on pinching, pressure, shocks, falls, and other external injuries, in consequence of which the cellular tissue had become compressed, and the glands indurated; a sensation of numbness accompanying these symptoms. Trembling of the limbs. Spasms and attacks of weakness, and other morbid phenomena in hysteric females. Epilepsy. Scrofulosis, especially with swelling and induration of the external glands. Nervous and serous apoplexy. Herpetic eruptions, with burning, smarting pains, especially on the forearms. Herpetic spots on the forearms; the skin looks bright red. Glandular swellings. Scirrhus and carcinoma. Scrofulous, herpetic, gangrenous ulcers. Painful nodosities. Malignant and painful ulcers, when these pains originate in the abuse of mercury, and become aggravated at night. Congestion of the brain, with giddiness. Inflammation of the eyes of different kinds, especially ophthalmia and dacryoadenalgia scrofulosa, with considerable photophobia. Scrofulous photophobia. Purulent otorrhœa. Prosopalgia. Status gastricus. Chronic disease and induration of the liver. Impotentia from onanism. Mesenteric atrophy of infants. Strangury and ischuria. Menostasia. Suppressed catamenia. Retarded appearance of the first catamenia. Dysmenorrhœa. Catamenia returning every fourteen days. Uterine spasms. Fluor albus. Galactorrhœa. Mastitis. Scirrhus of the mammæ from contusions. Dry, spasmodic, slightly irritable cough, with violent oppression of the chest and evening fever, especially in scrofulous individuals. Hooping-cough. Hysteric asthma. Asthma senile. Pneumonia nervosa, with inclination to suffocation. Phthisis tuberculosa. Phthisis florida, sicca et purulenta. Chronic affections of the heart, etc. etc.

Antidotes.—To poisonous doses, Pliny states that the antidote is Wine. According to Nicander, the Nettle (Urtica urens) is an antidote to Conium; also the Storax Calamita. To small doses, Coffea. Spirit. Nitros. Conium antidotes Acidum Nitricum.

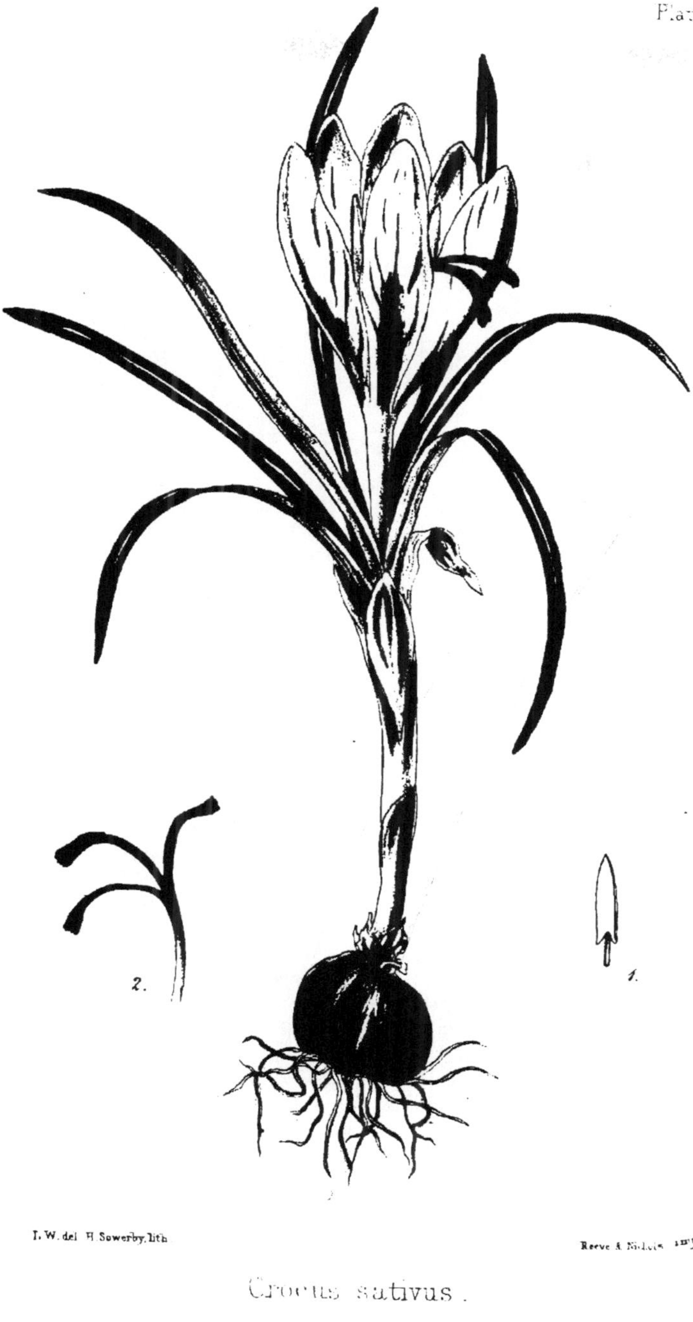

I. W. del H. Sowerby, lith

Reeve & Nichols imp

Crocus sativus.

XXVII.

CROCUS SATIVUS.

Common Saffron Crocus.

SYNONYMS.—Crocus, *Gerard. Emar.*, p. 151; *Raii Hist.*, p. 1176. Crocus verus sativus autumnalis, *Park. Parad.*, p. 167. Crocus sativus, *Bauh. Пιν.*, p. 65; *With. Bot. An.*, p. 37. Crocus autumnalis, *E. Fl.*, vol. i. p. 46.

FOREIGN NAMES.—*Fr.:* Safran. *Ital.:* Zafferano. *Span.:* Azafran. *Port.:* Açafrão. *Germ. and Dan.:* Safran. *Dut.:* Saffraan. *Swed.:* Saffran. *Russ.:* Schafran. *Arab.:* Zafran. *Pers.:* Aheer. *Tam.:* Khoongoommapor.

Nat. Order, IRIDIÆ.—TRIANDRIA, MONOGYNIA.

GEN. CHAR.—*Calyx* radical, of two unequal, membranous, tubular sheaths, single flowered. *Corolla* (perianthium) superior, tube cylindrical, upright, three or four times the length of the limb, which is regular, in six elliptic, oblong, equal segments, three of them partly internal. *Filaments* three, in the mouth six; the tube shorter than the limb. *Anthers* arrow-shaped, upright. *Germen* at the root inferior, roundish. *Style* thread-shaped, very long, rising as high as the stamens. *Stigmas* three, dilated upwards, variously folded, jagged, or many-cleft. *Capsule* membranous, of three cells and three valves. *Seeds* several, globular. The inferior corolla, with a very long, slender tube, and six-parted, equal, inflated, upright *limb*, and the three-plaited, many-lobed stigma, will distinguish this from other genera in the same class and order.

SPEC. CHAR.—*Stigma* protruding, drooping, in three deep, linear divisions.

HISTORY.—The earliest notice of Crocus is in Homer (*Iliad*, Book xiv., *Pope's Trans.*):

"And flaming Crocus made the mountain glow."

It is also mentioned in sacred history (Solomon's Song,

Fig. 1. An anther. 2. The stigma.

chap. iv., verse 14): "Spikenard and Saffron." It was called Carcom by the Hebrews, by whom it was much esteemed as a medicine and as a perfume. It is the Κροκος of the Greek physicians, Hippocrates, Theophrastus, Dioscorides, etc.; and the Zaffaran of the Arabians. It was held in great estimation in early days as a purgative, emollient, and discutient, and possessing aphrodisiacal properties. The Arabian physicians, Serapion, Rhases, and Avicenna, used it in uterine diseases, in cases of difficult labour, and as a deobstruent in obstructions of the liver. Later it has been at times employed by different physicians for a variety of diseases, as hysteria, hypochondriasis, melancholia, arthritic and rheumatic affections, dysmenorrhœa, chlorosis, asthma, spasms, etc., etc., and to promote uterine contractions in labour, without any decided or successful results. It is a popular remedy for assisting the eruption of exanthematous diseases. At present it is chiefly employed as a colouring agent, and is used considerably on the Continent, in the culinary art, to flavour and colour dishes.

DESCRIPTION.—The *root* (cormus) is roundish; its brownish coats reticulated, separating superiorly into distinct parallel fibres. *Leaves* linear, of a rich green colour, with a white central stripe, and surrounded at their base with long membranous sheaths. The *flowers* appear after the leaves, of a light purple, shorter than the leaves. The *anthers* are pale yellow; and the *stigmas* of a deep orange colour. It flowers in September and October (*Woodville and Pereira*).

GEOGRAPHICAL DISTRIBUTION.—A native of Asia Minor; according to Pereira, naturalized in England, France, and some other European countries. It is a doubtful native of the eastern parts of Europe. Woodville says that it is indubitably a native of England; although unknown to Ray, Miller, and several other subsequent botanists. All the different plants of this genus are considered by Linnæus as only varieties of the Crocus sativus.

Parts used in Medicine, and Mode of Preparation.—The dried Stigmata. For homœopathic purposes we prepare the Saffron as all dry substances, either by treating it at once in twenty parts of alcohol, or making the three first attenuations by trituration. Stapf (*Additions to Mat. Med., Amer. trans.*) orders the potencies to be prepared by triturating the crude substance up to the third potency, and afterwards carrying the potencies up to the thirtieth by means of succussion. The flowers are to be gathered in the morning, and the stigmata and part of the style taken for use, and dried on paper, either by kilns or by the sun. There are two kinds found in commerce, Hay Saffron and Cake Saffron. The former is to be taken for our use. According to Pereira (op. cit.), Hay Saffron consists only of the stigmata and part of the style; they are from an inch to an inch and a half long, brownish-red, the upper portion expanded and notched at the extremity (the stigma); the lower (style) narrow, capillary, and roundish. The odour is penetrating, aromatic, and of large quantities, narcotic. The taste is bitter and aromatic, and when chewed tinges the mouth and saliva yellow. One grain of good commercial Saffron contains the stigmata and style of nine flowers; hence, 4,320 flowers are required to yield one ounce of Saffron. The Cake Saffron is to be avoided, as being adulterated with safflower mixed with gum, and then rolled into cakes.

The best Saffron (according to Pereira) is the Spanish (*Crocus Hispanicus*), imported from Gibraltar, Cadiz, and Malaga. The next is the French (*Crocus Gallicus*), the produce of C. Gatenais and C. Orleanais. The chief adulteration is with safflower (*Carthamus tinctorius*), which may be detected by the slighter stain on the skin when rubbed; and also by placing the substance in hot water, when the *florets* of the safflower will be readily distinguished from the *stigmata* of the Crocus. Saffron also was formerly adulterated with the flowers of the marigold (*Calendula officinalis*), the pomegranate (*Punica granatum*), and with fibres of smoked beef; but all these are readily detected by infusing the suspected substance in hot water. Saffron owes its colour to a peculiar substance, called by Vogel and Bouillon-Lagrance, Polychroite, every hundred parts of Saffron containing sixty-five parts of this substance. Saffron formerly was grown in great quantities near Saffron Walden, in Essex.

PHYSIOLOGICAL EFFECTS.—J. Lusitanus (*apud Fric. de Venen.*, p. 394) says that blisters, headache, blindness, delirium, and loss of consciousness came on after a large dose of Saffron, and even that death has been produced; and that death ensued from a man inhaling a large quantity of the vapour of Saffron.

Borellus (*Hist. et Observ.*, Cent. iv.), says that headache and debility were produced by remaining some time in a room where there was much saffron. Tralles (*De Opis*, sect. i. p. 114) states that it inclines to apoplexy.

Riverius (*Op. Med., ed. Horstius*, p. 136, Fref. 1674) says that a great dose of Saffron given to a woman to increase the catamenia, produced death after the third day by uterine hemorrhage. Forster (*Gottinger Mag. Jahrg.*, i. st. 2) records a case of death produced by the vapour of Saffron. Alexander (*Exp. Ess.*, p. 88, 1763) took four scruples of Saffron without any deleterious effect; and Wibmer took a drachm without perceiving any sensible change.

MEDICAL USES (HOMŒOPATHIC).—Crocus was not proved by Hahnemann, but we find it mentioned in his Lesser Writings, translated by Dr. Dudgeon, p. 347. "It appears as if Saffron crocus (*Crocus sativus*), in its direct action, brought down the circulation and vital heat. Slow pulse, pale face, vertigo, and exhaustion have been observed. In this stage most probably occur the melancholy and headache that have been observed from its action; and in the second stage (the indirect secondary action) occur the senseless, extravagant gaiety, the stupefaction of the senses, the increased action of the arteries and heart, and lastly, the hemorrhage, which have been observed from its use. For this reason it may be useful in restoring flows of blood that have been checked, as a similarly acting remedy; as its power of increasing the circulation occurs first in the secondary action, consequently the opposite must take place in its direct action. It has been found useful as a similarly acting remedy in vertigo and headache, with slow pulse. In some cases of melancholia, with slow pulse, and in amenorrhœa, it appears also to be of service as a similarly acting remedy. It has (in its direct action) produced death by apoplexy, and is said to have proved efficacious in similar affections (probably in relaxed organisms). The phenomena of its secondary action point to much increased irritability of the fibre, hence probably the cause of its so readily producing hysteria."

The following are Dr. E. Stapf's observation, taken from the American translation of the *Additions to Hahnemann's Materia Medica Pura.* "This drug was a favourite article of the physicians of the sixteenth and seventeenth centuries. Latterly it has been employed much less frequently, and the few prominent effects which we know it is capable of producing have been merged in vague, general terms, such as stupefaction, heating, sopor, intoxication, insanity, exciting the blood, etc. It is evident that this imperfect knowledge is of very little avail in the treatment of disease, and that the virtues of Crocus, which certainly is an interesting drug, ought to be investigated in a more adequate manner. From the absence of all sound and comprehensive knowledge which prevails amongst physicians in regard to the remedial virtues of Crocus, in spite of the frequent and constant use which has been made of it by physicians in the treatment of disease, it is evident that the mere empirical use of Crocus has not sufficed to procure an adequate knowledge of its remedial powers, and that this knowledge can only be obtained by carefully proving the drug upon healthy persons. Further observations and experiments will no doubt make the list of symptoms more complete and useful; but the present symptoms are sufficient to point to many affections, especially of the female sex, in which Crocus may be used with success.

Formerly the third potency of Crocus had been used, it is true, with success, but sometimes occasioning, in irritable persons and in very violent diseases, a somewhat dangerous aggravation of the symptoms. To obviate this danger, the thirtieth potency is now generally employed, although the lower preparations may sometimes be useful in torpid individuals. The intelligent and observing physician will easily be able to discriminate.

Clinical Observations.—*Noack and Trinks* (op. cit.): "Saffron is especially applicable in predisposition to congestion of blood, and in inflammation, which arise chiefly in persons of the sanguineous temperament; in serene, merry, and gay dispositions. It suits especially in hysterical, clonic cramps, or a disposition to abortion in the climacteric years, but especially for typhus in the infantile organism. Those conditions, which are distinguished by a remarkable alternation from one state to another, give a specific indication for Crocus. Hemorrhage, characterised by dark, black, viscid blood. Chorea of an intermittent character, complicated with hooping-cough. Spasmodic yawning. Melancholia. Imbecilitas. Extasis melancholia. Violent heating and smarting pain in the eyes after surgical operations. (*Aconite* seems to be the chief remedy here, but in some persons of a mild temperament *Aconite* does not suit, and the violent shooting pain in the temple and eyes is relieved by *Ignatia*); the darting pains, with vomiting and lienteria, by *Asarum;* the burning pains by *Arsenicum;* the lancinating pains commencing in the temple, and accompanied by loss of appetite, by *Thuja occidentalis;* the broken-up lens, after depression, is absorbed by *Senega;* the disturbance of the eyesight after a surgical operation, particularly when objects appear to be covered with blood, is relieved by *Strontiana* (*Würzler*). Epistaxis, especially when the blood is thick and dark (also when red), and the nose bleeds easily either by exercise or blowing. Bleeding of the nose, which returns every day in hot weather. Frequent bleeding of the nose every day, preceded by pressure in the forehead. Bleeding at the nose, and critical periods in youth. Menstrual disturbance with fulness, headache, etc. Metrorrhagia after violent exertions, or stimulating drinks taken at the period of the menses, or from fright."

According to Hirzel, *Crocus* is more suitable for metrorrhagia, with erethism of the circulation, and *Secale* for hemorrhages from atony. According to Lobethal, *Crocus* corresponds to active hemorrhage; *Sabina* to hemorrhage with erethism, and *Secale* to torpid hemorrhage. According to Hartmann, the characteristic indication for *Crocus* is a dark, blackish, clotty, viscid blood, always accompanied with lancinating pains in the abdomen, and towards the small of the back. According to others, *Crocus* is indicated even when the labour-like pains are wanting, and the discharge of blood is either fetid or not. Different affections accompanying hemorrhage from the uterus, as frequent anxiety and flying heat over the whole body, with irritation of the skin, syncope, chilliness, etc. Lochia too excessive. (In some cases of elongation of the uvula, causing a tickling cough.)

ANTIDOTES.—Aconitum. Opium. The stupefaction and sopor caused by Crocus may probably be counteracted by Opium, or perhaps by Belladonna (*Stapf*). Forestus (*De Venen., in Schol.*, lib. iii. fol. 122) states that Crocus is an antidote in cases of poisoning by Aconitum napellus.

XXVIII.

CYCLAMEN* EUROPÆUM.

Sow-bread.

SYNONYMS.—Cyclamen Europæum, *Engl. Bot.*, t. 548; *Linn. Sp. Pl.*, p. 207; *With.*, vol. ii. p. 299. Cyclamen vernum, *Gray's Nat. Arr.*, vol. ii. p. 303. Cyclamen neapolitanum, *Bot. Reg.*, *U. S.*, 1838, t. 49; *Loud. Gard. Mag.*, vol. xiv. Cyclamen hedere folio, *Bauh. Πιν.*, p. 308; *Johns. Gerarde*, p. 843, f. 2. Artanita Cyclamen, *Blackw. Hist.*, p. 147. Cyclamen orbiculare, *Dodon. Pempt.*, 335. Cyclamen, *Lobel. Icon.*, 604.

FOREIGN NAMES.—*Fr.:* Cyclame, Pain de pourceau. *Ital.:* Pan porcino. *Span.:* Mazana de puerco. *Germ.:* Erdschuba, Schweinsbrod. *Dut.:* Werckens byoot. *Greek:* Κυκλαμινος. *Latin:* Tenæ rapum, Rapum porcinum, Tenæ malum.

Nat. Order, LYSIMACHIÆ, *Juss.*; RUTACEÆ, *Linn.*; PRIMULACEÆ, *Lindl.*—PENTANDRIA, MONOGYNIA.

GEN. CHAR.—*Calyx* inferior, bell-shaped, of one petal, divided half-way into five egg-shaped segments, permanent. *Corolla* of one petal, wheel-shaped; tube egg-shaped, longer than the calyx; mouth naked, prominent; limb much longer than the tube, in five deep, oblique, equal segments, which are reflexed upwards. *Filaments* very short in the tube. *Anthers* straight, acute, converging in the mouth of the corolla. *Germen* roundish. *Style* cylindrical, straight, rather longer than the lips of the anthers. *Stigmas* simple. *Capsule* globose, rather fleshy, of one cell, opening at the top, with five teeth. *Seeds* numerous, somewhat egg-shaped, angular, covering a central, roundish, egg-shaped, stalked, unconnected placenta or receptacle.

The superior, bell-shaped, five-cleft *calyx*, the monopetalous wheel-shaped *corolla*, with a naked prominent mouth and five reflexed segments, and the somewhat fleshy, one-celled, many-seeded capsule, will distinguish this from other genera in the same class and order (*Baxter*).

Fig. 1. Calyx. 2. Segment of corolla, showing the situation of the stamens. 3. Stamens attached to the base of the tube of the corolla. 4. A ripe capsule.

* From cyclos (Gr.), a circle, from the root being round.

Plate XXVIII

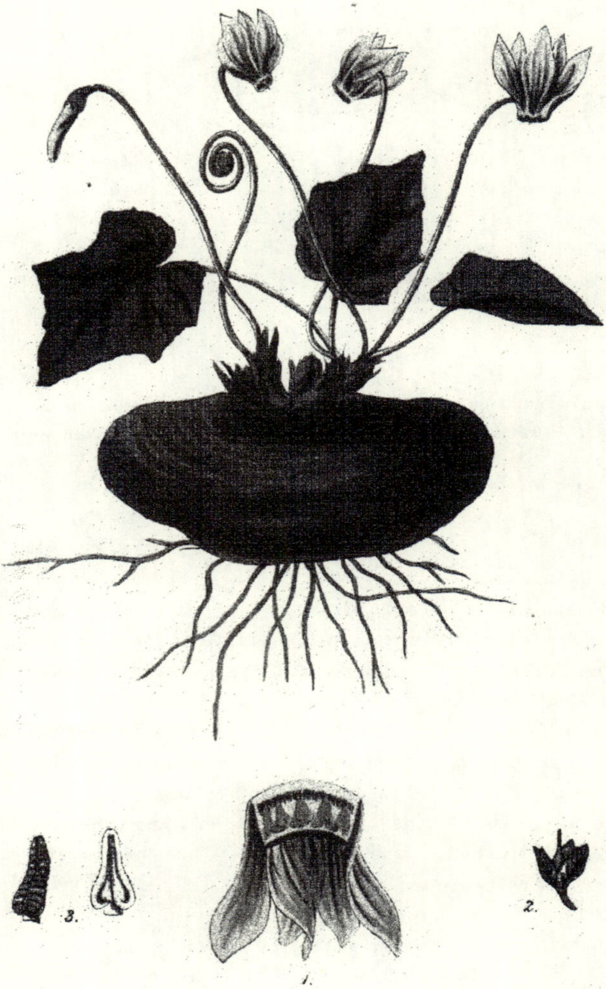

) del · H. Sowerby, lith.

Cyclamen Europæum

SPEC. CHAR.—*Leaves* heart-shaped, angular, finely toothed, their ribs and footstalk roughish, mouth of the corolla toothed.

The Cyclamen is the chief food of the wild boars in Sicily, hence the name, Sow-bread.

HISTORY.—Although at the present time entirely discarded from the allopathic pharmacopœias, Cyclamen was used extensively by the Greek, Latin, and Arabian physicians. Dioscorides (op. cit., ii. 193—4) recommended it as a phlegmagogue, hydragogue, emmenagogue, and alexipharmic; and as an errhine in diseases of the head. Galen (*De Simplicibus*, vii.) recommends it as an external application in hardness of the spleen; in jaundice, not only by purging but by evacuating the whole body by sweats; and also in amenorrhœa, both taken internally and applied as a suppository. Avicenna (ii. 271) copies from Galen, and recommends it as a cure for jaundice by sweating; the body to be covered by many clothes, so that the bile may be sweated out of the body. Mesne (*De Simplicibus*, xxvi.) states that it is a general purger of bile, when taken by the mouth; as an emmenagogue, and in induration of the spleen. Serapion (*De Temp. Simp.*, cap. 249) gives long extracts from Dioscorides, Galen, Armasius, Paulus, Aben Mesnai, etc., upon the virtues of this plant. Gerarde (*Hist. of Plants*, book ii. p. 695) says that "the roote hanged about women in their extreme travell with childe, causeth them to be delivered incontinent, and taketh away much of their paine." Also, "it scoureth the skin, and taketh away sunne burning, and all blemishes of the face, pilling of the haire, and markes also, that remaine after the small pockes and mesels; and given in wine to drinke, it maketh a man drunke." And writing of the dangers: "It is not good for women with childe to touch or take this herbe, or to come neere unto it, or stride over the same where it groweth, for the naturall attractive vertue therein contained is such, that without controversie they that attempt it in maner abovesaid, shall be delivered before their time, which danger and inconvenience to avoide, I have (about the place where it groweth in my garden) ſastened sticks in the ground, and some other stickes I have fastened also crossewaies over them, least any woman should by lamentable experiment finde my words to be true, by their stepping over the same."

Some authors state that the juice rubbed over the umbilicus will produce an evacuation; and it has been used in the same manner to produce abortion. Vicat (*Mat. Med.*, Leip., 1782) gave it in toothache. Bourgeris in amenorrhœa, and to promote the expulsion of the placenta.

DESCRIPTION.—Cyclamen is a perennial plant. The *root* is large, orbicular, compressed, brown, sending out many branched fibres. *Leaves* all radical, heart-shaped, angular, finely toothed; when full grown three inches and a half long, and two inches and a half broad, deep green, and spotted above, commonly reddish-purple underneath, smooth, on very long petioles. *Flowers* drooping, purplish, sweet scented, peduncles resembling the petioles, erect, with the flower spiral with the fruit. *Capsular* berry coriaceous, purple, opening first at the top and then entirely. *Seeds* large, rufous, kidney-shaped. After the flowers are over, the flower-stalks curl spirally, inclosing the germen in the centre, and lowering it to the earth, repose on the surface of the soil till the seeds are ready to escape.

GEOGRAPHICAL DISTRIBUTION. — Cyclamen is a native of the south of Germany, Austria, Italy, Sicily, Greece, Tartary, etc.; cultivated extensively in our gardens, and is now found in a wild state, but is not truly indigenous.

LOCALITIES.—In shady places, and on moist grounds. Grows in profusion round the temples of Pæstum, near Naples, where it was found by the author, in full flower, in August. The specimen from which the drawing was taken was found near Drumcondra, in Ireland.

PARTS USED IN MEDICINE, AND MODE OF PREPARATION.—For homœopathic purposes, we take the fresh roots gathered in the autumn, and express the juice, mix it with equal quantities of alcohol, and prepare as ordered for other medicinal substances, to the fourth attenuation only (*Quin, Phar. Hom.*)

PHYSIOLOGICAL EFFECTS.—In large doses, Cyclamen acts as an irritant; and is placed among that class of poisons by Boerhaave, because it purges violently. Bulliard (*Herb. de la France, Plant. vénén.*) states that the fresh root, in a dose of two drachms in a decoction of half a glass of water, caused violent vomiting and purging in a robust man. In the septentrional provinces of France, where this herb is common, it is employed frequently as a purge; but often followed by violent vomitings, sometimes of blood, cold sweats, accompanied with singing in the ears, swimmings of the head, and convulsive movements.

MEDICAL USES (HOMŒOPATHIC).—*Hahnemann's observations:* "An unfounded suspicion has existed from remote times that the action of this precious medicine is prejudicial and uncertain; but supposing that Dioscorides had really in view the plant to which we give its name, all that he says of it is merely from report. The Arabs used the root of Cyclamen under the denomination of Artanita, as an ingredient in a purgative unguent rubbed upon the body, which also contained several other violent aperients, and having associated it with such companions, they gave it the reputation of a drastic medicine, which it did not deserve. But as our homœopathic study admits nothing on the ground of tradition, and neither praises nor contemns anything without an unprejudiced examination, this much-abused root has fallen into my hands. And since we are unable to judge of the merits of a person from exterior circumstances, or the slight and superficial opinion of the multitude, so neither the external appearances of a medicine nor its reputed qualities afford any proofs of its true value. I have submitted it to the only safe test, that of trying it on persons in health; and it appears to be an excellent remedy in several desperate cases."

CLINICAL OBSERVATIONS.—*Noack and Trinks* (op. cit.): Acute and chronic eruptions of the skin. Dullness of the mind and memory. Arthritic toothache (*Ruckert*). Violent sneezing, with profuse discharge of mucus.

XXIX.

DIGITALIS PURPUREA.

Purple Foxglove.

SYNONYMS.—Digitalis purpurea, *Lin. Sp. Pl.*, p. 868; *Willd.*, vol. iii. p. 283; *Raii Syn.*, p. 283; *Ger. Em.*, p. 790. Digitalis, *Hall, Hist.*, vol. i. p. 143. Campanula sylvestris seu Digitalis, *Trag. Hist.*, 896. Digitalis speciosa, *Salisbury, Prodromus*, p. 100; *Gray's Nat. Arr.*, vol. ii. p. 325.

FOREIGN NAMES.—*Fr.*: Digitale pourprée, Gantes nôtre dame, Gantelée. *Ital.*: Digitello. *Span.*: Dedalera. *Port.*: Dedaleira. *Germ.*: Fingerhut, Schwulstkraut. *Dut.*: Vingerhooden. *Swed.*: Finger borrsört. *Dan.*: Rod fingerhat. *Russ.*: Naperstianka.

Nat. Order, LURIDÆ, *Linn.*; SCROPHULARIÆ, *Juss.*—DIDYNAMIA, ANGIOSPERMIA.

GEN. CHAR.—*Calyx* inferior, much shorter than the corolla, of one sepal, deeply divided into five roundish, pointed segments, permanent, the upper segment narrower than the rest. *Corolla* of one petal, bell-shaped. *Tube* large, cylindrical, and contracted at the base, dilated, and turned upwards. *Limb* small, with four unequal segments, the upper one recurved, slightly cloven; lower one largest. *Filaments* four, two long and two short, awl-shaped, arising from the tube of the corolla towards the base, bent, declining. *Anthers* deeply cloven, pointed. *Germen* egg-shaped, pointed. *Style* thread-shaped, as long as the stamens. *Stigma* cloven, pointed. *Capsule* egg-shaped, pointed, of two cells, and two cloven valves, with a double partition formed of the inflexed margins of the valves. *Seeds* very numerous, small, oblong, angular, attached to a central, oblong partition in each cell. Distinguished from other genera in the same class and order by the five-cleft calyx, bell-shaped, four-lobed *corolla*, turned underneath, bent *stamens*, and two-celled *capsule* (*Baxter*).

SPEC. CHAR.—Segments of the *calyx* egg-shaped, acute. *Corolla* obtuse; its upper lip or lobe scarcely cloven. *Leaves* downy.

Fig. 1. A section of the corolla, to show the position of the anthers. 2. Calyx, germen, and stigma.

Plate XXIX

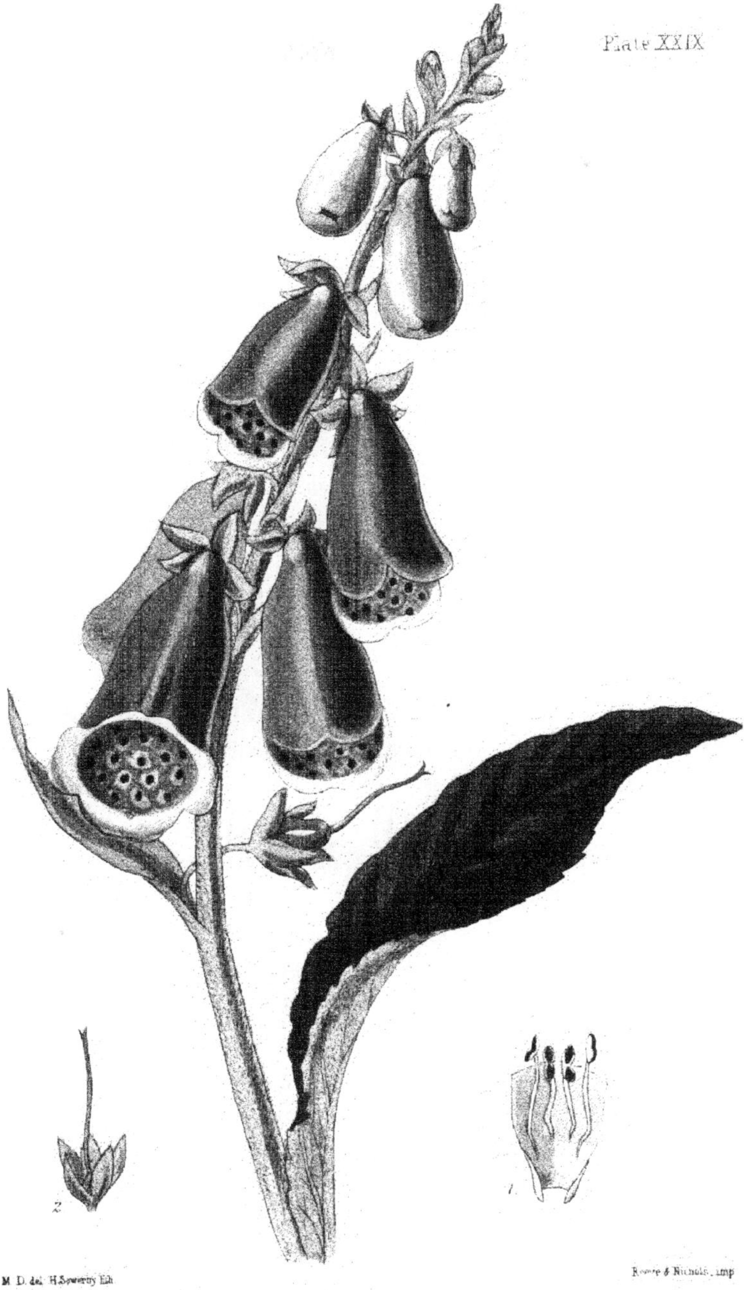

M. D. del. H. Sowerby lith.

Reeve & Nichols, imp.

Digitalis purpurea

History.—Pereira (*Elements of Mat. Med.*, vol. ii. p. 836) states that the term Foxen-ȝloƿe occurs in a MS. (*Glossarium Ælfrici*), probably written before the Norman Conquest (A. D. 1066), and in a MS. Saxon translation of L.' Apulius, both of which are among the Cottonian Manuscripts in the British Museum. The first authentic notice, however, is in Fuchsius (*Hist. Stirp.*, 1542), who gave this plant the name of Digitalis, from the German *finger-hut*, a finger-stall, from the corolla resembling the finger of a glove. It is singular that there is no record of this powerful medicinal drug in the writings of the ancient physicians, although by some it is supposed to be the Εφημερον of Dioscorides, and by others the Βαρχαρις of the same writer. The Digitalis purpurea, however, is not indigenous in Greece or Asia Minor. According to Sibthorp, the Ελλεβορος λευκος of Dioscorides is the Digitalis ferruginea, a very beautiful species of this order. Gerarde (*Hist. of Plants*, p. 647) says that Foxgloves some call in Greek Θρυαλλις, and make it Verbasci speciem, or a kind of Mullein; and as to its virtues, states that "Foxglove, boiled in water or wine, and drunken, doth cut and consume the thicke toughnesse of grosse and slimie flegme, and ranke humours. It openeth also the stopping of the liver, spleene and milt, and of other inward parts; the same taken in like maner, or boiled with honied water or sugar, doth scoure and clense the brest, ripeneth and bringeth forth tough and clammie flegme."

As a medicine, it has been used for a variety of diseases under the allopathic school. Formerly it was externally applied by fomentations and ointments; and so highly was it prized by the Italians, that they have the adage, "Aralda tutte le piaghe salda," Foxglove cures all wounds. It has been employed to reduce the frequency and force of the heart's action, to promote the action of the absorbents as a diuretic, and also for its specific influence over the cerebro-spinal system. In fevers (*Withering, Sachs, Maclean, Beddoes, Schönlein*, etc.) In inflammations, on account of its power of reducing the frequency of the pulse (*King, Clutterbuck, Reil, Jörg*, etc.) In acute rheumatism (*Geyser*, *Gapper*, etc.) In dropsy (*Withering*, *Darwin*, *Joret*, etc.), on account of its diuretic properties; and Dr. Withering remarks, "that this medicine seldom produces its desired effects in men of great natural strength, of tense fibre, warm skin, of florid complexion, or in those with a light and cordy pulse. On the contrary, if the pulse be feeble or intermitting, the countenance pale, the lips livid, the skin cold, the swollen belly soft and fluctuating, or the anasarcous limbs readily pitting under the pressure of the finger, we may expect the diuretic effects to follow in a kindly manner." Blackall recommends Digitalis in dropsy after scarlet fever, when the urine is thick, small in quantity, and bad smelling. In jaundice (*Mayer and Schönlein*). In phlegmasia alba dolens (*Kraus*). In delirium tremens (*Webster*, *Pearson*, *Huss*, etc.) In hydrocephalus (*Jörg*, *Sachs*, *Heineger*, *Hufeland*, etc.) In metrorrhagia (*Neumann*). In disposition to abortion, particularly for congestion of the uterus (*Burns*). In croup (*Constance*, *Jurine*, *Geyser*). In hæmoptysis (*Jahn*, *Jones*, *Geyser*). Acute inflammation of the pleura. Pneumonia and peripneumonia (*Maclean*, *Currie*, *Canning*, *Brera*, *Rasori*, *Jahr*, *Geyser*, etc.) Chronic catarrh (*Neumann*). Phthisis. Digitalis has been declared capable of curing pulmonary consumption, and numerous cases of supposed cures have been published. Bayle (*Bibl. Thérap.*, t. iii. p. 362) has collected from the writings of Sanders, Kinglake, Fowler, Beddoes (*Obs. on the Management of the Consumptive*, 1801), Drake, Mossman (*Essay to elucidate the Nat. Orig. and Connex. of Scroph. and Gland. Consump.*), Maclean, Ferriar (*on Digitalis*), Maginnis, Moreton, and others, reports of 151 cases treated by Foxglove. Of these, eighty-three are said to be cured, and thirty-five relieved. But a more accurate and extended experience has fully proved that this medicine possesses no curative and very slight palliative powers in genuine phthisis. It is totally incapable of preventing or of causing the removal of tubercular deposits, and has little, if any, influence in retarding the progress of consumption. The power of diminishing the rapidity of the circulation cannot be doubted; but this effect is, as Dr. Holland justly remarks, "of less real moment than is generally supposed" (*Pereira*, op. cit., vol. ii. p. 845). In palpitation of the heart (*Otto, Joret, Heisinger*). Organic diseases of the heart, with hydrothorax (*Kreysig*). Inflammation of the heart (*Davis*). In hypertrophy, with dilatation (*Schönlein*). In aneurism of the aorta, by lessening the force of the circulation, and allowing the coagulation of the blood in the sac, etc. etc. In insanity and melancholia (*Jones, Cox, Currie, Haas, Halloran*, etc.) In epilepsy (*Scott*). Amaurosis (*Horn*), etc. etc. (Vide *Noack and Trinks*, op. cit., p. 688).

"We have few indigenous plants, not one perhaps, which we have so often summoned to aid us in our distresses as the Foxglove; no plant, not even the colchicum, has been more the object of our fears, our hopes, our trust, and disappointment than this; we have been grateful for the relief it has afforded, and we have mourned the insufficiency of its powers. Could we rely upon its yielding the virtues it is considered to possess, or could we regulate or control its influence, it would exist unrivalled for beauty and worth amidst our island plants" (*Knapp, Journ. of a Nat.*, 2nd edit., p. 90).

DESCRIPTION.—This elegant and beautiful plant is a biennial, and flowers from June to August. The *root* is composed of numerous long and slender fibres. *Stem* from three to five, and even six feet high, upright, mostly simple, leafy, roundish, with several slight angles, pubescent, or downy. *Leaves* alternate, between egg-shaped and spear-shaped, crenate, downy, rugged, and veiny, of a dull green above, whitish underneath, tapering at the base into winged footstalks; root-leaves largest. *Flowers* large and handsome, in long terminal spikes or clusters, pendulous, and leaning all one way. *Bracteas* spear-shaped. *Flower-stalks* pubescent, thickest at the top, one-flowered; after the flower drops off becoming nearly upright; segments of the calyx egg-shaped, pointed, the upper segment narrower than the rest. *Corolla* of one petal, nearly bell-shaped, above an inch long, purple, sometimes white, marked in the inside with blood-coloured spots and hairs.

GEOGRAPHICAL DISTRIBUTION.—Indigenous in Great Britain, and in the temperate and southern countries of Europe.

LOCALITIES.—In this country, in pastures, woods, and on banks, in a gravelly or sandy soil. Common in most counties, but not in Suffolk or Norfolk. The white variety has been found wild in several parts of England: in Worcestershire, near Bromsgrove, and near Hartlebury; in Staffordshire, about Moxhall; and near Penmynydd, in Anglesey.

PARTS USED IN MEDICINE, AND MODE OF PREPARATION.—For homœopathic preparations, we use the fresh Leaves of the second year, gathered in the month of May, before the plant flowers. The juice is to be expressed, mixed with equal parts of spirits of wine, and diluted to the thirtieth attenuation. The leaves procured in the shops are sometimes adulterated with those of the Verbascum Thapsus and Symphytum officinale, but which adulteration is easily discovered by the spurious leaves being hairy on both sides.

PHYSIOLOGICAL EFFECTS.—*On Vegetables.* According to Marcet (*Ann. de Chim. et de Phys.*, vol. xxix. p. 200), a watery extract of Digitalis killed a haricot plant in twenty-four hours.

On Animals.—From an extensive series of experiments by Orfila (*Tox. Général*, vol. ii. p. 290) with the powder, extract, and tincture of the leaves, Foxglove appears to cause, in moderate doses, vomiting, giddiness, languor, and death in twenty-four hours, without any other symptoms of note; but in larger doses it likewise produces tremors, convulsions, stupor, and coma. According to Moiroud (*Pharm. Vétér.*, p. 334), two ounces of the extract given to a horse produced death in twelve hours.

On Man.—In small and repeated doses on the healthy organism, it produces headache, salivation, nausea, and vomiting; diarrhœa; increase of the action of the kidneys; violent constriction and sense of suffocation in the chest; hæmoptysis, cough, and perspiration; great sense of weariness; pain and heaviness in the limbs; alteration in the heart's action; the pulse not beating above half its natural beats, or becoming hard, small, and quick; palpitation; great sense of chilliness; depression of spirits, and fear of death, etc. (vide *Hahnemann, Materia Medica Pura*, pp. 220—223). Pereira (op. cit.) remarks that, from various observations, the influence of Foxglove over the circulation is not at all constant. In some cases the frequency of the pulse is augmented, in others depressed, while in some it remains unaltered, and in a considerable number it becomes irregular or intermittent. He also remarks that a great deal depends upon the position of the patient; when recumbent, the pulse is reduced in frequency much sooner and with more certainty than when in the upright position. Shrock (*Wibmer, Wirk d. Arzneim.*, vol. ii. p. 311) found that two grains of Digitalis produced in himself nausea, headache, small, soft, and quick pulse, dryness of the gums and throat, giddiness, weakness of the limbs, and increased secretion of saliva; some hours after he observed sparks before the eyes; his vision became dim, and he experienced a sensation of pressure on the eyeballs. In larger doses, and when too long continued, more serious and more unpleasant symptoms are produced; such as nausea, vomiting, and purging; coldness of the extremities; sense of faintness and giddiness; confusion of vision and ideas; external objects appear green or yellow; great sense of weight and pain in the head; weakness of the limbs; pulse is slow and irregular; and sometimes stupor, delirium, and convulsions. Salivation in one case (*Rust's Magazine*, vol. xxv. p. 578) lasting for three weeks. These symptoms are not only produced by taking too large a dose, but often by repeated small doses, owing to the power this drug has of accumulating in the system, whereby its poisonous or deleterious effects are manifested, after its continued employment as a remedial agent.

In large or poisonous doses.—The following cases will exemplify its action, which (as in all other medicinal or poisonous effects of plants on the human organism) are peculiarly interesting to the homœopathist.

"Dr. W. Henry was called, in October, 1809, to assist a female, an out-patient of the Manchester Infirmary, labouring under dropsy, who had taken an overdose of decoction of Foxglove. It was prepared by boiling two handfuls of the leaves in a quart of water, and then pressing the mass so as to expel the whole of the liquor. Of this, at seven a.m., she drank two teacupfuls, amounting in the whole to not less than ten ounces by measure. Before eight she began to be sick, and vomited part of the contents of her stomach. Enough, however, was retained to excite vomiting and retching throughout the whole of that and the following day, during which everything that was taken was instantly rejected. In the intervals of sickness she was excessively faint, and her skin was covered with a cold sweat. The tongue and the lips swelled, and there was a continual flow of viscid saliva from the mouth. Very little urine was voided on the day she took the Digitalis, and on the following days the action of the kidneys was entirely suspended. When Dr. Henry saw her, which was forty-eight hours after she had taken the poison, the tongue was white, the ptyalism continued, though in a less degree, and the breath was fetid. The pulse was low, irregular (not exceeding forty), and after every third or fourth pulsation, an intermission occurred for some seconds. She complained also of general pains in the limbs, and cramps in the legs. By the use of effervescing draughts, and ether, with ammonia, she gradually recovered her imperfect health. Dr. Henry remarks that she had not taken any mercury, and that the ptyalism was entirely the effect of Digitalis" (*Edin. Med. and Surg. Jour.*, vol. viii. p. 148).

"Six ounces of a strong decoction were taken as a laxative early in the morning. Vomiting, colic, and purging were the first symptoms; towards the afternoon lethargy supervened;

about midnight the colic and purging returned; afterwards general convulsions made their appearance, and a surgeon, who saw the patient at an early hour of the succeeding morning, found him violently convulsed, with the pupils dilated, and insensible, and the pulse slow, feeble, and irregular: coma gradually succeeded, and death took place in twenty-two hours after the poison was swallowed. The post-mortem appearances are very imperfectly recorded in this case, and this is the more to be regretted, as a hiatus here remains in the toxicological history of the drug, that much wants filling up" (*Christ. on Poisons*, 3rd edit. p. 825).

"It is sometimes customary in pharmaceutical laboratories, to leave tinctures upon the dregs, after they have stood a due time, and gradually to pour off the clear part for use; the dregs are afterwards pressed out, and the last portion of the tincture acquires, by this careless proceeding, double the strength of the first. A person suffering under hydrothorax, who had been in the habit of taking forty drops of tincture of Digitalis every night, went from home without his medicine, and was obliged to send to an apothecary in the country for an ounce of the tincture, of which he took his accustomed dose: its effects were much more violent than usual, and he died, exhausted by repeated fainting, in the morning" (*Christ.*, op. cit.)

Mr. Brande, in his *Elements of Pharmacy*, observes: "I know an instance of a person who suffered under anasarca of the legs, and who applied for relief at a dispensary, where he received a box of pills (containing Digitalis), one of which he was directed to take three times a day. On the evening of the third day he complained of great debility and faintness, and in the course of the night vomiting and fainting fits came on. In the morning he died, upon attempting to get out out of bed" (*Id.*, op. cit.)

"A man, fifty-five years of age, suffering from humid asthma, took about an ounce of Digitalis instead of a grain of the powder of the leaves. An hour after he ate some soup, which he immediately vomited. The vomitings continued, accompanied with vertigo, so that he could not stand upright nor distinguish objects. During the whole day he continued to suffer from violent bilious and mucous vomitings, accompanied with great depression and abdominal pains, which were diminished by two emollient injections. These symptoms continued the whole of the next day and night. The patient was still further depressed; the pulse was slow and intermittent; and this symptom continued with but little alteration to the *ninth day*, when it had completely disappeared. At this time the vision was still confused, the fire appeared to him of a blue colour; and on the fourteenth day this symptom disappeared" (*Obs. de M. Bidault de Villiers, Journ. de Med. Chir. et Pharm.*, Nov. 1817).

"A man, of weak constitution, attacked with anasarca and hydrothorax, swallowed by mistake four or five times more of the tincture of Digitalis than he was ordered. He was seized with nausea and vomiting of a little bile after most violent and repeated efforts, with great depression and sweating during the night. These symptoms, from the treatment pursued, gradually disappeared, and in about seven days all the effects had passed off, except some œdema of the feet" (*Beddoes' Contr. to Phys. and Med. Knowledge*).

M. Bidault de Villiers (op. cit.) says, that he took a pretty good pinch of the powder of the leaves of Digitalis, which he had prepared with great care, and the following symptoms ensued: an extreme bitterness in the mouth, which increased the secretion of saliva to a considerable extent, and which continued after he had got rid of the Digitalis from the mouth; and it was only after the sensation of bitterness had entirely disappeared that he perceived a slight acridity in the throat. It also caused a sort of desire to vomit, and likewise a slight palpitation of the heart, with dryness in the mouth.

"A healthy, robust, young man, affected with sore throat, was advised to take *throatwort tea*. Having filled a quart pitcher with the fresh leaves of the Digitalis purpurea, he poured upon them as much boiling water as the pitcher would hold. Of this strong infusion he took a teacupful on going to bed, which caused him to sleep soundly. In the morning he took a second cupful (the infusion being much stronger), and he then went to his employment. He soon felt dizzy and heavy, began to stagger, lost his consciousness, and at length fell down in a state of syncope. On being conveyed home, he vomited severely, and suffered extreme pain in the abdomen. When visited, he was conscious; complained of great pain in the head; the pupils were dilated, and the surface cold, pallid, and covered with copious perspiration. The pulse was low, about forty a minute, three or four feeble pulsations being succeeded by a complete intermission of several seconds, and each stroke, though weak, was given with a peculiar 'explosive shock.' There was still great pain in the abdomen, with incessant and violent vomiting, no diarrhœa, suppression of urine, and an abundant flow of saliva. Brandy and ammonia, with warmth, were employed, and after reaction had commenced, purgatives were administered. The man slowly recovered, but the pulse presented its peculiar beat and weakness for several days, and during this time the man could not bear the upright position" (*Wilson, Med. Gazette*, vol. xxxiv., p. 659).

"R. N., ætat. 60, subject to irregular gout and dyspepsia; considerable dyspnœa; legs œdematous, and spotted with a few petechiæ. Half an ounce of infusion of Digitalis was given daily for some time, and then in lesser quantities. During the use of no more than two drachms of the infusion daily, a pain came over one of his eyes. He complained of great disturbance of his brain, which he himself referred to the draughts, and within twenty-four hours this symptom was followed by a watery exhausting diarrhœa and low delirium. General convulsions speedily ensued, in which there was complete insensibility, and foaming at the mouth, with an almost total cessation of the action of the heart. From this state he was recovered by an opiate injection. Similar paroxysms returned two or three times during the next three weeks. In the intervals, he became forgetful, delirious, and felt much pain in his head. The anasarca totally disappeared, discovering the most excessive emaciation; his posture in bed became nearly natural, and in one of the convulsions he expired" (*Blackall, Observ. on the Nature and Cure of Dropsies*, p. 175).

"A man, aged 50, took the tincture in medicinal doses for about twenty days, which produced the following symptoms: the pulse, which during the former use of the medicine had lessened by ten or fifteen beats in a minute, sank to almost half its usual number. The patient was tormented by the most painful disquietude, so that even in the night he left the bed every moment; could not sleep, and with his eyes open conversed with persons who were not present. At the same time the pupils were dilated, the conjunctiva both of the eye and the lids was red. He had but little appetite, with great nausea, violent thirst, and dryness of the mouth. The alvine evacuations were scanty, secretion of urine increased; these phenomena, evidently the effect of Digitalis, showing its accumulative properties, disappeared in about six days" (*Med. Gaz.*, vol. xxxi. p. 270).

"Dr. Williams related, upon unquestionable authority, an instance of a drunken butcher having taken two ounces of the tincture of Digitalis in two doses, of an ounce each, in quick succession, without the slightest inconvenience ensuing" (*Med. Gaz.*, vol. i. p. 744).

Medical Uses (Homœopathic).—*Hahnemann's observations:* "Although the following catalogue of symptoms is far from complete, it is sufficient to prove that, in all the chronic diseases that physicians have succeeded in curing by Digitalis, they have constantly acted homœopathically, without being aware of it; but the infinitely greater number of cases in which they have failed with this powerful plant, must not be separated from those in which it has been directed against the pathological *names* of diseases, purely from conjecture. While they continue to act thus, homœopathy, according to its doctrine of analogies, applies it where alone it can be useful, an immense advantage over the ordinary method.

"A small part of a drop of the quintillionth or rather the decillionth dilution will often be found even too strong for homœopathic uses (*Mat. Med. Pura*).

"The purple Foxglove (*Digitalis purpurea*) causes the most excessive disgust at food. During its continued use, therefore, ravenous hunger not unfrequently ensues. It causes a kind of mental derangement, which is not easily recognisable, as it only shows itself in unmeaning words, refractory disposition, obstinacy, cunning, disobedience, inclination to run away, etc., which its continued use frequently presents. Now, as in addition to these, it produces in its direct action, violent headaches, giddiness, pain in the stomach, great diminution of the vital powers, sense of dissolution and the near approach of death, a diminution of the rapidity of the heart's motion by one-half, and reduction of the vital temperature, it may easily be guessed in what kind of madness it will be of service; and that it has, in fact, been useful in some kinds of this disease many observations testify, only their particular symptoms have not been recorded. In the glands it creates an itching and painful sensation, which accounts for its efficacy in glandular swellings.

"It produces, as I have seen, inflammation of the Meibomian glands, and is a certain cure for such inflammations. Moreover, as it appears to depress the circulation, so does it seem to excite the absorbent vessels, and to be most serviceable where both are too torpid. The former it assists by virtue of similarity, the latter by virtue of antagonism of action. But as the direct action of Foxglove persists so long (there are examples of its lasting five or six days), it may, as an antagonistically-acting remedy, take the place of a permanent curative agent. The last observation is in reference to its diuretic property in dropsy; it is antagonistic and palliative, but nevertheless enduring, and valuable on that account merely.

"In its secondary action it causes a small, hard, rapid pulse; it is not therefore so suitable for patients who have a similar (febrile) pulse, but rather for such as have a pulse like what Foxglove produces in its direct action—slow, soft. The convulsions it causes in large doses assign it a place among the anti-epileptic remedies; probably it is useful in epilepsy only under certain conditions, to be determined by the other morbid symptoms it produces. During its use, objects not unfrequently appear of various colours, and the sight becomes obscured; it will remove similar affections of the retina. Its tendency to produce diarrhœa, sometimes so adverse to the cure, is counteracted, as I have ascertained, by the addition of potash.

"As the direct action of Foxglove lasts occasionally several days (the longer its use is continued, the longer lasts the direct action of each dose, a very remarkable fact, not to be lost sight of in practice), it is evident how erroneously those act who, with the best intentions, prescribe it in small but frequently-repeated doses (the action of the first not having expired before they have already given the sixth or eighth), and thus, in fact, they give unwittingly an enormous quantity, which not unfrequently causes death.

"A dose is necessary only every three, or at most every two days, but the more rarely the longer it has been used. During the continuance of its direct action, cinchona bark must not be prescribed; it increases the anxiety caused by Foxglove, as I have found, to an almost mortal agony."

Clinical Observations.—*Noack and Trinks* (op. cit.): Digitalis influences especially the sympathetic ganglia and the cardiac plexus. It is especially serviceable in sanguine and indolent temperaments, and persons with soft muscles and blonde hair, as well as for scrofulous individuals. Gouty nodosities (*Schubert*). Icterus, with mucous vomiting. Icterus spasticus. Morbus cæruleus, with great anxiety. Sense of suffocation, especially on lying down. Increased action of the heart. Hoarseness and dry cough (*Schüler*). Hydrothorax. Ascites and Anasarca, from organic lesion of the heart (*Attomyr*). After scarlet fever (*Schrön*). Dropsy of the pericardium. Nervous fever, with profuse salivation (*Lobethal*). *Dementia*, with an alteration of the normal state of the pulse (*Hahnemann*). Melancholia. Swelling of the glands (*Hahnemann*). Mercurial eczema, with palpitation of the heart (*Schrön*). Inflammation of the Meibomian glands (*Hahnemann*). Catarrhal, scrofulous, and arthritic inflammation of the eyes. Photophobia in scrofulous children (*Hartlaub*). Amaurosis, especially when the patient sees objects of various colours. Tenesmus vesicæ. Diabetes. Pleuritis serosa (*Wurm*, *Fleischmann*). Angina pectoris. Palpitation of the heart. Carditis. Chronic endocarditis. Chronic and organic diseases of the heart, especially of the left side, and of the large vessels, especially hypertrophy, with or without enlargement of the left ventricle. Valvular diseases of the heart. Aneurisma aortæ, etc. etc.

Antidotes. — Large doses, Sweet Milk, with Fœnum græcum. Vegetable acids. Vinegar. Infusion of galls (*Dulong*). Ether (*Sachs*). Camphor (*Otto*). Cinchona (*Dupuy*). Opium (*Beddoes*). To small doses, Nux Vomica. Opium.

XXX.

DROSERA* ROTUNDIFOLIA.

Round-leaved Sundew, Red-rot, Youth-wort, Moor-grass.

SYNONYMS.—Drosera rotundifolia, *Engl. Bot.*, t. 868; *Linn, Sp. Pl.*, p. 402; *Sm. Fl. Brit.*, vol. vi. p. 346; *With.*, vol. ii. p. 410. Rorella rotundifolia perennis, *Raii Syn.*, p. 356. Ros solis folio rotundo, *Raii Syn.*, p. 356; *Johnson's Gerarde*, p. 1556. Drosera capillaris, *Poir.* Salsisora seu Sponsa solis, *Thal. Harcy.*, 116, 69, f. i.; Rorida sive Ros solis major, *Lobel.*, 8. iii.

FOREIGN NAMES.—*Fr.:* Drosère à feuilles rondes, Rosée du soleil. *Germ.:* Rundblättriger, Sonnenthau. *Ital.:* Rugiada del sole. *Span.:* Rociada. *Dut.:* Zonnedauw. *Russ.:* Solncz najatrawa. *Port.:* A Rossolina.

Nat. Order, DROSERACEÆ, *De Cand.;* GRUINALES, *Linn.*
PENTANDRIA, HEXAGYNIA.

GEN. CHAR.—*Calyx* inferior, of one sepal, with five deep-pointed, upright, permanent segments. *Corolla* of five petals, without appendages, rather longer than the calyx. *Filaments* five to eight, awl-shaped, as long as the calyx. *Anthers* small, roundish. *Germen* roundish. *Styles* six to eight, simple. *Stigmas* club-shaped. *Capsule* egg-shaped, of one cell, with from three to five valves. *Seeds* numerous, minute, inversely egg-shaped, rough, attached to the inside of each valve, chiefly in the middle.

(Herbaceous plants, with leaves clothed with beautiful glandular hairs.)

The five-cleft *calyx*, the *corolla* of five petals, and the one-celled, three-valved (sometimes four or five), many-seeded *capsule*, will distinguish this from other genera in the same class and order.

SPEC. CHAR.—*Leaves* radical, nearly orbicular. *Footstalks* hairy, longer than the limb. *Scapes* naked, upright, four or five times higher than the leaves. *Seeds* chaffy (*Baxter*).

HISTORY.—It was supposed by some of the physicians of the

Fig. 1. A separate flower. 2. The stamens, germen, and pistils. 3. The calyx. 4. A capsule. 5. A transverse section of the same.

* From δροσερος, dewy, because the plants appear as if covered with dew, in consequence of being covered with glandular hairs.

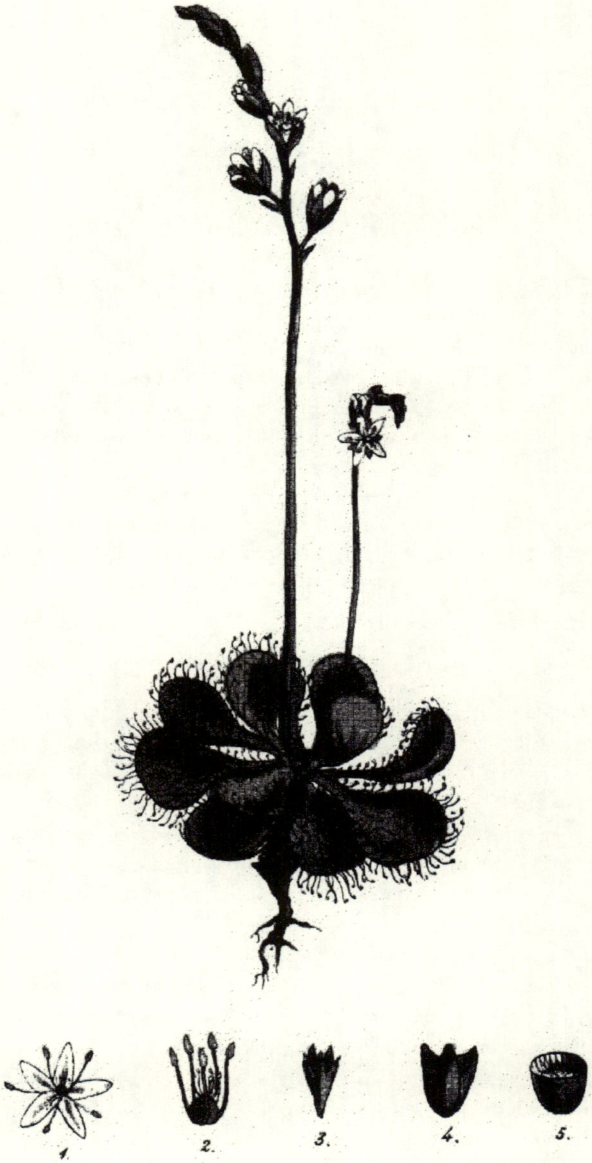

Drosera rotundifolia.

werby lith.

sixteenth century, that the permanent moisture of the Sundew would be an excellent remedy to restore vital moisture in persons labouring under consumption. Gerarde, however, states that those who took this distilled water died sooner than those who were treated by other means. "The later phisitians have thought this herbe to be a rare and singular remedie for all those that be in a consumption of the lungs, and especially the distilled water thereof; for, as the best doth keep and hold fast the moisture and the dew, and so fast that the extreme dry heat of the sun cannot consume and waste away the same; so, likewise, men thought that heerwith the naturall and lively heate in mens bodies is preserved and cherished. But the use thereof doth otherwise teach, and reason sheweth the contrarie; for, seeing it is an extreme biting herbe, and that the distilled water is not altogether without this biting qualitie, it cannot be taken with safetie: for it hath also been observed that they have sooner perished that used the distilled water hereof, than those that abstained from it and have followed the right and ordinary course of diet."

Quincy (*Engl. Disp.*, p. 71, 1742) states that the secretion from the Sundew is reported to cure the toothache if held in the mouth; to cure madness if hung about the neck; tied about the wrist to cure ague; and to promote delivery, if rubbed on the abdomen. The Droseras constituted the sole ingredient of the famous Aqua rosala, or Spirit of Sundew, and which was formerly extolled as a specific in plague and convulsions. The juice, mixed with milk, is used in Italy as a cosmetic. As a medicine it has been used in plica polonica (*Bonfiglio*). In megrim and ophthalmia (*Boerhaave*). In different kinds of coughs, arising from bronchial attacks, phthisis, and other diseases of the lungs (*Forest, Schenck, Holland, Valentin, Chomel*). In chronic asthma and palpitation of the heart (*Osiander, Volk. Arz.*, 1838).

Description.—Drosera rotundifolia is a perennial plant, flowering in July and August. The *root* is fibrous. *Stem* almost always entirely wanting. The *leaves* are numerous, on hairy footstalks, depressed, nearly circular, of a purplish-red. The whole *disk*, but especially the margin, beset with red, inflexed hairs, which discharge from their ends a drop of viscid, acrid fluid. The *scape* is from two to six inches in height, upright, naked, round, and smooth, terminated by a simple (sometimes bifid) cluster of flowers, which is drooping or revolute when growing. *Bracteas* awl-shaped, deciduous, one under each partial stalk. *Flowers* white, with five petals, five stamens, and six pistils. The *pistils* are said to be always double the number of the valves of the capsule in every known Drosera. The flowers are seldom seen in an expanded state. Linnæus says that they only open at nine in the morning, and close at noon. The leaves have a peculiar property of entrapping insects, like the Dionea muscipula.

Geographical Distribution.—The Drosera rotundifolia is indigenous in Great Britain, France, Germany, Italy, and other parts of Europe. Wildenow enumerates ten species, which are found in Asia, North and South America, New Holland, and the Indian Archipelago.

Localities.—In mossy, turfy bogs. In this country it is found generally among sphagnum.

Parts used in Medicine, and Mode of Preparation.—For homœopathic purposes we take the whole plant, gathered in July; express the juice, and treat it like other fresh plants. Hahnemann declares that succussion increases to a great extent the medicinal power of the juice of Drosera, and therefore great care must be taken in preparing this drug.

Physiological Effects.—*On Animals.* Ray (op. cit.) mentions that this plant is supposed to produce intestinal disease in sheep; hence the origin of one of its provincial names, *Red-rot.* Viborg (*Abh. für Thier Arzt.*) gave Drosera to a sheep daily for three weeks, without producing any deleterious effect.

On Man.—The whole plant is acrid, and sufficiently caustic to erode the skin. Burdach (*Arzneim.*, vol. iii. p. 105, 1820) states that the juice produces shuddering, sense of constriction at the chest, rawness in the throat, cough, hæmoptysis, pain in the bowels, sweat, and diminished secretion of urine.

MEDICAL USES (HOMŒOPATHIC).—*Hahnemann's observations:* "Drosera is one of the most powerful medicinal plants of our country. It was formerly used externally, but without success, in cutaneous affections, and it seems also to have been taken with greater advantage internally. Modern practitioners who, according to custom, have tried only large doses, have not ventured upon giving it internally, fearing to kill their patients, and have therefore rejected it.

"I first used the trillionth dilution, but have since proceeded as far as the decillionth.

"A very small portion of a drop of this liquor, that is to say, one or two globules, are a dose under homœopathic conditions. "Thus, for example, a single dose suffices for the homœopathic cure of the epidemic hooping-cough."*

CLINICAL OBSERVATIONS.—*Noack and Trincks* (op. cit.): Drosera appears to be especially serviceable in phlegmatic temperaments, in chilly individuals, and such as are predisposed to the hemorrhoidal and inflammatory diathesis. Drosera may be useful in diseases prevailing during an epidemic of hooping-cough. Intermittent fevers, with much shivering. Pallor of the face, and icy coldness of the hands and feet, with bilious vomiting, followed by heat and violent headache. Constant sneezing, with dryness of the eyes and nose (*Caspari*). Pain in the face (prosopalgia), increased by contact and movement (*Jahr*). Bloody diarrhœa during hooping-cough (*Hartlaub*). Hooping-cough in the second and third stage. Hooping-cough, with bleeding from the nose and mouth. Hooping-cough after

* "The cure is certain to take place in seven or nine days, care being taken not to give a second dose soon after the first. It is necessary to abstain from giving any other medicinal substance whatever, which would infallibly prevent the good effect of the first dose, and even cause serious consequences, as experience has proved to me."

measles. Hooping-cough, in alternation with Cina and Sulphur (*Tietzel*). Hooping-cough, with much rattling of mucus in the bronchial tubes (*Schrön*). (*Knorre* states that Drosera is only useful in the convulsive stage of hooping-cough). Chronic bronchitis. Chronic hoarseness after repeated catarrhs. Incipient laryngeal phthisis, etc.

ANTIDOTE.—Camphor.

Plate XXXI.

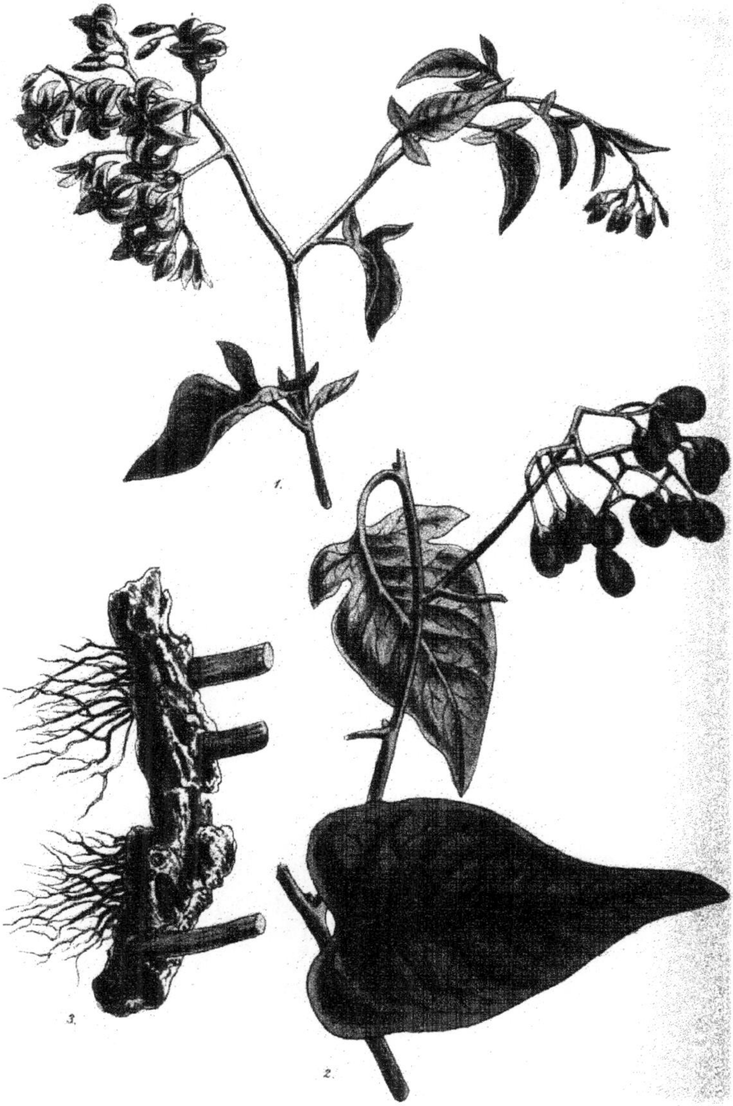

H Sowerby lith.

Dulcamara,
(Solanum Dulcamara.)

XXXI.

DULCAMARA.*

(SOLANUM DULCAMARA.)

Woody Nightshade, or Bitter-sweet, Fellon-wood.

SYNONYMS.—Solanum lignosum seu Dulcamara, *Raii Syn.*, vol. i. p. 265. Solanum, *Hall Hist.*, vol. i. p. 242. Dulcamara flexuosa, *Meneh. Meth.*, 514. Amara dulcis, *Ger.*, 3506. Vitis sylvestris, *Matth. Vulgr.*, vol. ii. p. 619; *Camer. Epi.*, 986. Solanum Dulcamara, *Linn. Sp. Pl.; Wild.*, vol. i. p. 1028. Solanum scandens seu Dulcamara, *Bauh. Πιν.*, 176. Glycypigros sive Amara dulcis, *F. Bauh.*, vol. ii. p. 109. Solanum caule flexuoso frutescente, foliis supremis tripartitis et cordato lanceolatis, *Hal. Stirp. Helv.*, 575; *Flor. Dan.*, t. 607. Dulcamara flexuosa, *Gray Nat. Arr.*, vol. ii. p. 331.

FOREIGN NAMES.—*Fr.:* Douce-amère, Morelle. *Ital.:* Morella, Solatro. *Span.:* Dulcamara. *Port.:* Dolçamarga. *Germ.:* Bittersuss. *Dan.:* Bittersöde. *Dut.:* Bitterroet. *Russ.:* Paslen sladkogorski, Binki.

Nat. Order, LURIDÆ, *Linn.;* SOLANEÆ, *Juss.*—PENTANDRIA, MONOGYNIA.

GEN. CHAR.—*Calyx* inferior, of one sepal, in from five to ten, more or less deep, acute segments, permanent. *Corolla* of one petal, wheel-shaped, tube very short, limb much longer, reflex, plaited in four, five, or six sharp-pointed, equal, rather deep segments. *Filaments*, four, five, or six, short, awl-shaped. *Anthers* much longer, oblong, angular, converging, sometimes unequal, opening by two pores at the apex. *Germen* roundish. *Style* thread-shaped, longer than the stamens, deciduous. *Stigma* blunt, simple, or notched. *Berry* roundish, or egg-shaped, smooth, with a hollow dot at the end of two (occasionally more) cells, with a fleshy receptacle to each, connected with the partition. *Seeds* numerous, roundish, compressed, imbedded in pulp, sometimes minutely dotted. *Embryo* (according to De Candolle) spiral; distinguished from other genera by a monopetalous, inferior corolla; in the same class and order, by the calyx of from five to ten segments, the wheel-shaped *corolla*,

---

Fig. 1. The flowering stem. 2. The fruit. 3. The root.

* From *dulcis*, sweet, and *amara*, bitter, owing to the peculiar flavour of the plant when chewed.

the anthers opening by two pores at the extremity, and the roundish berry of two or more cells (*Baxter*).

SPEC. CHAR.—*Stem* shrubby, zigzag, without thorns. *Leaves* heart-shaped, upper ones hastate. *Clusters* cymose.

HISTORY.—According to Pereira, the first undoubted notice of Dulcamara occurs in the works of Tragus (*Spreng. Hist. Rei Herb.*, vol. i. p. 227). Dodonæus and Hardouin (*ad Plin. H. N.* t. xxv. p. 68) consider that the Κυκλαμινος ετερα of Dioscorides is the Solanum Dulcamara. Sprengel (op. cit.) states it to be the same as the Cilocatra of the Abbess Hildegard of Bilgen; whilst others again (*Christ. Disp.*) have confounded the Αμπελος ἀγρία, or Vitis sylvestris of Dioscorides, with the Bitter-sweet. As a medicine it was first brought into notice by Boerhaave, who recommended it in phthisis, peripneumonia, scorbutus, icterus, jaundice, as a sudorific and tonic. Murray (*App. Med.*, vol. i.) orders the juice from the younger branches to be used, and says that it promotes all the secretions. Haller observes that it partakes of the milder powers of Belladonna. Bergius (*Mat. Med.*, 131) "pellens urinam, sudorem menses, lochia sputa mundificans;" he chiefly recommended it in rheumatismus, retentio mensium, et lochiorum. It was recommended in different diseases of the skin, by Linnæus, Carrere, Rayoux, and others; and Sir Alexander Crichton states that out of twenty-three cases of lepra græcorum, only two resisted its action. Bateman also declares that it is a most effectual remedy in this disease; and Rayer (*Treat. of Dis. of Skin, Willis*) has used it with advantage in eczema and psoriasis, Pereira (op. cit.) found it useless in these diseases. De Haen (*Val. Med. Tom.*) employed it in cramps and convulsions. Carrere and Starke, in coryzas and diseases produced by damp and wet. Chronic catarrh by Vogt. In hysteria and hypochondriasis by Geoffroy, Hartmann, Boecler, Kühn, etc. In fluor albus by Carrere and Kühn; and by others in catarrhal fever, blennorrhœa, inflammation (erysipelas) of the skin, ischuria, hemorrhoidal affections, etc. etc. Dr. Pearson (*Synop. Mat. Med.*) gave an infusion of the stalks with benefit in humoral asthma and dropsy.

Description.—This beautiful and well-known shrub flowers from June to August. The *root* is woody. The *stem* shrubby, somewhat climbing branches, thinly set with small, pointed tubercles, slightly angular, and growing, when supported, to the height of from eight to ten feet. The *branches* are alternate, the younger ones of a purplish hue, the lower ones covered with a greyish-green bark. The *leaves* are alternated, acute, on leaf-stalks, generally smooth, the lower ones egg or heart-shaped, the upper ones more or less perfectly halbert-shaped; all entire at the margin. *Flowers* in branched clusters, either opposite to the leaves or terminal, purple, with two green tubercles at the base of each segment. *Anthers* yellow, large, united into a pyramidal or cone-shaped figure. Dr. Withering observes that the anthers, on the first opening of the flower, are easily separable, but that afterwards they become drier, and tear whilst endeavouring to disunite them. *Berry* egg-shaped, bright red, glossy, bitter, and poisonous. Ray mentions a hairy variety growing on the southern coast of England. Baxter states his having seen this variety at Dorton, in Oxfordshire. The white-flowered variety has been noticed about Glasgow by Mr. Hopkirk, and near Oxford by Miss Baxter.

Geographical Distribution.—In most parts of Europe, Greece, and as far north as Norway.

Localities.—Very general in moist hedges and thickets, on the banks of ditches, and sometimes on old walls. More rare in Scotland and Ireland.

Parts used in Medicine, and Mode of Preparation.—Quin (*Phar. Hom.*) orders the juice from the young branches and leaves of the plant, when it commences to flower. Jahr orders the fresh juice expressed from the plant before the flowering season. But Murray (*App. Med.*, vol. i. p. 424) states that the sensible qualities of the plant are strongest in the autumn, when the leaves are falling, and on this account it should be gathered in the autumn rather than the spring. The roots are said to possess the same properties as the annual stems. These stems when fresh have a heavy, unpleasant odour, which they entirely lose by drying. Their taste is at first bitter, afterwards slightly acrid and sweet.*

PHYSIOLOGICAL EFFECTS.—*On Animals.* Thirty of the berries were given to a dog, which soon became mad, and died in the space of three hours; and upon opening the stomach, the berries were found to have undergone no change by the powers of digestion (*Floyer, Pharm.*, p. 86). Others have stated that no effect has been produced by these berries. M. Duval (*Hist. Mat. Méd. et Econ du Solanum*) having given very large doses, both to animals and man, without their producing any deleterious effect.

On Man.—In large doses, Solanum Dulcamara will produce nausea, vertigo, syncope, diarrhœa, etc. Dr. Crichton found that, in delicate people and hysterical women, it frequently produced syncope, with slight palpitation of the heart, accompanied occasionally by nausea and giddiness. Chevalier (*Hist des Drogues*, t. ii. p. 229) states that narcotism was produced in a man, merely by carrying a bundle of this plant on his head.

The following cases illustrate the poisonous action of the berries. Two children, one five years, the other three and a half years of age, ate a few berries of the Dulcamara; an hour after they were seized with excruciating pains in the intestines; great heat in the throat and chest; could not bear the slightest pressure on the abdomen; much nausea, thirst, and prostration of strength; pulsations at the wrist very frequent; breathing painful and hurried; evacuations, after administering castor oil, green, slimy, and extremely offensive. These symptoms gra-

* The berries are poisonous, and possess very active properties; a preparation from them would be worthy of trial. The active principle of Dulcamara is an alkali, Solania, which exists in the plant, combined with malic acid.

dually disappeared, and the children were quite recovered in two days.

A child, after having swallowed some of the berries, was seized with the same symptoms, only accompanied with violent vomiting and purging, with contraction of the abdominal muscles, and a profuse secretion of saliva, but after appropriate treatment recovered. Two other children died, from being left without medical aid for twelve hours after they had swallowed the berries (*Wheeler in Med. Bot.*, vol. i.)

MEDICAL USES (HOMŒOPATHIC).—*Hahnemann's observations:* "The Bitter-sweet produces in large doses, among other symptoms, great swelling of the affected parts, and acute pains and insensibility of them, also paralysis of the tongue (and of the optic nerves ?). In virtue of the last powerful action, it is not to be wondered at that it has cured paralytic affections, amaurosis, and deafness, and that it will render still more specific service in paralysis of the tongue in moderate doses. In virtue of the two first properties, it is a main remedy in chronic rheumatism, and in the nocturnal pains from the abuse of mercury.

"In consequence of its power of causing strangury, it has been useful in obstinate gonorrhœa; from its tendency to bring about itching and shooting in the skin, it shows its utility in many cutaneous eruptions and old ulcers, even such as arise from the abuse of mercury. As it causes in large doses spasms of the hands, lips, and eyelids, as also shaking of the limbs, we may easily understand how it has been useful also in spasmodic affections. In nymphomania it will probably be of use, as it acts so specifically on the female organs, and has the power of causing, in large doses, itching and pains in these parts (*Hahnemann's Less. Writ., Dudgeon,* 1851).

"It has been found curative in the following affections: boring and burning pain in the forehead; sensation as of a board being in front of the forehead; scrofulous ophthalmia; incipient amaurosis; crusta lactea; cough, with hoarseness; catarrh of the bladder, with difficulty of micturition; a sort of hooping-cough consequent upon cold; rending pain in the limbs consequent upon cold," etc. etc. (*Hahnem. Cron. Krank.*, vol. iii.)

Clinical Observations.—Dulcamara is especially serviceable in phlegmatic, torpid, scrofulous, psoric, debilitated constitutions, and individuals with restless, irritable disposition. Dulcamara is especially indicated in pains which increase in proportion as the affected parts are kept quiet. It is also indicated in individuals liable to constant attacks of cold, and in all affections originating in sudden cold, owing to damp or cold air, or wet. Also in metastases of rheumatism, and cutaneous diseases. Acute and chronic affections of the mucous membranes, with abnormal secretions. Acute and chronic rheumatism. Paralysis, especially from metastases. Dropsy following ague. Hydrargyrosis. Lichen simplex. Sequelæ of measles. Acute and chronic urticaria. Nettle-rash, with fever. (Knorre states that Dulcamara is specific against chronic urticaria). Pemphigus, with violent thirst, etc. Impetigo figurata. Crusta lactea et serpiginosa. Suppurating, humid, corrosive herpes, forming dry crusts. Eczema after getting wet. Warts, especially on the face. Rheumatic fever (with Acon., Puls., and Bry.) Cephalalgia, especially after getting wet; especially violent stupifying headache, with tearing pains in the limbs. Cephalalgia after a fainting fit. Ophthalmia neomontanum. Angina tonsillaris from cold. Status pituitosus. Rheumatic irritation of the intestinal canal. Inflammatory swelling of the inguinal glands, brought on by cold, especially when moving the feet, and trying to walk. Catarrhal, rheumatic, and mucous diarrhœa, brought on by cold or wet. Chronic diarrhœa after a cold. Catarrh of the bladder. Ischuria, especially when consequent on a cold, or after having drank cold liquids. Gonorrhœa secundaria in scrofulous individuals. Fluor albus rodens. Asthma humidum. Hoarseness, and sense of confusion in the head after a violent cold. Hooping-cough, especially when it has become moist, and the more severe symptoms have been removed by other remedies. Incipient phthisis. Violent tearing pains in the limbs, especially in the feet, with much perspiration. Rheumatism of the joints, etc. etc. (*Noack and Trinks*, op. cit.)

Antidotes.—To large doses, Carbonate of Potassa. To small doses, Belladonna. Ipecac. Mercurius. Dulcamara is an antidote against Cuprum.

XXXII.

EUPHORBIA OFFICINARUM.

Officinal Euphorbium, or Spurge.

Synonyms.—Euphorbia tenella planta, *Lob. Icon.*, ii. t. 25. Euphorbium, *Raii Hist.*, 872. Euphorbium polygonum spinosum cerei effigie, *Isn. Act. Acad. Scien.*, n. iv. t. 10, p. 385, 1720. Euphorbia officinarum, *Lin. Sp. Pl.*, 647; *Plench. Icon.*, t. 365.

Foreign Names.—*Fr.:* Euphorbe. *Ital. and Span.:* Euforbio. *Germ.:* Euphorbien-harz, Wolfsmilch. *Dut.:* Euphorbium. *Swed.:* Preustkäda. *Dan.:* Euphorbium gummi. *Arab.:* Ahalnafsah, Fasfryun. *Tam.:* Shadry kulliepaal.

Nat. Order, Tricoccæ, *Linn.;* Euphorbiæ, *Juss.*—Monœcia, Monandria.

Gen. Char.—*Flowers* collected in monœcious heads, surrounded by an involucrum, consisting of one leaf with five divisions, which have externally five glands alternating with them. *Males* naked, monandrous, articulated, with their pedicle surrounding the female, which is in the centre. *Females* naked, solitary. *Ovarium* stalked. *Stigmas* three-forked. *Fruit* hanging out of the involucrum, consisting of three cells, bursting at the back with elasticity, and each containing one suspended seed (*Lindley*).

Spec. Char.—Aculeated, naked, many-angled. *Prickles* in pairs, spreading, equal.

History.—This plant is the Δενδρον ευφορβιον of Dioscorides (lib. iii. cap. 96), and is supposed to derive its name from Euphorbus, the physician of Juba, king of Mauritania and Numidia. Euphorbus was brother to Musa, physician to Augustus Cæsar. Cæsar raised a statue to Musa. Juba named

---

Fig. 1. The corolla. 2. The germen and pistils.

Plate

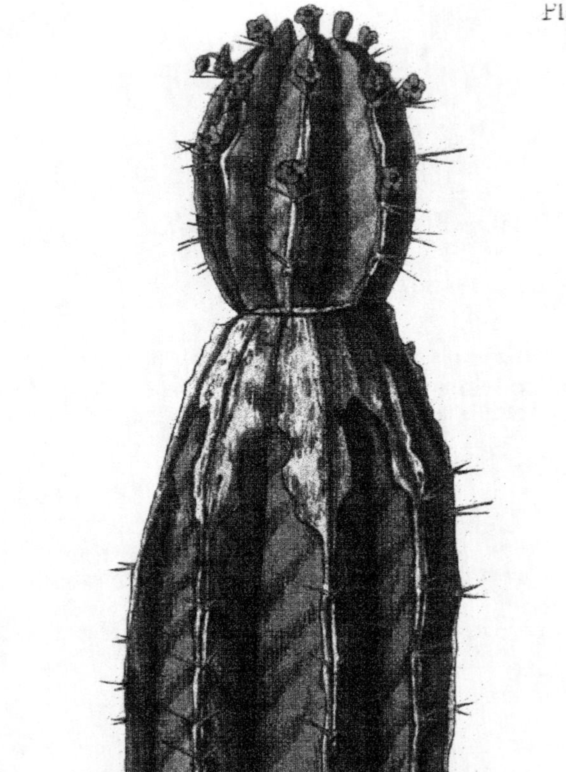

2.

Euphorbia officinarum.

this plant after Euphorbus, "ubi jam Musæ statua? periit! evanuit! Euphorbi autem perdurrat, perennat, nec unquam destrui potest" (*Crit. Bot.*, 89).

The following is Pliny's account of this plant. "No longer ago than our forefathers' days, Juba, king of Mauritania, found out a herb, Euphorbia, which he so called after his own physitian, Euphorbus, brother to that learned Musa, physitian to Augustus Cæsar, who saved the life of the said emperor, as heretofore I have declared. These two brethren physitians joined together in counsell, and gave direction for to wash the body all over in much cold water, after the hot baine or stouve, thereby to knit and bind the pores of the skin; for before their time the maner was to take in hot water only, as we may see plainly in the poet Homer. But now to return up to our herb, Euphorbia: the foresaid king Juba, wrote one entire book (at this day extant), wherin he doth nothing els but expressly set forth the commendable vertues and properties of this one herb. He found the same first upon the mountain Atlas, where it was to be seen (saith he) bearing leaves resembling Branc-ursin, so strong and forcible it is, that those who receive the juice or liquor issuing from it must stand a good way off; for the maner is to lance or wound it first, and then presently to retire backe, and so at the end of a long pole to put under it a paile or trey made of kids or goats leather for a receptory, into which there runneth forth out of the plant a white liquour like unto milke, which, when it is dried and growne together, resembleth in shew a lumpe or mass of frankincense. They that have the gathering of this juice called Euphorbium find this benefit thereby, that they see more clearly than they did before: an excellent remedy this is against the venom of serpents, for what part soever is stung or wounded by them, make a light incision upon the crown [of the head], and apply thereto this estimable liquor, it will surely cure it. But in that country the Getulians who commonly do gather

Euphorbium, for that they border upon the Mount Atlas, sophisticate it with goats milke. Howbeit, fire will soon detect this imposure of theirs, for that which is not right but corrupt, when it burneth, doth yield a lothsome fume and stinking sent." (*Nat. Hist., Holland's Trans.*, b. xxv. cap. vii. p. 222, 1634).

Neither Dioscorides nor Galen take any notice of its cathartic properties, but Pliny does, as does also Ælius, Paulus, and the Arabian physicians. Mesne particularly recommends it in diseases of the joints; it was also employed in ascites, rheumatism, ague, paralysis, and caries before exfoliation; and later, in ulcers, warts, chronic ophthalmia, amaurosis, deafness, diseases of the hip-joint (*Cheselden*). Sciatica, (*Henman*). It was used in dropsy and podagra in Mogador. At present it is seldom employed allopathically in this country, except in veterinary medicine.

Description.—The *stem* of this plant rises four or five feet in height, simple or branched towards the top, erect, angled, or furrowed with eight or more longitudinal fissures. The *branches* go off first horizontally, and then ascend; they are more distinctly angled than the stem, the angles notched and furnished with prickles, which are everywhere in pairs; these branches are everywhere destitute of leaves. The *involucres* are sessile, and arise at the extremities of the branches in the axil of the spines. The involucre is monophyllous, bell-shaped, persistent, and divided into eight or ten teeth or segments, of which the four or five outer are thick, yellow, obtuse, spreading; four or five alternate and inner ones, smaller, obtuse, entire, and directed inwards. *Barren or male flowers*, about twelve, each consisting of a single capillary *filament*, which supports a globular two-lobed *anther*. *Fertile or female flower*, a single naked pistil. The *germen* roundish, three-lobed, supporting a short, simple *style*, crowned with three spreading, obtuse *stigmas*. The *capsule* is tricoccous, elastic, and contains three roundish seeds (*Hooker*). The genus Euphorbia comprises a very numerous tribe of singular plants; upwards of two hundred are described by Wildenow; one hundred and twenty are cultivated in our botanic gardens, and fourteen species are natives of Britain.

Geographical Distribution.—The Euphorbia officinarum is a native of Africa, about Mogador, the coast of Barbary, and the Atlas range. The different species are distributed all over the world.

Parts used in Medicine, and Mode of Preparation.—The Gum-resin. The officinal Euphorbium is the concrete juice of the plant, obtained by making slight incisions in the branches with a knife, from which a milky juice exudes, which, by exposure to the air and the heat of the sun, hardens and forms a whitish, yellow solid, generally pierced with two holes by the prickles of the plant. This drops off in September, is collected, and forms the Euphorbium of commerce.* The recent juice is of so acrid a nature, that the people who collect it are obliged to tie a cloth over their mouth and nostrils to prevent the small, dusty particles from annoying them, as they produce incessant sneezing.

Bruce says, "the tree-gum which is found in the shops consists of irregular, yellowish, slightly friable tears, almost odourless." When triturated with water, only one part in seven of the Euphorbium is dissolved. Alcohol takes up one part in four, and forms a clear, straw-coloured solution, which is rendered milky by the addition of water.† For homœopathic purposes: one part of the gum-resin, reduced to powder, and to which ninety-nine parts of sugar of milk is added; these are mixed together, the three first attenuations made by trituration, then diluted to the thirtieth attenuation.

* The plants are only cut once in four years, as the quantity exuded is so great that it is sufficient for the supply for that time.

† The concrete juice imported into Europe, and sold as Euphorbium officinalis, is the produce of several species, but more particularly of the Euphorbium Canariensis; others, as the Euphorbia Esula and E. Lathyris, are quite as violent in their effects.

PHYSIOLOGICAL EFFECTS.—*On Animals generally:* Euphorbium acts on horses and dogs as a powerful acrid substance, irritating and inflaming the parts with which it is placed in contact, and by sympathy affecting the nervous system. When swallowed in large quantities, it causes gastro-enteritis (two ounces are sufficient to kill a horse); when applied to the skin, it acts as a rubefacient and epispastic. Farriers sometimes employ it as a substitute for cantharides for blistering horses, but cautious and well-informed veterinarians are opposed to its use (*Pereira*, op. cit.)

On Man.—Messrs. Herring, the wholesale druggists in London, informed Dr. Christison that their workmen are subject to headache, giddiness, and stupor, if they do not carefully avoid the dust when reducing this substance to powder.

When Euphorbium dust is inhaled, and also applied to the face, it causes sneezing, redness and swelling of the face, and great irritation about the eyes and nose. In one person it always produced a sense of intoxication, and another was made temporarily insane by it, and who, during the fit, insisted on saying his prayers at the tail of the mill horse.

A man was engaged at a mill where Euphorbium was being ground, and remained in the room longer than was considered prudent; suddenly he darted from the mill-room, and ran with great velocity down two pair of stairs; on arriving at the ground-floor or yard, he became insensible and fell. Within five minutes I saw him; he was lying on his back, insensible and convulsed; his face was red and swollen; his pulse frequent and full, and his skin hot. I bled him, and within half an hour he became quite sensible, but complained of great headache. He had no recollection of his flight down stairs, which seems to have been performed in a fit of delirium (*Pereira*, op. cit.)

Pyl (*Aufsäl und Beobacht.*, vol. i. p. 79) states that when powdered Euphorbium is applied to the skin, it causes itching pain and inflammation, succeeded by vesication. A teaspoonful of the tincture of Euphorbium was administered to a man by a farrier, in the dark, through mistake for rhubarb; burning heat in the throat and then in the stomach, vomiting, irregular hurried pulse, and cold perspirations were the leading symptoms. The person died in three days; gangrenous spots were found in the stomach, and the coats tore with the slightest touch (*Furnival, in Brande's Journ.*, vol. iii. p. 51). In the case related in the *Philosophical Transactions* for 1760, many of the symptoms are attributable to the Camphor.

Dr. Christison states that probably all species of Euphorbium possess the same properties as the E. officinarum. Orfila found the E. Cyparissias and E. Lathyris produced precisely the same effects. Dr. Hood relates the case of a child who ate some of the seed of the E. Lathyris (or Caper Spurge), soon after he vomited severely, which is the usual effect. Drowsiness, however, succeeded, and after a few returns of vomiting, which was promoted by an emetic, deep sleep gradually came on, broken by convulsions, stertorous breathing, and sighs; sensibility was somewhat restored by blood-letting and the warm bath; after which the tendency to sleep was interrupted by frequent agitation and exercise in the open air; the vomiting then recurred for a time, and the child got well.

The seeds of this species (Caper Spurge) are used by the inhabitants of the northern Alps, in doses of fifteen grains, as an emetic.

Sprœgel applied the juice of E. Lathyris to his face, which produced an eruption like nettle-rash; and he also found that it caused the hair to drop out, and warts to fall off (*Orfila*, vol. i. p. 712).

Scopili mentions that the Euphorbia Esula produced death in a woman in half an hour after she had swallowed thirty grains of the root; and also, that he witnessed gangrene and death follow the application of the same plant to the abdomen. The same author states that in a person who allowed his closed eyelids to be rubbed with the juice of this species, inflammation followed, and was succeeded by the loss of the eye.

It was with the Euphorbia Tiraculli that Hyder Ali, in his ferocious wars against the English in India, ordered the wells to be poisoned (*Quart. Rev.*, vol. xviii.)

Medical Uses (Homœopathic).—Stapf has proposed to employ Euphorbium in the following cases: Chronic disease of the bones and mucous membrane. Cutaneous eruptions. Chronic ophthalmia, with painful affections of the eyelids, which itch violently, and are humid and agglutinated. Dim-sightedness, weakness of the eyes, and optical delusions. Tearing pain in the teeth, and a feeling as if the tooth was drawn out, increased by contact. Malignant affections of the throat. Salivation. Hydrargyrosis. Chronic abdominal affections. Colic, with violent burning pains, and sense of distension of the intestines. Affections of the rectum and bladder, with tenesmus, and painful sensations in those organs. Cough, with constant tickling in the throat, or in the middle of the chest. Asthma. Painful affections of the extremities. Erysipelas vesiculosum faciei (*Haubold*). Breaking of the teeth (*Ruckert*). Pulsating, boring toothache, as if the teeth were screwed together. Very painful abscess at the root of the eye-teeth, sensitive to the touch, with erysipelatous swelling of the cheek. Cardialgia in the morning, soon after getting up, with painful cramps in the scrobiculus cordis, increased after the mid-day meal. Vomiting of mucus and water. Pain in the back, and drawing rheumatic pain between the shoulders, and through to the pit of the stomach and chest; afterwards shortness of breath, with palpitation on lying down; together with violent throbbing, bursting headache. Constipation, and frequent flying heats, alternating with shivering.

Antidotes.—To large doses, emollient and demulcent drinks. Clysters of mucilaginous, amylaceous, or oleaginous liquids. To small doses, Camphor.

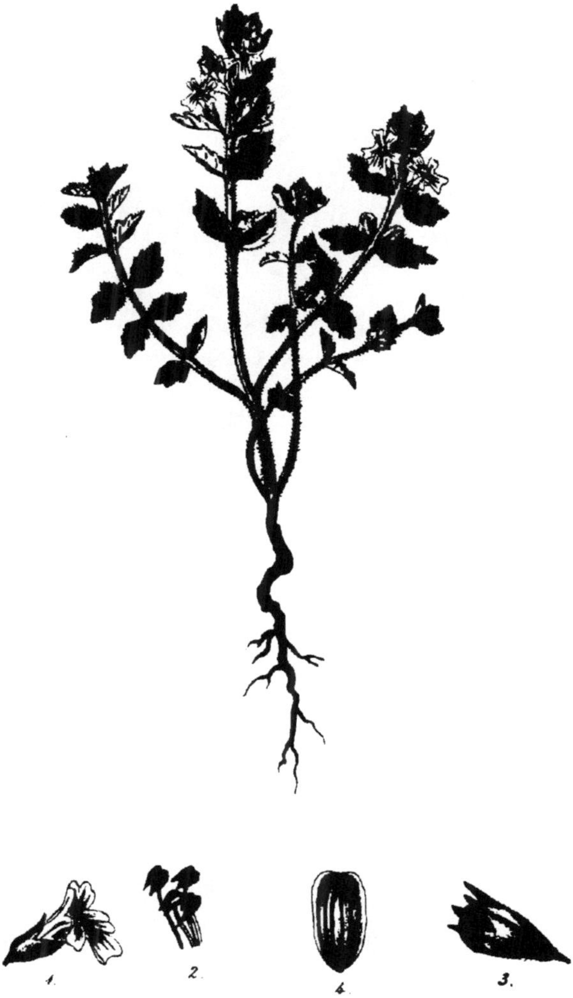

Euphrasia officinalis.

Frederic Reeve imp

XXXII.

EUPHRASIA* OFFICINALIS.

Eyebright.

SYNONYMS.—Euphrasia sive Euphrasine oculari, *Icon. Plant.*, p. 496. Euphragia alba, *Brunself.* Euphrasia candida, *Schœr.* Euphrasia, *Râii Syn.*, p. 284. Euphrasia officinalis, *Linn. Sp. Pl.*, p. 841, etc.

FOREIGN NAMES.—*Fr.:* Eufrasie, Eufrase. *Ital.:* Eufragra, Eufrasina. *Germ.:* Augentrost, Heinkraut, Milchdienst. *Hung.:* Æffrasi.

Nat. Order, RHINANTHACEÆ, *Dec.;* SCROPHULARINEÆ, *Lindl.;* PEDICULARES, *Juss.*—DIDYNAMIA, ANGIOSPERMIA.

GEN. CHAR.—*Calyx* inferior, of one sepal, tubular, cylindrical, ribbed, permanent; the margin in four deep, nearly equal, pointed teeth. *Corolla* of one petal, ringent, open; tube as long as the calyx, cylindrical; upper lip slightly concave, with several notches; lower lip spreading, divided into three, more or less, unequal, obtuse, cloven, or inversely heart-shaped lobes. *Filaments* thread-shaped, directed towards the upper lips. *Anthers* incumbent, large, of two roundish lobes, pointed at the base; the points of the lower anthers elongated into straight, bristly spines. *Germen*, egg-shaped. *Style*, thread-shaped, as long as the stamens. *Stigma* blunt, undivided. *Capsule* oblong, blunt, compressed, emarginate (notched at the summit), of two cells, and two membranous valves. *Seeds* several, very small, elliptical, compressed, furrowed, or striated on each side. The four-cleft calyx, spinous anthers, two-celled capsule, and furrowed or striated seeds will distinguish this from other genera in the same class and order (*Baxter*).

SPEC. CHAR.—*Leaves* egg-shaped, furrowed, sharply toothed.

HISTORY.—F. Bauhin (*Phytop.*, p. 442) states that, although Dalechampius gave the derivation of Euphrasia from the Greek, yet there is no notice of this herb in the works of Dioscorides,

---

Fig. 1. The corolla. 2. Stamens. 3. Calyx. 4. Seed.

* From Ευφροσυνη, expressive of joy and pleasure.

Galen, Pliny, nor even by the Arabian physicians. He says that it was known as a remedy for the eyes about two hundred years ago; he wrote this in 1580. Arnaldus Villanovanus, who died in 1313, was the author of "Vini Euphrasiati tantopere celebrati." How long before him Euphrasia was in repute for eye diseases is impossible to say; but in Gordon's "Liticium Medicinæ," published in 1305, among the medicines for the eyes, Euphragia is one, and is used both outwardly in a compound, distilled water, and inwardly as a syrup (*Alston, Mat. Med.*, vol. vii. p. 139). Euphragia is not mentioned in the "Schola Salernitana," compiled about 1100. The earliest notice of Euphrasia, as a medicine, is in the works of Tragus (*Sprengel*, op. cit.) It was employed as a remedy in diseases of the eyes, by Fuschius, Dodonæus, Haller, and others, and has been a vulgar remedy in these diseases from time immemorial throughout the whole of Europe. Fuschius recommended it in suffusions and cataracts. The Highlanders of Scotland make an infusion of it in milk, and anoint the patient's eyes with a feather dipped in it. Hoffmann employed it in jaundice. Hildanus, Villanova, and Velebt, in weakness of the eyes. In 1836, Kramehfeld (*in Ozann's Jour.*) employed it with success in rheumatic and catarrhal inflammation of the eyes and eyelids; in cough, hoarseness, earache, and headache, which have supervened on catarrhal affections, and glandulous, catarrhal, and scrofulous blepharophthalmia.

It has been immortalized by Milton, who probably, owing to his infirmity, tried this plant to give him back that which he had lost. He makes the archangel Michael employ it to remove the film from the eyes of our first parents, occasioned by eating the forbidden fruit:

"But to nobler sights.
Michael from Adam's eyes the film removed,
Which that false fruit that promised clearer sight
Had bred; then purged with Euphrasy and rue
The visual nerve, for he had much to see."

Paradise Lost, book ii.

In Shenstone, also, we have the virtues of this plant described:

> "Yet Euphrasy may not be left unsung,
> That gives dim eyes to wander leagues around."

Description.—Euphrasia officinalis is an annual plant. Flowers from June to September. The *root* is fibrous and whitish. The *stem* from one to six inches high, upright, square, leafy, downy, either simple or branched. *Leaves* sessile, almost entirely opposite; small, egg-shaped, downy; slightly ribbed and furrowed; serrated or indented teeth, pointed. *Flowers* axillary, solitary, very abundant, inodorous, forming a leafy spike or raceme at the tops of the branches and stems. *Calyx* angular, hairy, four-toothed, teeth nearly equal, spear-shaped, pointed. The *corolla* varies much in size, as well as colour, being commonly white, with deep purple streaks, and a yellowish palate. *Anthers* violet or brown, armed with two spines at the base. *Germen* a little hairy at the top. *Style* pubescent on the upper part. *Stigma* fringed with very minute glands round the edge. *Capsule* four-cornered at the bottom, compressed above, slightly notched at the end, a little hairy towards the top, and marked with black dots. *Seeds* few, somewhat angular; thin at the edges, strongly striated or furrowed at the sides.

"No gem can equal this brilliant and lasting ornament of the turf. When summer, with her gay companions, has divested the woods and fields; when the completion of the harvest has robbed the landscape of its richer features, the grassy downs are still glowing with the tufted Euphrasia, which, scattered around, yet reminds us, by its beautifully varied white, of snow, a chill though beneficial attendant of approaching winter. Its whiteness is tastefully varied with purple and pale yellow; as a hint which, though unwelcome, is kindly and delicately conveyed."

Geographical Distribution.—Over all Europe. North America, etc.

Localities.—On heaths, downs, and on mountainous meadows, common.

Parts used in Medicine, and Mode of Preparation.—The Whole Plant, gathered in July. The expressed juice is to be mixed with equal parts of alcohol. It is, however, so viscid, that it is generally necessary, after beating the Euphrasia into a smooth and homogeneous paste, to mix it with a small quantity of the same alcohol, in order to extract the juice.

Physiological Effects.—*On Man.* Lobel states that it produces inflammation of the eyes, and that a friend of his nearly lost his eyesight by the use of it.

Langhammer states that it produces violent headache, with pressive, shooting pains; with dimness of sight and myopia; engorgement of the vessels of the sclerotic; painful pressure and lachrymation in the eyes; sense of constriction in the superior eyelids, with painful rheumatic feelings in different parts of the face; enuresis; painful sensations in the lower extremities, with lassitude over the whole body, accompanied by frequent cold; the sleep interrupted by frequent, anxious dreams.

Other observers, viz. F. Hahnemann and Wislicenus, have noticed similar effects.

Medical Uses (Homœopathic).—Hahnemann remarks, that it was not without reason that this plant received the name it bears, and that it has fallen into unmerited disuse in the present day.

Clinical Observations.—*Noack and Trinks* (op. cit.): Bad consequences from contusions, blows, and falls (as far as the eyes are concerned) (*Jahr*). Scrofulosa mucosa (*Leon Simon*). Blenorrhœa oculorum (*Diegs, Lobethal*). Catarrhal, rheumatic, and scrofulous ophthalmia, the greater the segregation of mucus, the more appropriate the remedy (*Lobethal*). Inflammation of the eyes from smoke (*Frank*). Ophthalmia. Swelling and agglutination of the lids. Ichorous and bloody discharge from the eyes. Running catarrh in the day; obstruction at night. Ophthalmia, with frontal headache and pressive pain in the temples. Severe inflammation of the eyes, with insupportable pain. Photophobia and distension of the eyelids. Burning in the eyes. Nightly agglutination of the lids. Ophthalmia. Catarrhalis inveterata et neglecta. Inflammation. Dimness of sight, and spots on the cornea (*Rummel, Knorre, Weber*). Lachrymation. Traumatic ophthalmia (*Baudis*). Amblyopia amaurotica. Slow speech, with paralytic stiffness of the tongue and cheeks (*Jahr*). Figwarts, after the removal of condylomata by alternation of Acid. nitric. and Thuja (*Schlender*). Moist cough remaining after influenza (*Balogh*). Cramps in the calves of the legs (*Jahr*).

ANTIDOTES.—Belladonna. Camphor. Pulsatilla.

XXXIII. 34

GUAIACUM OFFICINALE.

Guaiac.

Synonyms.—Guaiacum, foliis fere impetiolatis, bijugatis, obovatis et leniter radiatis; pinnis et ramulis dichotomis, *Browne's Jamaica*, p. 225. Lignum vitæ, or Guaiacum, *Hughes' Barbadoes*. Guaiacum Americanum primum, fructu aceris, sive legitimum, *Breyn. Prodr.*, vol. i. p. 31. Pruno vel Euonymo affinis arbor, folio alato buxeo, subrotundo, flores pentapetalo cæruleo racemoso, fructu aceris cordato, cujus cortex luteus corrugatus, semen unicum majusculum nigricans, nullo ossiculo tectum operit, *Sloane's Jamaica*, vol. ii. p. 133. Guaiacum flore cæruleo, fructu subrotundo, *Plum. Nov. Gen.*, p. 39. Guaiacum, magna matrice, *Bauh. Πιν.*, p. 448. Lignum sanctum. Lignum Indicum. Palus sanctus.

Foreign Names.—*Fr.:* Gaïac. *Ital.:* Guaiaco, Legno sancto. *Span.:* Guayaco, Palo santo. *Port.:* Guaiaco. *Germ.:* Pockenholz, Frangosenholz. *Dut.:* Pokhut. *Swed.:* Pockenholt. *Dan.:* Pockenholt, Guajah. *Russ.:* Bakaut.

Nat. Order, Zygophyllaceæ, *Lindl.;* Rutaceæ, *Juss.;* Gruinales, *Linn.*—Decandria, Monogynia.

Gen. Char.—*Calyx* five-partite, obtuse. *Petals* five. *Stamens* ten. *Filaments* naked, or somewhat appendiculate. *Styles* and *stigma* one. *Capsule* somewhat stalked, five-celled, five-angled, or by abortion, two or three-celled. *Seeds* solitary in the cells, affixed to the axis, pendulous. *Albumen* cartilaginous, with small chinks. *Cotyledons* somewhat thick. *Trees* with a hard wood. *Leaves* abruptly pinnate. *Peduncles* axillary, one-flowered (*D. C.*)

Spec. Char.—*Leaves* bijugate. *Leaflets* obovate or oval, obtuse (*D. C.*)

History.—Guaiacum was first introduced into Europe by the Spaniards, in the year 1508, from the West Indies, very soon after the discovery of America, and was supposed to be a per-

---

Fig. 1. The stamens and germen. 2. The pericarps. 3 and 4. Transverse and longitudinal sections of the germen.

Plate XXXIV.

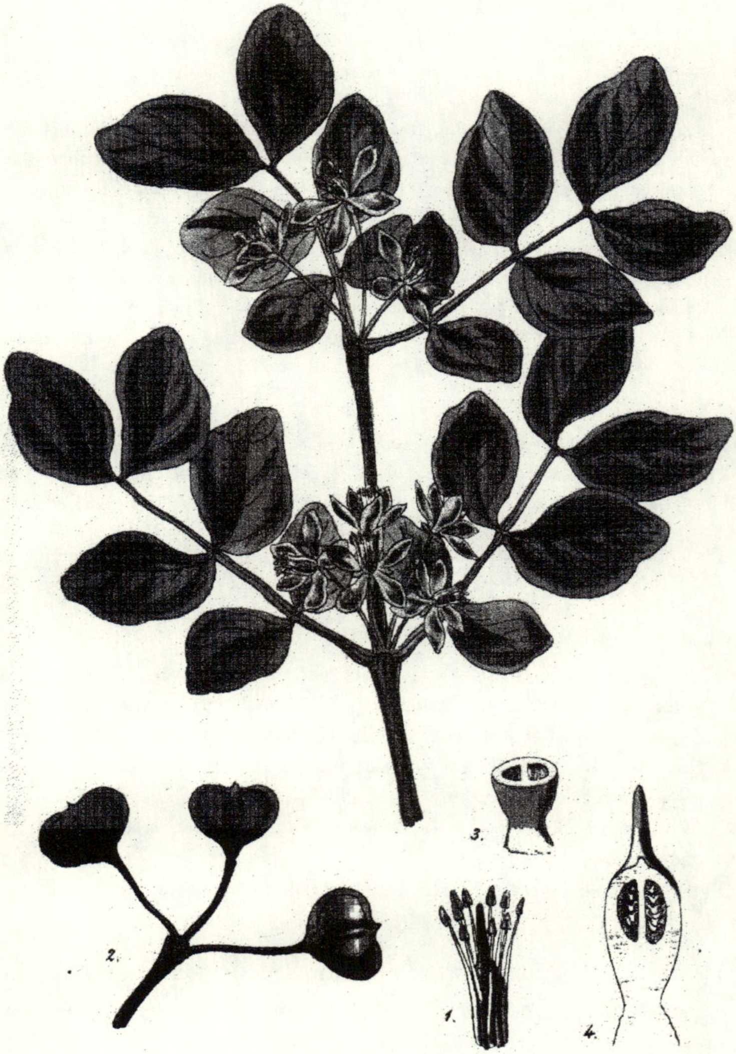

H. Sowerby del. et lith. Guaiacum officinale F. Reeve, imp.

fect specific for lues venerea, gaining such repute as to have been sold at seven gold crowns a pound. However, as it often failed in curing this disease, it fell into disuse, and was almost entirely superseded by mercury. "Although its utility was much overrated by many, it is, on the other hand, by no means the inert agent which some strenuous mercurialists will have it to be." The general virtues of Guaiacum, as stated by Bergius, is mundificans, sudorifera, diuretica, subcalefaciens, stomachica; and its use to be in syphilis, arthritis, morbi cutis, odontalgia. It was also employed by Mead and Pringle in rheumatism, both acute and chronic. By Cullen, and many others, in arthritis vaga, atonica, in gouty affections of different kinds, and various rheumatic combinations. By Schönlein in herpetic exanthemata and herpes circinatus. By Murray, Jahn, and Stark in deafness and confusion in the head, rheumatic prosopalgia. By Bell in toothache and angina tonsillaris. By Hufeland in giddiness from gout or syphilitic causes. By Desmarchais in sciatica. By Dr. Dewees in dysmenorrhœa. As a preventive of gout by Emerigon, of Martinico. In chronic skin diseases; in scrofula; and in chronic pulmonary catarrh, especially of gouty subjects, etc. etc.

Description.—The Guaiacum tree grows to the height of from thirty to forty feet, and near a foot in the diameter of its trunk. The *branches* numerous, divaricated, knotty, leafy at the ends. The *bark* very smooth, variegated with green and white. The *wood* hard and ponderous, dark olive-brown within, whitish towards the bark, having a peculiar acid, aromatic scent, and well known in England by the name of Brazil-wood, or Lignum-vitæ. The *leaves* are opposite, abruptly pinnate, consisting only of two pairs of obovate or roundish, obtuse, entire, smooth, pale, rigid leaflets, various in size, with several radiating veins. *Flowers* pale blue, on simple, axillary, clustered stalks, shorter than the leaves. The tree was first cultivated in this country by the Duchess of Beaufort, in 1669.

GEOGRAPHICAL DISTRIBUTION.—The Guaiacum tree is a native of the West India islands, but especially of Jamaica, St. Domingo, and St. Thomas, and the warmer parts of the continent of America.

PARTS USED IN MEDICINE, AND MODE OF PREPARATION.—The Gum-resin, which is obtained from the wood of the tree. The process usually followed in procuring this is, in heating billets several feet long, which have been previously perforated from end to end, and collecting the resin which slowly flows out from the depending extremity. Guaiac is imported in irregular lumps of various sizes. It often contains chips of wood. Its surface is brownish-red, or brownish-yellow when recent, but becomes greenish under exposure to light. It is brittle, presents a splintery, vitreous fracture, and possesses some translucency. Its powder, at first greyish, gradually acquires a greenish tint. It emits a somewhat basalmic odour while triturated, and has a faintly-bitter, sweetish taste, followed by a pricking in the back of the throat, which is very strong and unpleasant if it be tasted in powder.

The wood commonly called Lignum-vitæ is largely imported into this country from St. Domingo, for making block-sheaves, wooden pulleys, and many other objects, for which it is peculiarly fitted by its extraordinary hardness and toughness. It is remarkably tough and dense in its texture, and quickly sinks in water. It consists of a broad grey and yellow alburnum, and a dark, dirty greyish-green, or greenish-black duramen, the latter of which is the denser and heavier of the two. The Guaiac wood of the chemist consists of the shavings and turnings from the workshops of the turners. It has an acrid, aromatic taste, attended with a singular pricking in the throat, which is excited most strongly by the alburnum. It is scarcely subject to adulteration. It is known to be genuine by its sinking in water; by the chips being a mixture of yellowish and greenish shreds, and by its peculiar taste.

Dr. Hancock considers that the whole medicinal property of

Guaiac exists in the wood, and that the gum-resin is a peculiar substance called Guaiacine.

Quin (op. cit.) orders, for homœopathic preparation, one part of the resin to be dissolved in twenty parts of alcohol. Jahr orders the three first attenuations to be made by trituration.

Physiological Effects.—When Guaiacum is given in large doses, or to plethoric or excitable individuals, it produces dryness of the mouth, sensation of heat at the stomach, nausea, loss of appetite, and a relaxed condition of the bowels; it also produces, in some cases, great perspiration, and by continued use it has caused a mild salivation (*Burdach, Syst. d. Arzneim.*, bd. ii. s. 283). It increases the menstrual and hemorrhoidal discharges; and in very large doses, it causes heat and burning in the throat and stomach, vomiting, purging, pyrexia, and headache.

Kraus (*Heilmittel*, 612) mentions a measle-like eruption over the whole body, as being produced by large doses of the wood.

Pearson noticed that its continued use occasions heartburn, flatulence, and costiveness.

Medical Uses (Homœopathic).—*Hahnemann's observations:* "The homœopathic physician will find, in the few symptoms of Guaiacum, indications quite sufficient to show with certainty the value of this remedy in cases analogous to them, and will not be induced, by the indiscriminate praises of the common Materia Medica, to use it in *nominal* gout or rheumatism, without previously ascertaining whether its symptoms agree with those of the disease in question. It has been found serviceable in the following affections. Attacks of cephalalgia. Swelling of the eyes. Painful straining in the ears. Sensation as if mucus were in the throat, causing a feeling of nausea. Repugnance to milk. Constipation. Stitches in the chest. Arthritic lancination in the limbs, the pains being excited by the slightest motion, and accompanied by heat in the affected parts, especially when the patient had been injured by mercury.

Clinical Observations.—*Noack and Trinks* (op. cit.): Guaiacum has been found useful in mercurial rheumatism and in gout. Attacks of headache and megrim. Dolores osteocopi. Gastric affections, accompanied with hæmatemesis (*Attomyr*). Amaurosis arthritica, etc.

Plate XXXV.

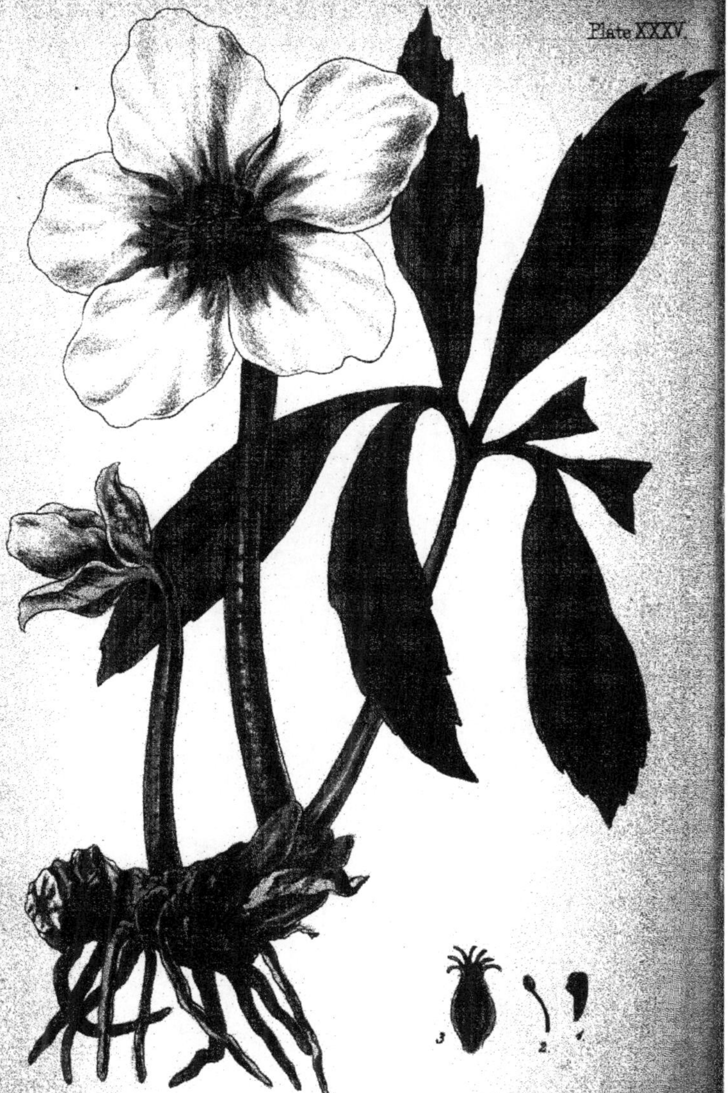

Helleborus niger.

XXXIV.

HELLEBORUS NIGER.

Black Hellebore, Christmas Rose.

SYNONYMS.—Helleborus niger legitimus, *Clus. Hist.*, 274. Helleborus niger flore roseo, *Bauh. Πιν.*, 186. Helleborus niger verus, *Gerarde, Herb.*, 975; *Raii Hist.*, 697. Helleborus niger, *Linn. Sp. Pl.*, 783. Melampodium, *Old Pharm.*

FOREIGN NAMES.—*Fr.:* L'Hellébore à fleurs roses, Hellébore noir, Rose de Noël. *Ital.:* Elleboro nero. *Span.:* Helleboro negro. *Germ.:* Schwartze Nieswurz, Schneerose. *Dut.:* Zwartnieskruid. *Swed.:* Schwartprustrot. *Dan.:* Sortnyserod. *Russ.:* Tschernija tschemeritza. *Arab.:* Khurbuc usivud.

Nat. Order, MULTISILIQUÆ, *Linn.;* RANUNCULACEÆ, *Juss.;* HELLEBOREÆ, *Decand.*—POLYANDRIA, POLYGYNIA.

GEN. CHAR.—*Calyx* permanent, of five roundish, obtuse, large sepals. *Petals* from eight to ten, very short, tubular, narrowest in the lower part, nectariferous. *Stamens* from thirty to sixty. *Ovaries* from three to ten. *Stigmas* terminal, orbicular. *Capsules* coriaceous. *Seeds* oval, disposed in two rows, on a linear, double-notched receptacle. Fetid, stiff, coriaceous, nearly smooth herbs, with divided leaves.

SPEC. CHAR.—*Scapes* leafless, bearing one to two flowers.

HISTORY.—It was for a long time supposed that this plant was the Ελλεβορος μελας of the Greek physicians, but the researches of Tournefort and Sibthorp prove the true black Hellebore of the ancients to be a distinct species from our Helleborus niger, and denominated by them Helleborus officinalis. Hahnemann* has endeavoured to show that, by a different reading of the Greek text, we may consider these plants identical; yet the opinions of such well-known botanists are quite conclusive as to

---

Fig. 1. A petal. 2. A stamen. 3. Germen, etc.

* On the Helleborism of the Ancients, translated by R. E. Dudgeon, M.D.

the distinctive characters of the two species.* The term Melampodon, used by some of the old Dispensatories for this drug, has arisen from its having been mistaken for the Veratrum album, the true Ελλεβορος of the ancients, the drug by which Melampus cured the daughters of Proetus, king of the Argivans. In Hahnemann's most erudite essay on the Helleborism of the Ancients, he proves that Veratrum album was not denominated ελλεβορος λευκος until after the discovery of the Helleborus niger, but that it was termed by them *Hellebore*, κατεξοχην, thereby denoting that it was their sole and well-known evacuant; and if this be the case, the old proverb "Naviget Anticyram," send a madman a voyage to Anticyra, will apply equally to the Veratrum album as to the Helleborus niger.

In early times it was used in mania and dropsy, from its peculiar drastic properties, the ancient physicians considering that it got rid of the black bile, which was supposed to cause these diseases. Paracelsus extols its virtues in gout, skin diseases, epilepsy, and jaundice. It was found especially serviceable in torpid, phlegmatic individuals, especially when the pelvic circulation was languid. Dr. Mead and others employed it with great success as an emmenagogue, and it has been found useful by many physicians in hypochondriasis and hysteria; headaches, with somnolency, which are increased by movements, etc. etc.

Description.—The Helleborus niger is a perennial plant, flowering from December to March; hence its name, Christmas Rose. The *leaves* are pedate, large, composed of five, six, or more leaflets, of a deep green colour, smooth, and dotted with red. The *leaflets* are ovate-lanceolate, smooth, shining, and coriaceous, with the distal half of each slightly serrated. The *flower-stalk* is a scape, six or eight inches in length, erect,

* This can be only interesting as regards the history of the plant, *practically* it does not signify. The Helleborus niger is the plant which Hahnemann and others proved, and it is that species we must describe.

round, variegated with red, and supporting one or two flowers. The *bracteas*, or *floral leaves*, are ovate, and indented at the edges. The *calyx* (*corolla?*) consists of five large, roundish, concave sepals, at first white, or of a pale rose colour, deepening by age, and finally becoming green, after the impregnation of the seed. The *petals* are tubular and two-lipped. The *filaments* are numerous, from thirty to sixty in number, capillary, and supporting yellow anthers. The *germens*, about six or eight in number, become pods, containing many black, shining seeds. "Few plants are more elegant; the large, concave flowers, white, with a tinge of blush-colour, are finely contrasted with the ample dark and shining foliage. The roots are perennial, creeping, very black externally, with numerous long, simple, perpendicular fibres." The distinctive characters between the Helleborus niger and Helleborus officinalis, or orientalis, seem to be, that in the officinalis the flower-stalks do not rise above the leaves, but are branched, bearing five or six drooping, concave flowers, white, turning purplish as they fade; the leaves are truly pedate, and their lobes elliptical, twice the breadth of the Helleborus niger. The properties of the orientalis are much more active, but the effects much the same.

Woodville says: "If any arguments were required to evince the necessity of botanical accuracy in discriminating medicinal plants, the Helleborus niger would furnish us with many facts in which such arguments might be deduced; for a great number of instances are recorded of the effects of this plant, by which it since appears that other plants were mistaken for it, and actually employed; of these we may enumerate the Helleborus viridis, Adonis vernalis, Troillus Europæus, Actæa spicata, Astrantia major, and Aconitum Napellus; and as the roots of these plants possess very different powers, we cannot be surprised that the medical history of this root is not only confused and contradictory, but calculated to produce very mischievous and even fatal consequences."

Geographical Distribution.—Most parts of Europe, especially in Austria, Carniola, Italy, and Greece; Burgundy, Vosges, Pyrenees, Alps, etc.

Localities.—On rocky and woody mountains.

Parts used in Medicine, and Mode of Preparation.—The Fresh Root, which is dug up about Christmas, and prepared as all other fresh plants. The root has been adulterated with the roots of other plants, as the Aconitum neomontanum, Adonis vernalis, Helleborus viridis, Troillus Europæus, Actæa spicata; these may be distinguished by their paler colour. Both the virtues and properties of the root are impaired by keeping.

Physiological Effects.—*On Animals.* Experiments on animals have shown, that when administered in doses of two or three drachms to dogs, death ensues in the course of sixteen or eighteen hours. Smaller animals are killed by its exhibition in much less time: for example, ten grains of the extract introduced into the windpipe of a rabbit destroyed life in six minutes; but with this, as with many other poisons, the effects are greater when applied to serous surfaces, and inserted into wounds, than when taken into the stomach.

Six grains of powdered Hellebore were sprinkled over a wound made in the interior of the thigh of a small, young dog; there were no visible symptoms at the expiration of eight hours; the next day, twenty hours after the operation, the animal was lying down on its side in a state of great dejection. He was quite sensible to external impressions; he could be moved like an inert mass of matter, but could not by any means keep himself on his legs. He died three hours after; no sensible lesion was perceived in the digestive canal or in the lungs (*Orfila*, op. cit.)

In all cases the leading symptoms are, efforts to vomit, giddiness, palsy of the hind legs, and insensibility.

On Man.—Black Hellebore is a local irritant; given in small doses, it increases the secretion and peristaltic motion of the intestines, and acts as a stimulant to the pelvic circulation. In larger doses, it often occasions sickness, cold sweats, and lowers the state of the pulse. In excessive or poisonous doses, it acts as a narcotic acrid poison, and causes vomiting, purging, burning pain in the stomach and intestines, cramps of the lower extremities, cold sweats, faintness, paralysis, and death.

Two persons took a decoction of this root in cider; three quarters of an hour after taking it, alarming symptoms were developed, without exciting suspicion of the real cause. One of the men, therefore, took another dose, when vomiting, delirium, horrible convulsions, accompanied with immediate coldness, supervened, and death at last ensued. On dissection, sixteen hours afterwards, the appearances in each were found precisely similar, except that in the one who took the largest quantity they were more strongly marked; the lungs were gorged with blood; the mucous membrane of the stomach was considerably inflamed, of a blackish-brown colour, and reduced almost to a gangrenous state; the œsophagus and intestines were natural (*Beck's El. of Med.*)

A man, who appeared to be nearly fifty years old, being in the hospital on account of melancholia, was about to depart, when he took some extract of black Hellebore, by which he was considerably purged. In the beginning of the night, at the seventh or eighth hour after taking it, he was attacked by vomiting and pains in the abdomen, which were allayed by warm broth; about the fifth hour of the night those symptoms returned, and were again relieved. He lay down an hour afterwards, having vomited two or three spoonfuls of a greenish matter. So quietly did he rest that none of the patients in the nearest beds heard him; but at the eighth hour they were attracted to his bedside by a peculiar noise from his mouth, and found him dead. He had taken about half a drachm of the extract, a quantity which had been administered to others with impunity. He had, however, neglected to drink copiously of whey, a precaution it was customary to recommend. On examination, the stomach, œsophagus, and intestines were inflamed, but not violently in any part; the whole cerebrum was soft (*Morgagni de Sed. Morb.*, vol. i. ix.)

Medical Uses (Homœopathic).—*Hahnemann's observations:* "The symptoms of this plant, which have been observed by myself and my pupils, are but few in number; nevertheless, one may consider them as a first step made in a new path. It appears that Helleborus niger may be useful in certain kinds of fevers, in those diseases characterised by swellings, and in certain affections of the mind. When the morbid conditions that this plant occasions have been more completely studied, we shall know what were the diseases for the cure of which many places in Greece were so celebrated; for the plant that the ancients employed was a species of Hellebore very similar to this, but with flowers of a pale red colour."

Clinical Observations.—Schrön says that Helleborus niger appears to exert its specific action on serous membranes; it increases the action of the circulatory organs, and especially of the heart, in a most extraordinary manner. It also appears to be especially serviceable in fat, plethoric constitutions, and in the phlegmatic and choleric temperaments. General dropsy. Acute dropsy, with swelling of the face and whole body, etc. General anasarca, especially after scarlet fever. Knorre recommends large and frequent doses in chronic dropsy. Mullenbein recommends it in dropsy after ague, the ague having been cured by Arsenicum. Helleborus niger and Scilla maritima seem to be especially serviceable in the dropsy of children, more than in grown-up persons. Retroceded measles, with metastasis to the membranes of the brain. Tinea capitis, with swelling of the cervical glands. Hydrocephalus acutus in the second stage; when the child screams, throws the head backwards, with convulsive movements of the limbs, especially the right arm and left foot. Aconite, Belladonna, Rhus, Arnica, and Helleborus, in the high potencies, had failed in giving relief in this case. Tincture of Hellebore, ten drops, in ℥j of distilled water, given at first every five minutes, increasing the interval between the dose to every half-hour, and then to every forty-eight hours, cured the child (*Hartlaub*). Hydrocephalus, after scarlet fever, with Aconite, Belladonna, etc. Aphthæ on the tongue (*Frank*). Stomacace. Aphthæ, with increased secretion of saliva. Constipation after gastrodynia in obstinate cases. Paralysis of the bladder, with excessive distension. Painful micturition, drop by drop. Complete suppression of urine for three days, with painful desire, with emission of drops of blood. Œdema of the limbs. Coldness of the whole body. Slow pulse. Yellow colour of the skin. Dry tongue. Much thirst (*Morzbauer*). Œdema scrotalis rheumaticum. Hydrothorax, especially after scarlet fever.

ANTIDOTES.—To large doses, Oxymel (*C. Gesner*). To small doses, Camphor. China. Ohlkauth says that magnetic passes relieved the violent spasms which had been excited by Helleborus niger.

XXXV.

HYOSCYAMUS * NIGER.

Common Henbane, Black Henbane, Hogbean.

Synonyms.—Hyoscyamus vulgaris et niger, *Bauh. Πιν.*, p. 169. Hyoscyamus vulgaris, *Raii Syn.*, vol. i. p. 274. Hyoscyamus, *Hall Hist.*, vol. i. p. 254. Hyoscyamus niger, *Gerarde Em.*, p. 353. Hyoscyamus lethalis, *Salisb. Prodr.*, p. 131. Hyoscyamus flavus, *Fuchs. Hist.*, 833, f. Hyoscyamus niger, *Linn. Sp. Pl.*, p. 257.

Foreign Names.—*Fr.:* Jusquiame, ou Hanebane potelée. *Ital.:* Beleno, Veleno. *Span.:* Miemendro, Velheno. *Port.:* Yosciamo. *Germ.:* Bilsenkraut. *Dan.:* Honsebane. *Swed.:* Bolmort, Honsable. *Russ.:* Belena. *Arab.:* Sickrau.

Nat. Order, Luridæ, *Linn.;* Solaneæ, *Juss.*—Pentandria, Monogynia.

Gen. Char.—*Calyx* inferior, large, permanent, of one sepal, tubular, swelling below, five-cleft above, segments pointed. *Corolla* of one petal, funnel-shaped, irregular; tube cylindrical, short; limb rather spreading, in five deep, blunt, rounded segments, one of which is broader than the rest. *Filaments* awl-shaped, from some part of the tube of the corolla, inclining, somewhat unequal in length. *Anthers* heart-shaped, incumbent. *Germen* roundish. *Style* thread-shaped, reclining, the length of the longer stamens. *Stigma* capitate. *Capsule* egg-shaped, filling the body of the calyx, blunt, somewhat compressed, and marked with a longitudinal furrow at each side, of two cells, opening transversely by a convex lid. *Receptacles* (*placentas*) oblong, convex, attached to the perpendicular partition. *Seeds* numerous, inversely egg-shaped, curved, dotted, covering the receptacles.

The monopetalous, inferior, funnel-shaped *corolla*, the capitate *stigma*, and the two-celled *capsule*, opening at the apex by a transverse aperture, will distinguish this from other genera in the same class and order (*Baxter*).

Spec. Char.—*Leaves* clasping the stem, sinuated. *Flowers* sessile.

Fig. 1. The corolla, showing the position of the stamens. 2. Style and stigma. 3. Seed-vessel.

* From υος, a hog, and κυαμος, a bean. Hogs are said to eat the fruit, which bears some resemblance to a bean.

Plate XXXVI.

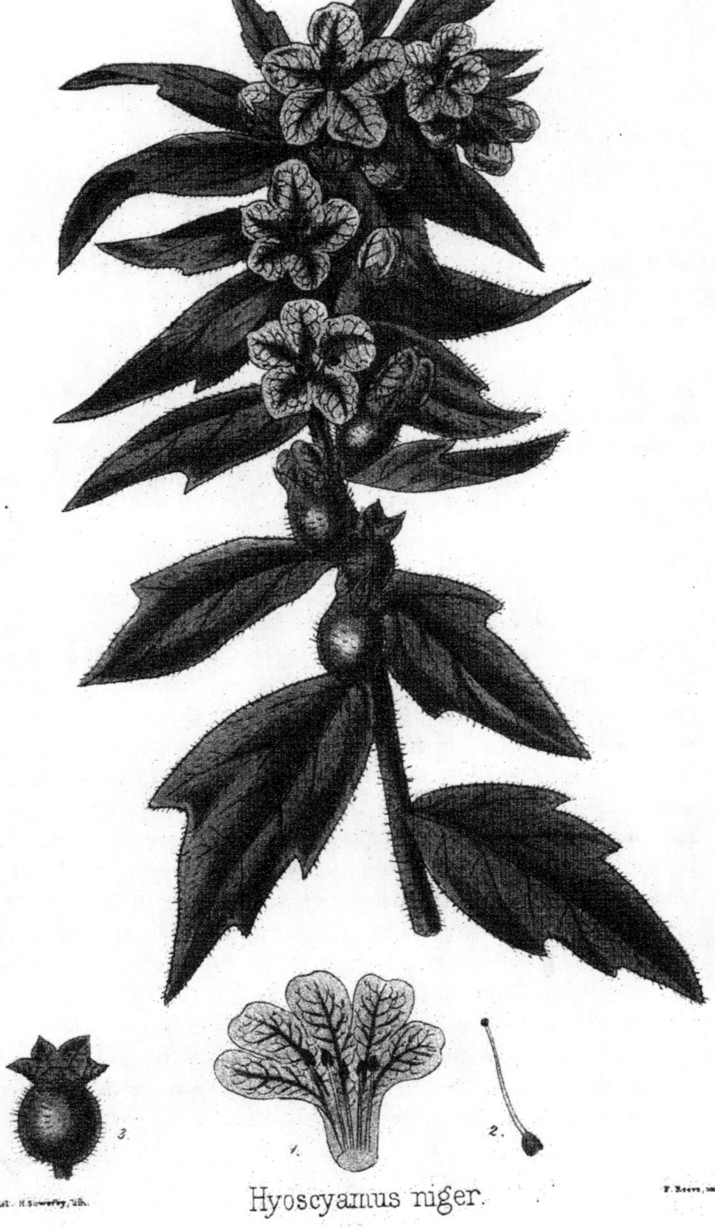

E.H.del. H.Sowerby, lith.

Hyoscyamus niger.

F. Reeve, imp

History.—Hyoscyamus niger is the Υοσκυαμος μελας of Dioscorides. He described three species, which were distinguished by the colour of their seeds; but he considered that the Hyoscyamus albus was the only one fit for medicinal purposes. The black (Hyoscyamus niger) he rejects as being highly poisonous. According to Sprengel, the Hyoscyamus described by Hippocrates is the Hyoscyamus albus.

The following is Pliny's account of Henbane (*Holland's Trans.*, ed. 1601, p. 215): "Moreover, unto Hercules is ascribed Henbane, which the Latines call Appollinaris; the Arabians, Altercum or Altercangenon; but the Greeks, Hyoscyamus. Many kinds there be of it, the one beareth black seed, flowers standing much upon purple, and this hearbe is full of prickes; and in very truth, such is the Henbane that groweth in Galatia. The common Henbane is whiter, and brauncheth more than the other, taller also than the poppie. The third kind bringeth forth seed like unto the grains of iris. All the sort of these alreadie named trouble the braine, and put men besides their right wits: besides that they breed dizzinesse of the head. As touching the fourth, it carieth leaves soft, full of down, fuller and fatter than the rest: the seed also is white, and it groweth by the seaside. Physicians are not afraid to use this in their compositions, no more than that which has red seed. Howbeit, otherwiles, this white kind especially, if it bee not throughly ripe, prooveth to be reddish, and then it is rejected by the physicians. For otherwise none of them all would be gathered, but when they bee fully drie. Henbane is of the nature of wine, and therefore offensive to the understanding, and troubleth the head. Howbeit, good use there is, both of the seed it selfe as it is in substance, and also of the oile or juice drawne out of it apart. And yet the stalk, leaves, and roots are employed in some purposes. For mine owne part, I hold it to be a dangerous medicine, and not to be used but with great heed and discretion. For this is certainely knowne, that if one take in drinke more than four leaves thereof, it will put him beside himself. An oile (I say) is made of the seed thereof, which if it be but dropped into the eares is ynough to trouble the braine. But strange it is of this oile, that if it be taken in drinke it serveth as a counterpoison. See how industrious men have ben to prove experiments, and made no end of trying all things, insomuch as they have found meanes, and forced very poysons to be remedies."

The Arabian physicians followed Dioscorides in their description and application of this plant, and reject the Hyoscyamus niger as a medicinal drug; but this latter has gradually taken the place of the white during the last two hundred years, until at the present time the Hyoscyamus albus is scarcely known in the Dispensatories and Pharmacopœias of modern times. Dr. Grey thinks that the Hebenon of Shakespeare, "with juice of cursed Hebenon," was a poetical modification of Henbane. That it was considered as a poison in Shakespeare's time we have sufficient evidence. In Drayton's "Barons' Wars," we have "the pois'ning Henbane and the mandrake dread." It was a belief also, even of the medical professors of that day, that poison might be introduced into the system by being poured into the ear. Ambrose Paré, the celebrated French surgeon, was charged with having administered poison in this way to Francis II. It has also been supposed that Shakespeare's Hebenon is the juice of ebony. (Vide note to Knight's Shakespeare, Hamlet, act i. sc. v.) But the Observations of Pliny, as mentioned above, translated by Holland in 1601, and the knowledge that Hyoscyamus will produce an eruption like tetters on the skin, would not escape the observation of Shakespeare; hence it may be concluded that "Hebenon" is Henbane.

As a medicine it fell into disuse, until the time of Baron Störck, in 1772, who published several cases of different diseases, in which an extract prepared from the juice of this plant had been found very efficacious. These diseases were, internal spasms and convulsions, palpitations of the heart, madness, melancholy, epilepsy, inveterate headaches, hæmoptysis, and a troublesome cough which accompanied the last-mentioned complaint. It has since then been employed in allopathic medicine as an anodyne, soporific, antispasmodic, and sedative. In laryngismus stridulus, and convulsions in children (*Hufeland, Collin, Marshall Hall*, etc.) Dysentery (*Robert Boyle*). Induration of the lymphatic glands (*Himly, Sachs*, etc.) Febris nervosa versatilis (*P. Frank*). Delirium tremens (*Brock, Müller*). Dementia and melancholy (*Störck, Greding, Fothergill*, etc.) Giddiness (*Marcellus*). Affections of the eyes (*Philoxenes*). Ulceration of the iris (*Himly*). Iritis (*Schmidt*). Scrofulous photophobia (*Wutzer*). Amaurosis (*Lelle, Molinelli*). Violent otitis (*Zoilus*, etc.) Neuralgia of the face (prosopalgia) (*Harrison*). Odontalgia rheumatica (*Dürr*). Gastralgia (*Harrison*). Croup (*Thribolet*). Hooping-cough in second stage (*Schäffer, Hillary*, etc.) Angina pectoris, etc. etc.

Description.—This plant is biennial, and flowers from June to August. The *root* is spindle-shaped. *Stem* from one to four feet high, upright, round, tough, branched, woolly towards the top, very leafy. The *leaves* are alternate, sessile, or stem clasping, soft, and pliant, somewhat egg-shaped, sinuated, with sharp lobes, downy, and viscid, exhaling a powerful and oppressive odour, like all the rest of the plant. *Flowers* numerous, from the bosoms of the crowded upper leaves, almost entirely sessile. *Calyx* a little distended on the under side, woolly at the base, the tubular part enlarging and enclosing the seed-vessel. *Corolla* of a pale, yellowish-brown, beautifully netted with purple veins, and a dark purple eye or base. *Filaments* white. *Anthers* and *style* of a fine, deep purple. *Capsules* in two rows, all turned to one side, enclosed in the permanent calyx, and forming a kind of unilateral, leafy spike. Each capsule contains a great number of small *seeds*, which find egress by the rounded convex top coming off like the lid of a box.

The plant, in the first year of its duration, has no stem. The leaves are all radical, each having a footstalk or pedicle. The leaves are woolly, but possess little of the odour of the mature plant. The leaves of the first year die in the autumn. The leaves of the second year are large, long, and deeply inverse, sessile, and nearly embrace the stem, and having decurrent lobes, which are of a more delicate texture than the blade of the leaf. These lobes are important points to observe in examining a specimen. The leaves are very clammy and fetid, having an odour very similar to that of the black currant; these are the true medicinal leaves, and they should be gathered as soon as the flowers are blown.

GEOGRAPHICAL DISTRIBUTION.—Over the whole of Europe, some parts of Asia, and North America.

LOCALITIES.—On roadsides, amidst rubbish, and on the *débris* of hill-slopes. It has been naturalized in this country, and is supposed to have been brought here by the Romans.

PARTS USED IN MEDICINE, AND MODE OF PREPARATION.—The Whole Plant, gathered in the months of May, June, and July. The juice is expressed and treated like that of all other fresh plants.

PHYSIOLOGICAL EFFECTS.—*On Animals.* Orfila (op. cit.) states that Hyoscyamus acts on dogs as on man, producing dilatation of the pupil, weakness of the posterior extremities, staggering, and insensibility. It has been supposed to be very hurtful to birds, particularly of the gallinaceous kind; hence the name Henbane, but goats and swine eat it with impunity. Moirond (op. cit.) states that, given in large quantities to horses, it causes only slight dilatation of the pupil, spasmodic movements of the limbs, and increase of the pulse.

On Man.—In small and repeated doses, it allays nervous irritability, irritation, and preternatural sensibility in any organ. In large doses, it causes headache, giddiness, dimness of sight, dilatation of the pupil, a greater or less tendency to sleep, and painful delirium. In some cases these symptoms are followed by thirst, nausea, griping, and either purging or constipation; and in a few instances, febrile heat and irritation of the skin. Very large doses are apt to be followed by delirium rather than sleep. In poisonous doses, it causes loss of speech, dilatation of the pupil, disturbance of vision, distortion of the face, coma, and delirium, generally of the unmanageable, sometimes of the furious kind, and paralysis, occasionally with convulsive movements. Irritation of the stomach and bowels, manifested by nausea, vomiting, pain, and purging, is occasionally induced (*Pereira*, op. cit.)

Boerhaave experienced a sensation of trembling and drunkenness whilst preparing a plaster, into the composition of which Henbane entered.

Wepfer relates that several monks made a repast on the roots of the wild endive, among which were mixed by mistake two roots of Henbane. In a few hours some experienced vertigo, others a burning of the tongue, lips, and throat; severe pains were also felt in the iliac region, and in all the joints. The intellectual faculties and the organs of vision were perverted, and they gave themselves up to actions which were mad and ridiculous. In other cases, a haggard countenance, dilatation of the pupils, difficulty of breathing, small and intermittent pulse, loss of speech, trismus, and temporary loss of intellect have been the principal symptoms; while the extremities have been observed to be cold and nearly paralysed (*Orfila*, vol. ii. pp. 135 et seq.)

Two soldiers ate the young shoots dressed in olive oil. They presently became giddy and stupid, lost their speech, and had a dull, haggard look. The pupils were excessively dilated, and the eyes so insensible that the eyelids did not wink when the cornea was touched; the pulse was small and intermitting; the breathing difficult, the jaw locked, and the mouth distorted by *risus sardonicus*. Sensibility was extinct, the limbs were cold and palsied, the arms convulsed, and there was that singular union of delirium and coma which is usually termed tymphomania. As the palsy and somnolency abated, the delirium became more extravagant (*Cloquet in Christ.*, op. cit.)

Six persons ate the roots of Henbane by mistake for parsnips: several were delirious, and danced about like maniacs; one appeared as if he had got drunk; and one woman became profoundly and irrecoverably comatose.

Dr. Patouillat, of Toncy, in France, saw nine persons who were poisoned by this root; some were speechless and convulsive, others occasionally howled. In all there was a protrusion of the eyes, contortion of the mouth, and delirium (*Phil. Trans.*, vol. xl. p. 446).

It is related that a tailor, under the influence of this plant, could not thread his needle; his needle seemed to have three points (*Lancet*, 1846, p. 479).

Professor Foderé (*Méd. Légale*, vol. iv. p. 23) gives an account of the effect of the Hyoscyamus albus on the crew of a French corvette. The plant was boiled and distributed among the whole ship's company; they were all soon seized with giddiness, vomiting, convulsions, colic, purging, and delirium of an active kind. They were all relieved by emetics and purgatives.

Dr. Archibald Hamilton (*Ed. Phys. and Lit. Ess.*, vol. ii. p. 268) has described a case which was caused by the seeds of this plant. A young medical student, who took twenty five grains of the seeds, was seized in half an hour with lassitude and somnolency, convulsive movements of the arms, incoherency, total insensibility of the skin, and loss of recollection. These symptoms continued for thirty-two hours, and then slowly receded.

Medical Uses (Homœopathic).—*Hahnemann's observations:* "The fact that Henbane (Hyoscyamus niger), in large doses, diminishes remarkably the heat of the body, and relaxes its tone for a short time in its direct action, and therefore is an efficacious palliative remedy when given in moderate doses inwardly, and outwardly in sudden attacks of tension of the fibres and inflammation, does not fail to be considered in this place. This is not the case, however, with the observation that this property only enables it to palliate very imperfectly, in any dose, chronic affections, with tension of fibre; in the end, however, it rather increases than diminishes them, by its indirect, secondary action, which is exactly the opposite of its primary action. On the other hand, it will help to assist the power of the strengthening remedy in chronic relaxation of the fibres, as in its primary action it relaxes, and in its secondary action it tends all the more to elevate the tone, and that in a durable manner. In *large* doses, it likewise possesses the power of producing hemorrhage, especially bleeding from the nose, and frequently relieving catamenial flux, as I and others have ascertained. For this reason it cures chronic hemorrhages, in small doses, in an extremely effectual and lasting manner. The most remarkable thing is the artificial disease it produces in very large doses, suspicious, quarrelsome, spitefully-calumnious, revengeful, destructive, fearless mania, hence Henbane was termed by the Ancients, Altercum; and this is the kind of mania it specifically cures, only that in such cases a tenseness of fibre sometimes hinders its effects from being permanent. Difficulty of moving and insensibility of the limbs, and the apoplectic symptoms it produces, it may also very probably be capable of curing. In large doses it produces, in its direct primary action, convulsions, and is consequently useful in epilepsy, probably also in the loss of memory usually accompanying it, as it has the power of producing want of recollection. Its power of causing, in its direct action, sleeplessness, with constant tendency to slumber, makes it in chronic sleeplessness a much more permanent remedy than the frequently merely palliative opium, especially as it at the same time keeps the bowels open, although only by the indirect secondary action of each dose, consequently in a palliative way. It causes dry cough, dryness of the mouth and nose, in its direct action; it is therefore very useful in tickling cough, probably also in dry coryza. The flow of mucus from the nose and the flow of saliva observed from its use only belong to its indirect secondary action. The seeds cause convulsions in the facial and ocular muscles; and by their action on the head, cause vertigo, and a dull pain in the membranes lying under the skull. The practical physician will be able to take advantage of this. Its direct action lasts scarcely twelve hours" (*Hahn. Lesser Writ.*)

Clinical Observations.—*Noack and Trinks:* Hyoscyamus niger appears particularly efficacious in nervous constitutions; in those irritable, nervous states, with variability and fickleness; in hysteria and hypochondriacal conditions, arising from grief, fear, fright, or anger; and in many spasmodic affections, particularly in women and children; in spasms and convulsions in children, from worms or from teething; and in pregnant females. Epilepsy from fright. Chronic hemorrhages. Redness of the skin. Brown spots on the skin. Large pustules, like small-pox. Chronic sleeplessness. Puerperal fever. Febris nervosa versatilis, with delirium and spectral delusions. Typhus fever. Delirium tremens. Nymphomania. Melancholia. Inflammation of the brain. Toothache, produced by cold. Grinding of the teeth during sleep, in children. Vomiting of blood after cold, with pain at the scrobiculus cordis on being touched. Painful stitches over the abdomen. Painless diarrhœa of lying-in women. Spasmodic stricture at the neck of the bladder, with violent tenesmus. Metrorrhagia. Irritable cough. Dry night cough. Rheumatic typhoid pneumonia, etc. etc.

Antidotes.—To large doses, Vinegar. Medoro states that a large dose of lemon-juice acts immediately as an antidote to Hyoscyamus; Christison doubts this. To small doses, Belladonna. Camphor. Opium. Stramonium. Hyoscyamus acts as an antidote to Belladonna and Cina.

END OF VOL. I.

Spotted something that isn't quite right?

Let us know and we'll fix it for future reprints. And as a thank you for your diligence, we'll send you a free Sothis book of your choice.

publisher@sothis.press

This page intentionally left blank

Made in United States
Orlando, FL
05 November 2026

90241900R10219